BIOPHARMACEUTICS
AND
PHARMACOKINETICS

BIOPHARMACEUTICS
AND
PHARMACOKINETICS

Jayant S Kulkarni
Research Scientist
Reliance Life Sciences Pvt. Ltd., Mumbai

AP Pawar
Professor, Department of Pharmaceutics
Bharati Vidyapeeth Deemed University
Poona College of Pharmacy, Pune

VP Shedbalkar
Head—Bioequivalence
GVK Biosciences Pvt. Ltd., Hyderabad

CBSPD

CBS Publishers & Distributors Pvt Ltd

New Delhi • Bengaluru • Chennai • Kochi • Kolkata • Lucknow • Mumbai
Hyderabad • Jharkhand • Nagpur • Patna • Pune • Uttarakhand

Biopharmaceutics and Pharmacokinetics

ISBN-13: 978-81-239-1307-0
ISBN-10: 81-239-1307-9

Copyright © Authors and Publisher

First Edition: 2006
Reprint: 2007, 2008, 2009, 2011, 2012, 2016, 2017, 2018, 2019, 2020, 2022, 2023, **2025**

Published by **Satish Kumar Jain** and produced by **Varun Jain** for

CBS Publishers & Distributors Pvt Ltd

4819/XI Prahlad Street, 24 Ansari Road, Daryaganj, New Delhi 110 002, India.
Ph: 011-23266838, 23289259   Website: www.cbspd.com
                               e-mail: delhi@cbspd.com

Corporate Office: 204 FIE, Industrial Area, Patparganj, Delhi 110 092
Ph: 011-4934 4934   Fax: 011-4934 4935
                            e-mail: publishing@cbspd.com; publicity@cbspd.com

Branches

- **Bengaluru:** Seema House 2975, 17th Cross, KR Road, Banasankari 2nd Stage, Bengaluru 560 070, Karnataka, India
  Ph: +91-80-26771678/79   Fax: +91-80-26771680   e-mail: bangalore@cbspd.com
- **Chennai:** 7, Subbaraya Street, Shenoy Nagar, Chennai 600 030, Tamil Nadu, India
  Ph: +91-44-26680620, 26681266   Fax: +91-44-42032115   e-mail: chennai@cbspd.com
- **Kochi:** 42/1325, 1326, Power House Road, Opp KSEB, Power House, Ernakulam Kochi 682 018, Kerala, India
  Ph: +91-484-4059061-65,67   Fax: +91-484-4059065   e-mail: kochi@cbspd.com
- **Kolkata:** 147, Hind Ceramics Compound, 1st Floor, Nilgunj Road, Belghoria, Kolkata-700056, West Bengal, India
  Ph: +033-25633055, 033-25633056   e-mail: kolkata@cbspd.com
- **Lucknow:** Basement, Khushnuma Complex, 7 Meerabai Marg (Behind Jawahar Bhawan), Lucknow-226001, UP, India
  Ph: +0522-4000032   e-mail: tiwari.lucknow@cbspd.com
- **Mumbai:** PWD Shed, Gala no 25/26, Ramchandra Bhatt Marg, Next to JJ Hospital Gate no. 2, Opp. Union Bank of India, Noorbaug, Mumbai-400009, Maharashtra, India
  Ph: 022-66661880/89   e-mail: mumbai@cbspd.com

Representatives

• Hyderabad	0-9885175004	• Jharkhand	0-9811541605	• Nagpur	0-8692091830
• Patna	0-9334159340	• Pune	0-9664372571	• Uttarakhand	0-9716462459

Printed at Glorious Printers, Jhilmil Industrial Area, Delhi, India

Preface

The authors are pleased to bring out the First Edition of *"Biopharmaceutics and Pharmacokinetics"*. This book is written specially keeping in mind the syllabi for Pharmacy, Medical and Nursing students. This text will also be useful to scientists working in the Pharmaceutical Industry.

Biopharmaceutics and Pharmacokinetics is increasingly becoming an important subject, especially in the new drug discovery and development. In addition, bioequivalence studies are becoming more and more important because of the increasing importance of generic products in pharmaceutical market. Also, with the increasing number of Clinical Research Organizations, a new field of Bioequivalence/Pharmacokinetics is emerging as a rewarding and challenging career option for medical and Para-medical students. Importantly as India is becoming the center of attraction for global pharmaceuticals for clinical research, new research and career opportunities are becoming available in this field.

Here an attempt has been made by us to write the text in a way, which would enable the readers to conceptualize the idea behind the words. The book covers not only the basics but it also introduces the new emerging trends in the field of biopharmaceutics/pharmacokinetics.

The entire book is divided into 13 chapters encompassing basic ADME, pharmacokinetic models, and applications of pharmacokinetics and bioequivalence studies. Efforts have been made by us to make the text "reader friendly." Simple illustrations are drawn to simplify mechanisms of drug absorption, distribution, metabolism and other biopharmaceutical aspects. New developments in respective areas e.g. *in vitro* systems, chronopharmacokinetics etc. have also been introduced. We have tried not to burden the text with too many mathematical details, but mathematical expressions are integral part of biopharmaceutics/pharmacokinetics. Hence wherever applicable, we have tried to explain the step-wise derivation of the final mathematical formulas for the easy understanding. In addition, schematics and representative graphs have been included which would definitely help the readers in understanding these concepts. Considering the importance of Bioanalysis in biopharmaceutics, a chapter has been included to introduce basic concepts in bioanalysis. In addition, special attention has been given in Chapter 12 and 13 so as to familiarize the readers regarding the various requirements of bioequivalence studies, including the regulatory point of view.

The authors would like to place on record our sincere thanks and gratitude to all our colleagues, friends and family members, who have been the source of inspiration in the preparation of this text.

The authors are indebted to Mr. Nilesh Patil (Lecturer in Mathematics, R. C. Patel College of Pharmacy, Shirpur, Maharashtra) for his invaluable contribution towards the mathematical inputs, especially "Laplace Transformation". We also acknowledge various sources for basic ideas and our sincere gratitude to many researchers whose findings have helped us in putting together this text.

The authors have made every attempt to ensure an error free text. But if there are any errors that have gone unnoticed, we are solely responsible for the same.

Last but not the least, the authors are thankful to Mr. H. S. Poplai, General Manager, CBS Publications and Distributors, New Delhi, for his expert assistance, kind co-operation and patience in bringing out this book.

The authors would appreciate any suggestions from fellow teachers, students and researchers in improving this book (biopharm@ rediffmail.com).

Dr. Jayant S. Kulkarni
Dr. Atmaram P. Pawar
Dr. V. P. Shedbalkar

Contents

1

Absorption of Drugs

1.1 INTRODUCTION

The major route of drug administration is oral route, where drug enters in to gastrointestinal (GI) tract and from different regions of it enters into blood circulation. The other routes for drug administration include oral cavity, rectum, skin, nose, eye, respiratory tract, vagina etc. Though the sites of absorption varies, the absorption is often controlled by same set of barriers, these include mucous, lipoidal membrane, transport process, and cell junctions. Parenteral routes involve the administration of a drug directly into blood circulation e.g intravenous, intra-arterial, etc.

Absorption is the process of movement of drug from its site of administration to the blood stream. The therapeutic response of the drug depends on the rate and extent of drug absorption and its concentration at the site of action.

1.2 CELL MEMBRANES

After administration, drug must surmount one or more biological membranes to reach at and interact with the site of action. Such a movement of drug across the membranes is termed as drug transport.

Each cell in the body is made up of different internal environment from that of its external environment. For example, there is vast difference in the ionic content of animal cells and circulating blood plasma. Throughout the life span of a cell this difference is maintained by a surface structure called *cell membrane* or *plasma membrane*. The main purpose of this membrane is to control the movement of solutes and this function of regulating the movement of solutes across the membrane is called as *permeability*.

In the molecular organization of the membrane (*fluid mosaic model*), few characteristics can be observed (Fig. 1.1):

(1) The membrane is made up of continuous bilayer of lipids into which proteins are embedded in a "mosaic" arrangement

(2) Various proteins are present peripheral to the bilayer and on the inner surface

(3) Oligosaccharide chains (glycolipids and glycoproteins) are present only at the outer surface of the membrane.

1.2.1 Cell Membrane Composition

In general, cell membrane is made up of proteins, lipids and carbohydrates. *In cell membranes, except myelin in neurons, there is higher protein:lipid ratio, in myelin lipid component predominates.* Oligosaccharides are mainly bound to proteins (glycoproteins) and lipids (glycolipids). The basic phospholipid bilayer structure and certain functions are common to almost all biomembranes. But each type of membrane also has certain distinctive functions, which are mainly determined by the unique set of proteins associated with that particular membrane.

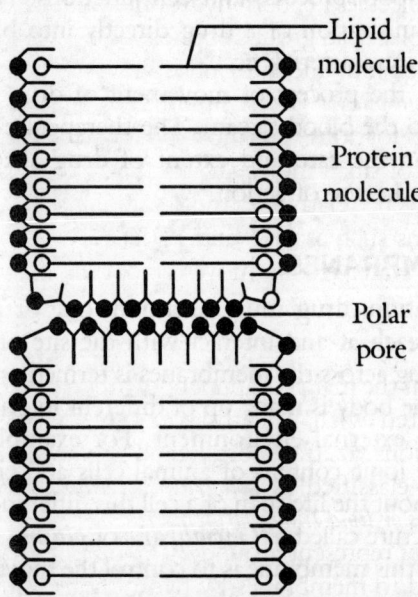

Fig. 1.1. Molecular organization of the cell membrane

Membrane Lipids

The most commonly found lipid components in most membranes are phospholipids, cholesterol and glucolipids. Phospholipids are amphipathic molecules i.e. they have hydrophilic and hydrophobic parts. Phospholipids are mainly constituted by phosphotidyl choline, phosphotidyl ethanolamine and sphingomyelin. There are also neutral phospholipids i.e. no net charge at neutral pH. Neutral phospholipids have a tendency to tightly pack in the bilayer. There are also acidic phospholipids present in the membrane e.g. phosphotidyl inositol, phosphotidyl serine, phosphotidyl glycerol etc. Acidic phospholipids are negatively charged and associate with proteins via lipid-protein interaction. Cholesterol and its derivatives are also important class of membrane lipids. Cholesterol is mainly present in the plasma membrane of mammalian cells and not prokaryotic cells. In spite of being hydrocarbon in composition, cholesterol is amphipathic in nature because of interaction between its hydroxyl groups and water.

Sphingomyelin is also an important class of membrane lipids. Sphingomyelin contains sphingosin, an amino alcohol with a long unsaturated hydrocarbon chain.

It is important to note that membrane lipids are amphipathic (amphiphilic) molecules i.e. both hydrophilic and hydrophobic moiety are present. As polar head groups of phospholipids like to be in contact with water, in aqueous medium phospholipids form a bimolecular sheet called as *lipid bilayer*. These lipid bilayer membranes have a very low permeability for ions and most polar molecules. Except water, the permeability of small molecules is correlated with their solubility in non-polar solvent relative to their solubility in water. Thus, the movement of ions such as Na^+ and K^+ is very slow across the lipid bilayer, however water readily moves across the bilayer.

Membrane Proteins

Proteins represent the main component of most biological membranes and are associated with lipid bilayer. Proteins mediate various membrane functions viz. transport, ligand recognition etc. Membrane proteins can be classified as *integral (intrinsic) proteins, peripheral (extrinsic) proteins or lipid linked proteins.*

Integral proteins represent around 70 % of membrane proteins and are tightly bound to membranes by hydrophobic interactions. These proteins span the lipid bilayer and can be separated only by disrupting the membrane. Also these proteins may be present in the form of glycoproteins e.g. glycophorin A.

Peripheral proteins can be separated by relatively mild treatments e.g. pH change, high ionic strength salt solutions. These proteins do not bind to lipids but are associated with integral proteins e.g. cytochrome C found in mitochondria, spectrin, etc.

Lipid linked proteins are covalently attached to lipids e.g. prenylated proteins are covalently attached to isoprene units such as farnesyl or geranylgeranyl residues or glycosyl phosphotidyl inositol-liked proteins.

Note that the molecular organization of lipids and proteins is highly asymmetrical in the membrane. Although lipid bilayer is impermeable to hydrophilic substances, in reality many hydrophilic substances are known to cross the cell membrane with relative ease. This is mainly because of the various transport proteins present in the membrane. This selective permeability of the membrane plays very important role in the drug action. Because, to produce pharmacologically significant effects, drugs have to cross many membranes in the body.

1.3 MECHANISMS OF DRUG ABSORPTION

Drug is rarely administered in its pure form. Instead, for the convenience of handling and administration, it is usually formulated in the suitable dosage form. Dosage forms such as mixtures, syrups, elixirs, suspensions, granules, tablets or capsules are the commonly administered dosage forms for administration of drug by oral route. In such cases the bioavailability of a drug is influenced chiefly by:

(*i*) Release of drug from the dosage form.

(*ii*) Dissolution of absorbable form of the drug in GI fluid,

(*iii*) Partitioning of drug across the GI membrane.

(*iv*) Extent of biotransformation of drug during its transport.

After oral administration drug can cross gastrointestinal membranes via two routes, intracellular and intercellular (Fig. 1.2). The various mechanisms of the drug absorption are as follows:

(a) Passive Transport

Passive diffusion is the primary process by which drugs are transported from the gastrointestinal tract to blood. It is also called as *nonionic diffusion*. Molecules have a natural tendency to move from high concentration to low concentration. Thus, drug molecules are passively transported because of concentration gradient between gastrointestinal tract and the blood. For this movement no work is expended by the system but only the kinetic energy of the molecules is utilized, hence this type of movement is called as *passive diffusion*.

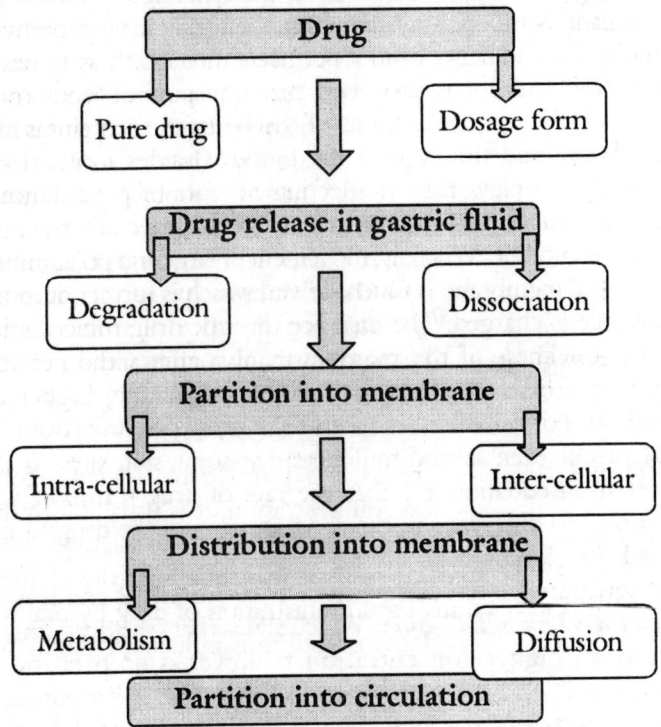

Fig. 1.2. Steps involved in the absorption of a drug

Consider the following equation:

Net rate of penetration = $P \cdot SA \cdot (C_{GIT} - C)$ ...(1.1)

where, P = Permeability

SA = Surface area

$C_{GIT} - C$ = Difference in the concentration of the drug molecule in the gastrointestinal tract and the blood.

It is apparent that increase in the surface area will increase the rate of penetration. The net rate of penetration will vary according to the permeability, which is dependent on molecular size, lipophilicity and charge of the drug molecule. Molecular size plays a vital role in the movement of solutes through the membrane. It appears that small water-filled pores are present in the bilayer. Very few substances e.g. small atoms such as K^+ and Cl^- can pass from GI tract into the blood by the pore route. This is called as *convective transport or filtration* and is important for drugs having M.W. less than 100. Movement of water through these pores helps in the transport of few substances by this route and is called as *solvent drag*. Generally drug molecules are large molecules and hence cannot permeate through these pores. Thus for drugs molecules it is proposed that transport depends on their ability to leave the aqueous fluids of the GI tract, then partition into GI membrane and finally into the blood. Besides molecular size, lipophilicity also plays role in affecting net rate of penetration. The small, lipid-soluble, un-ionized drug molecules are easily transported across the membrane. Whereas, movement of large and polar molecules across the cell membrane is much slower, which is further decreased if the molecule is charged. The distance that the drug molecule has to travel i.e. thickness of the membrane, also affects the net rate of penetration. Lesser the thickness of the membrane, higher is the permeability. For cell membranes this thickness may vary from 0.005 to 0.01 μm or even several millimeters at some skin sites. It is also apparent from equation 1.1 that the rate of drug transport will be proportional to difference in the concentration of the drug in the GI tract and the blood.

The equation 1.1 can be rewritten as equation 1.2 and it is called as *Fick's First Law of Diffusion*. Which states that "the drug molecules diffuse from higher concentration to lower concentration until equilibrium is achieved, and the rate of diffusion is proportional to the concentration gradient across the membrane." It can be mathematically expressed as:

$$\frac{dQ}{dt} = \frac{(D \cdot SA \cdot K_{m/w})}{h(C_{GIT} - C)} \qquad \qquad ...(1.2)$$

where, $\dfrac{dQ}{dt}$ = rate of drug diffusion (rate of penetration); amount/time

          D = diffusion coefficient of the drug through the membrane; area/time

       SA = surface area; area

    $K_{m/w}$ = partition coefficient of the drug

$C_{GIT} - C$ = difference in concentration of the drug molecule in the gastrointestinal tract and the blood

h = thickness of the membrane across which diffusion is taking place; length

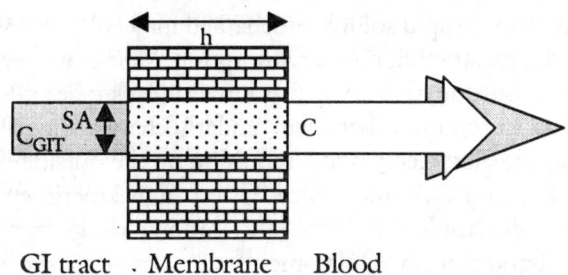

GI tract . Membrane   Blood

Fig. 1.3. Principle of Fick's first law of diffusion

It is important to note that the diffusion of the drug will continue till the equilibrium state is achieved, where concentration of drug molecule is same on both sides of the membrane. Even at equilibrium there will be movement of drug molecule across the membrane but net flux will be zero. When drug is administered, initially difference between drug concentration in GI tract and blood will be large. As the drug is diffused into the blood, because of constant circulation, it will be removed from the site of absorption and will be distributed to various body tissues and cells. Hence a concentration gradient ($C_{GIT} - C$) will always be maintained at the site of absorption. This is called as *sink condition*.

The justification for significance of lipid-water partition coefficient of drug lies with the nature of membrane through which drug travels. The presence of drug in its solution state in GI tract shows better absorption. The partitioning of drug from aqueous GI fluid to lipoidal barrier and again second partitioning from this lipoidal layer into aqueous blood circulation is involved in drug absorption. The drug that has sufficient affinity for the membrane could partition readily into membrane. A drug with high lipid solubility would tend to remain in the intestinal wall and resist partitioning into the blood stream. Therefore, balanced lipoidal-water affinity is needed for absorption into the wall and transfer from wall into the blood. Since the unionized form of drug exhibits greater lipid solubility, the membrane is preferentially permeable to the unionized species.

(b) Electrochemical Diffusion

The diffusion of uncharged molecules is called as *nonionic* diffusion, whereas diffusion of ionic molecules as a function of potential difference or electrical gradient across the membrane is termed as *electrical or ionic diffusion*. The ionic drugs cross the membrane much more slowly than do lipid soluble, uncharged molecules. Nevertheless, ionic drugs demonstrate significant absorption. Membrane is positively charged on the outside surface whereas intracellular surface is negatively charged. Due to repulsion between similarly charged molecules, the cationic drugs exhibit electrostatic repulsion on the outside surface of the membrane and only molecules with a high kinetic energy can cross the barrier. Inside the membrane, cationic drugs interact with negatively charged intracellular membrane, creating the electrical gradient, in turn causing *electrical diffusion*. An *electrochemical diffusion* is the function of both electrical field and the concentration difference across the membrane. This process continues until equilibrium is attained.

(c) Ion-pair Transport

The zwitterionic drugs ionize over the entire pH range of the GI tract, e.g. ampicillin, amoxicillin, tetracycline. As discussed above, smaller ionic drug can travel through water-filled pores. However, zwitterionic drugs are too large to pass through the water-filled pores and are too lipid insoluble to partition through lipoidal membrane. Such drugs cross the membrane by forming ion-pair with endogenous ions of the GI tract. The charge is utilized to form ion-pair and the resulting molecule gets partitioned into the lipoidal membrane. Though these drugs are ionic, they show passive absorption and exhibit maximum partition coefficient when the net charge on the molecule is at its minimum.

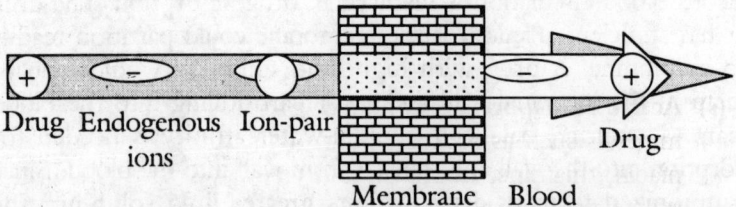

Drug Endogenous Ion-pair
ions

Membrane Blood

Drug

Fig. 1.4. Ion pair transport of cationic drug

(d) Carrier Mediated Transport

Most of the drugs are absorbed by passive diffusion down the chemical, electrical or electrochemical gradient. When the concentration of drug is equal on both sides of the membrane, the net absorption is zero and the state is said to be as *equilibrium absorption state*. In carrier mediated system, drug-carrier complex brings about drug transport. Carrier may be an enzyme or some other type of biological agent capable of forming a complex with the drug at the surface of membrane. The drug -carrier complex moves across the membrane and releases the drug on the serosal side. The free carrier then returns to its initial position to carry another drug molecule. The carrier system is one-way transport system. However, due to structural similarity two or more solutes may compete for the same carrier and preferential absorption of one solute over other is possible. This fact is positively utilized in cancer treatment e.g. 5-fluorouracil and 5-bromouracil have structural resemblance to the naturally existing pyrimidines. Hence these drugs get absorbed via the pyrimidine transporter. The carrier-mediated transport may be active or passive.

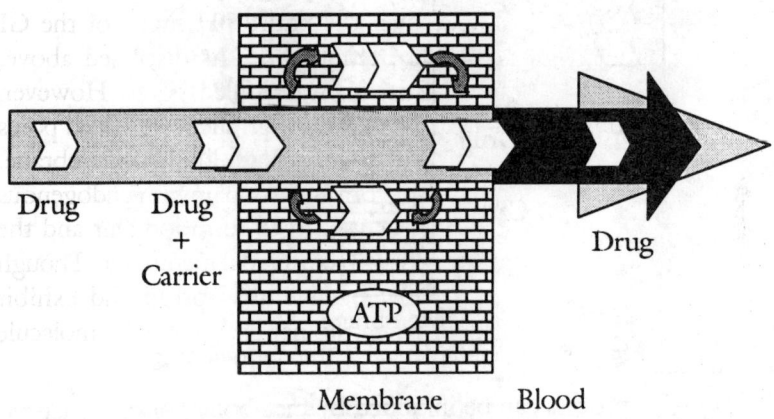

Drug   Drug + Carrier   Drug

ATP

Membrane   Blood

Fig. 1.5. Active transport of drug

(*i*) **Active Transport:** Many nutrients such as sugars, amino acids, minerals such as sodium, potassium, iron, and vitamins like niacin, thiamine, riboflavin and vitamin B_6 get absorbed via active transport system. Methyldopa, 5-fluorouracil, 5-bromouracil, nicotinamide are examples of drugs which utilize active transport systems. The characteristics of active transport include:

(*i*) Drug is transported from *uphill*, that is, against concentration gradient or electrochemical gradient.

(*ii*) The process requires energy.

(*iii*) Maximum absorption of drug occurs from the location of higher carrier density. Hence the number of drugs show good absorption from the proximal portion of the small intestine.

(*iv*) It involves carriers for a drug with specific chemical structural properties. Therefore the transport may be competitively inhibited by other chemicals (food/drug) of similar characteristics. For example, preferential absorption of levodopa in place of tyrosine and phenylalanine by the same carrier (Fig. 1.6).

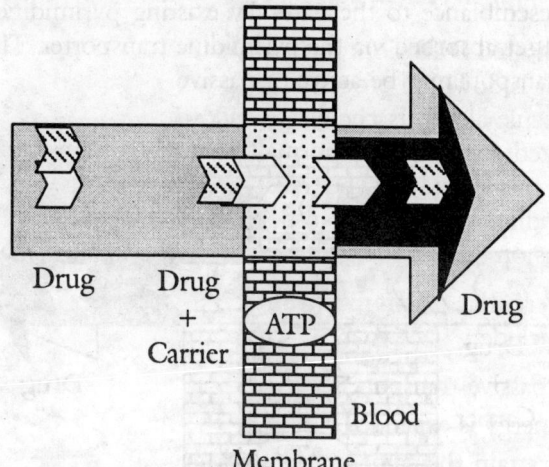

Fig. 1.6. Competitive active transport of drug

(*v*) The process can be inhibited by metabolic poisons, such as sodium fluoride, cyanide, dinitrophenol etc.

(*vi*) Rate of passive absorption is a linear function of drug concentration at the site whereas carrier mediated transport shows linear dependence on concentration at low concentrations only. At higher drug concentration the carrier mechanism becomes saturated, therefore it is termed as *a capacity limited process* (Fig. 1.7).

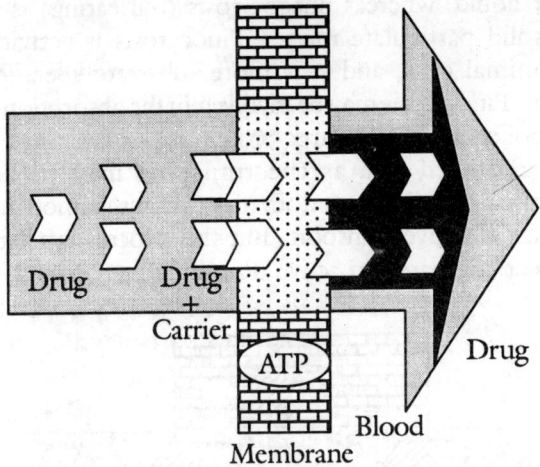

Fig. 1.7. Saturation of active transport of drug

(*ii*) **Facilitated Diffusion:** It is also a carrier mediated drug transport but it is downhill process. This process involves transport of a molecule along its chemical or electrochemical gradient. It is utilized for ions that normally would not pass through the lipid bilayer but may be transported by membrane proteins by providing hydrophilic transport channels. It is faster than passive diffusion.

The differential points between active transport and facilitated diffusion include:

(a) it is passive transport,

(b) no energy is expended,

(c) may attain the same concentration inside the cell as that on outside and

(d) the process is not inhibited by metabolic poisons.

Examples are glucose, vitamins such as thiamine, riboflavin and vitamin B_{12}.

(e) Endocytosis

This process is characterized by engulfment of the solute by membrane and subsequent release. This process is divided into pinocytosis and phagocytosis. Pinocytosis (cell drinking) involves the capture of extracellular liquid, whereas phagocytosis (cell eating) is absorptive uptake of solid particulate matter. Pinocytosis is activity of most nucleated animal cells, and it is more substrate specific than the phagocytosis. Pinocytosis may be involved in the absorption of vitamin B_{12}, Sabin polio vaccine and large protein molecules. Since metabolic activity is required and as the transport may be against an electrochemical gradient, endocytosis shows some of the same characteristics as active transport. But this process is relatively slow and inefficient compared to active transport.

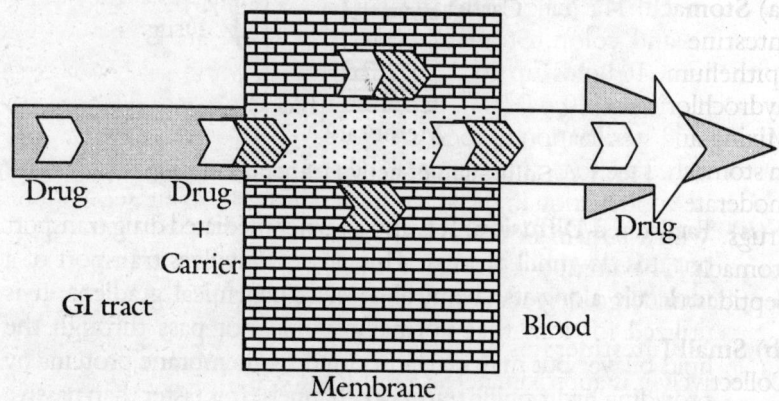

Fig. 1.8. Facilitated diffusion

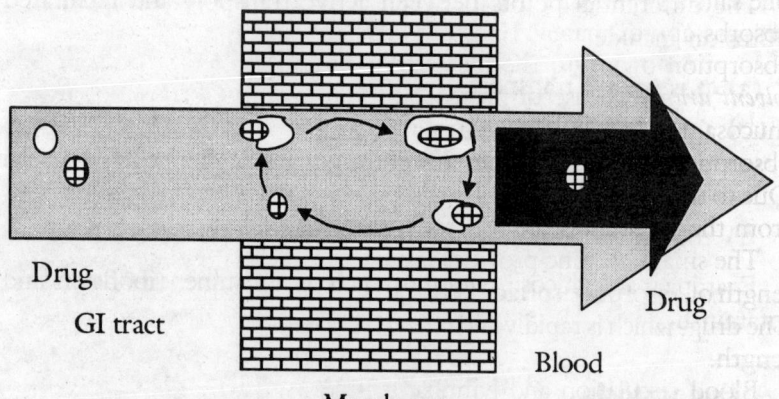

⊗ = Phagocytosis of solid, ○ = Pinocytosis of liquid

Fig. 1.9. Mechanism of endocytosis

Like pinocytosis there is another process which is highly selective for specific molecules or particles and this process is called *as receptor-mediated endocytosis* e.g. transport of hormones, cholesterol, iron etc. Through the same process some viruses can sneak into and infect cells e.g. HIV

1.4 FACTORS INFLUENCING DRUG ABSORPTION

(A) Physiological Factors

1. Gastrointestinal Physiology

(a) **Stomach:** The major compartments of GI tract are stomach, small intestine and colon. Stomach is lined with a relatively smooth epithelium. It holds up to 1 to 1.5 L of gastric juice containing hydrochloric acid (0.4-0.5%), pepsin, mucus and various electrolytes. Mixing and sterilization of food are the two main activities occurring in stomach. Due to less surface area and shorter gastric residence it has moderate contribution in the absorption of drugs. Mostly, weak acidic drugs, which remain in unionized state, demonstrate absorption in stomach. The number of drugs including antibiotics, proteins and peptides undergo degradation because of the acidic environment.

(b) **Small Intestine:** It is divided into duodenum, jejunum and ileum. Collectively it is approximately 23 feet long with surface area of about 300 m^2. The jejunum is more vascular than the duodenum and has larger and more numerous villi than the ileum. It contains bile acids, bile salts and enzymes like maltase, nuclease, lipase, etc. The intestine absorbs approximately 10 L of water per day. The increase in drug absorption owing to the increase in water absorption is termed as *solvent drag*. Because of presence of villi, microvilli and folds in the mucosa, the small intestine provides largest effective surface area for absorption. Secondly, carrier density is highest in the small intestine. Due to these reasons, most drugs in solution are absorbed more rapidly from the small intestine.

The small intestine provides lager *reserve length*; it is defined as the length of absorptive surface available after the drug has been absorbed. The drug, which is rapidly and effectively absorbed, has a larger reserved length.

Blood circulation and lymphatic circulation are the two drainage systems operating for drug absorption. The material absorbed through veins undergo first pass metabolism. In the ileum, the Peyer's patches (lymphatic follicles) are larger and more numerous than rest of the intestine. Lymphatic route by passes the portal metabolism, but this route is restricted to extremely lipophilic drugs and the drugs formulated in oily vehicles show a greater absorption by this route.

(c) Colon: Colon is 125 cm long and can be divided into the caecum and ascending, transverse, descending and sigmoidal colon, rectum and anus. The conservation of water and electrolytes and formation of solid stool ready for defecation are the main functions of colon. Unlike intestinal mucosa, colonic mucosa lacks well-defined villi, which reduces the absorptive surface area. The longer residense time of drug in viscous colonic content may provide sustained release of drug. A significant portion of drug enters into colon if a drug demonstrates inefficient absorption from the upper part of GI tract. It can be used as an important site for the absorption of some drugs that undergo degradation in upper GI tract. Drug can be targeted to colon in two ways, proximal colon have to be delivered via oral route and the distal colon via anus. Colon is rich in different bacteria species and enzymes. Drug may undergo metabolism by these bacteria resulting in either inactive or toxic metabolite.

2. pH of Gastrointestinal Tract

An unionized form of a drug due to its lipid solubility has faster absorption than the ionized form from any particular site of GI tract. For example, absorption of NSAIDs, sulphonamides (weak acids) is favored in stomach and absorption of weak basic drugs like antihistamines and antidepressant is favored in small intestine. The weak acidic drugs such as furosemide (pK_a = 3.9), ibuprofen (pK_a = 4.4) are relatively insoluble in the gastric content but have faster dissolution in the upper small intestine The pH of GI fluid varies considerably from 1.3 to 7.5. The average pH values at different location of GI content in the fasted and fed state in healthy human are summarized in Table 1.1.

Table 1.1: The average pH values at different locations in GI tract

Location	Average pH in the fasted state	Average pH in the fed state
Stomach	1.3	4.9
Duodenum	6.5	5.5
Jejunum	6.6	5.2-6.0
Ileum	7.4	7.5

3. GI Transit

The total GI transit time is highly variable ranging from 6 hrs to 5 days. In general the total residence time can be divided as gastric residence (~2 hrs), small intestine residence (~3 hrs) and remaining in colon.

(a) **Gastric Emptying:** Gastric residence of drug may have significant effect on absorption of weak acidic drugs. But in overall sense this region shows poor absorption. Since small intestine is a comparatively better absorption site, any factors that promote gastric emptying increase the absorption rate of drugs.

Factors affecting gastric emptying are as follows:

(*i*) *Circadian Rhythm*: Gastric emptying is rapid in daytime than during night.

(*ii*) *Sex*: In females gastric emptying is slower than males.

(*iii*) *Food*: The presence and type of the food mainly determine the gastric residence of dosage form. Food intake prolongs gastric retention time (GRT). Broadly the effect of type of food on rate of gastric emptying can be ranked as carbohydrates > proteins > fats. Greater is the energy content of the meal; longer is the duration of emptying. Hot or cold food reduces gastric emptying.

(*iv*) *Medicines:* Intake of alcohol, antacids, and anti-cholinergic drugs can also delay gastric emptying. Prokinetic drugs like cisapride, mosapride increase gastric emptying.

(*v*) *Disease State*: Gastric emptying is delayed by various disease conditions including atropic gastritis, gastric carcinoma, pyloric stenosis, pancreatitis, and gastric ulcer. Diseases like duodenal ulcer, celiac disease, stress may accelerate it.

(*vi*) *Dosage Form*: The gastric emptying of liquid dosage form is much faster, exponential and less variable compared to solid and non-disintegrating unit dosage forms. The particles greater than 1-2 mm get reduced by the normal digestive process and have emptying similar to liquids. Interdigestive housekeeper wave empties the non-digestible particles at the end of digestive phase. In general the gastric emptying time of liquid formulation is 1-2 hours, large non-disintegrating units given after meal show emptying at around 2 to 3 hours, the pellets and microspheres empty more slowly in fed condition, as they are in the dispersed state. Low density spheres and 'floating dosage forms' empty more slowly, may be 8 hours or longer (more than 10 hours) if administered after a heavy meal.

(b) Intestinal Motility: The intestinal residence is comparatively constant; 3 ± 1 hour. The mixing movement because of motility increases the dissolution rate of drug and brings drug into intimate contact with the large absorptive surface area of the small intestine. The single unit can be retained in ileocaecal valve for long periods (4-12 hours) before being carried into the colon.

(c) Colonic Residence: Longer travel distance and longer residence are contributing factors for drug absorption from colon. However, only the ascending colon provides favorable conditions for drug absorption. The consolidation of fecal matter gradually increases the viscosity of the colonic content with a resulting difficulty of drug release from the dosage form and diffusion of released drug to the absorbing surface. The number of factors such as diet, stress, disease condition and drug change colonic residence of drug. Food, especially fibrous food decreases colon transit time. Diarrhoea decreases gut transit time, changes electrolyte content and luminal pH resulting in the changes in absorption of drug.

4. Absorption Sites

Drugs have a particular site for maximum absorption. The following table summarizes the comparative drug absorption from different regions of GI tract.

Table 1.2: Comparative absorption from different parts of GI tract

Drug	Stomach	Jejunum	Ileum	Colon
Furosemide	****	–	**	*
Isradipine	**	**	****	****
Nifedipine	**	**	–	****
Omeprazole	–	*	**	***
Phenytoin	–	*	**	***
Theophylline	***	**	–	**

5. Protein Binding

Free drug concentration in body is responsible for pharmacodynamic properties of drug. The drug bound to proteins in blood (plasma), membranes or tissue is difficult to diffuse, absorb, reach to the site of action and interact with receptors. The rate of biotransformation and elimination are also decreased because of protein binding. Albumin is the main component, which binds to a wide variety of drugs. The protein binding is usually reversible and it releases drug from the protein until drug in the extravascular water equilibrates with free drug in the plasma. Binding may be competitive where one drug displaces another drug e.g. aspirin displaces penicillin. Infants and adults show difference in plasma protein binding and tissue binding of drugs, e.g. local anesthetics, sulfaphenazole.

6. Presystemic Metabolism

Liver is the primary site of drug metabolism. In addition, presystemic metabolism of drug can occur in GI tract or in membrane. Reduction in amount of absorbed dose by biotransformation of drug in liver before its entry into blood circulation is termed as *first pass metabolism*. After oral administration of drug, almost entire absorbed dose is exposed to the liver. If a drug is subject to rapid metabolism in liver, then a reduced absorbed dose reaches in blood circulation. For some drugs bioavailability may be reduced to such an extent so as to render the GI route of administration ineffective. The examples include alprenolol, imipramine, lignocaine, pethidine, phenacitin, and propranolol.

7. Circadian Rhythm

The functions of body including body secretions and pharmacokinetics display its own time schedule per day and over entire life period; this is called as *circadian cycle*. Diseases such as bronchitis, ischemic heart attacks, rheumatoid arthritis, and allergic rhinitis display circadian dependent symptoms in early morning hours. Acidity gradually increases from 4 pm and it is maximum at mid night. Patients suffering from sleeping disorder need second dose of sedatives at around 2 am.

NSAID, theophylline, nifedipine, oral nitrates, and propranolol have been reported to have higher C_{max} and shorter t_{max} when administered in the morning than evening. It was correlated with the faster gastric emptying which carry drug to efficient absorption site of small intestine and greater GI perfusion in the morning. Such variation in pharmacokinetics was mainly observed in case of lipophilic drugs. Atenonol, a hydrophilic drug has not shown such rise in bioavailability after oral administration at morning time.

8. Patient Factors

(a) **Age:** In general, processes involved in bioavailability of the drug such as absorption, distribution, metabolism and elimination decline with age. On the other side, young children may also not absorb some drugs readily and they may not have certain systems completely developed.

(b) **Sex:** The relative proportion of muscular and adipose tissue in the individuals may alter the absorption, distribution and clearance of drug. The pregnant females may react differently to a drug. In pregnancy, the total body water increases (6-8 L); secondly variations in hormones, weight distribution may have direct or indirect effect on drug distribution. Also, during the luteal phase of the menstrual cycle and during pregnancy when progesterone levels are high there is a delay in GI transit.

(c) **Body Weight:** Whether the body weight is lean body mass or fat mass significantly affects drug distribution. Patient with smaller volumes of body fluids and of lighter weight usually have higher blood drug levels.

(d) **Activity and Posture:** The activity and posture dependent changes in plasma volume or blood flow rate may show variation in pharmacokinetics of certain drugs.

(e) **Food:** In general drug absorption is maximum from the empty stomach. Food reduces rate of absorption of drug but does not changes the extent of absorption, e.g. aspirin, acetaminophen, phenobarbital sodium and rifampin. Absorption of certain drugs such as vitamin B_2 is increased in the presence of food.

The volume of fluid available for disintegration and dissolution of dosage form is low in stomach in fasted state. A meal can raise the pH to 3 to 5, whereas food such as milk can raise it to 6. This is important for weak acids and bases, since the ionization of drug is dependent on the pH of GI content. Food increases GI secretions, GI motility and splanchnic blood circulation. The reasons behind enhancement of absorption of drug in presence of food are:

(*i*) Increased gastric residence and by enhanced segmental contractions associated with an increase in mixing efficiency. The latter reduces the diffusion layer thickness and maintains greater concentration gradient.

(*ii*) The prolonged gastric residence in presence of food increases concentration of lipid soluble unionized form of weakly acidic drug.

(*iii*) Bile salts due to their surface tension lowering property have manifold effects such as increase in the permeability of the intestine, increase in solubility and rate of dissolution of some poorly soluble drug or decrease agglomeration of powders.

On the other hand, the acid secreted in response to food may enhance the degradation of drug causing incomplete drug absorption. The presence of viscous chime can act as a physical barrier reducing drug access to the absorbing surface. Pellets, disintegrated particles empty more slowly in the presence of food, since they are dispersed in a large volume of meal. Foods containing polyvalent metals and fibers also have negative effect on absorption of certain drugs. The polyvalent metals form complex with drugs like doxycycline, tetracycline, whereas fibers entrap drugs.

Table 1.3: Effect of food on absorption of some drugs

Unaffected	Increased	Delayed	Reduced
Chlorpropamide	Carbamazepine	Acetaminophen	Ampicillin
Ethambutol	Diazepam	Cephalosporins	Atenolol
Oxazepam	Griseofulvin	Diclofenac	Penicillin
Tolbutamide	Propranolol	Furosemide	Warfarin

(**f**) **Medicines:** As compared to small intestine, the absorption of drug from stomach is considered to be relatively insignificant. Therefore, any drug that influences the rate of gastric emptying can change drug absorption. Anticholinergic drugs inhibit or reduce gastric secretions and the antacids usually elevate gastric pH. The increase in gastric pH may increase the solubility of acidic drugs and decrease the solubility of basic drugs. Anti-diarrhoeal formulations containing kaolin and pectin reduce drug absorption due to adsorption of drug on their high surface area. Heamatinic formulations containing ferrous sulphate may form chelates with antibiotics such as tetracycline and doxycycline.

(g) **Disease Conditions:** The GI secretions and GI transit differ during different disease conditions such as GI ulcer, acidity, achlorhydria, Diarrhoea, constipation etc. Analgesics like aspirin, paracetamol have good absorption from small intestine. Since gastric emptying is delayed in migraine, the absorption of these analgesic drugs is also delayed during migraine attacks. In cystic fibrosis, the pancreatic secretions are significantly reduced, which results in lowering the buffer capacity of small intestine. Iron and folic acid show poor absorption after gastrectomy. Intestinal inflammatory conditions such as Crohn's disease and Celiac disease cause malabsorption of drug and nutrients. Post surgery reduced absorption of sulphasalazine from colon is associated with decrease in azo reductase bacteria, which cleave azo linkage in colon to release the active metabolic 5-aminosalicylate.

(B) Physicochemical Factors
1. Drug Solubility

Formation of drug solution in the body fluid is a prerequisite for the drug absorption after its administration. The differences in bioavailability of various commercial brands of phenytoin have been reported as a result of poor solubility. Therefore various attempts were made to improve solubility of phenytoin, these includes conversion in crystal form, micronization, co-precipitation with PVP, complex with cyclodextrins, solid dispersion with PEG etc.

Since body fluids are aqueous in nature, the water-soluble drugs are best candidates for better absorption. But aqueous solubility of the drug is not the only way to achieve rapid and complete drug absorption. The powder properties, ionic properties, lipophilic-hydrophilic properties, molecular size and ability to get soluble in body fluid are some of the other important parameters, which influence absorption.

The drugs are usually orally administered in doses ranging from few micrograms to 1 g. After oral administration the complete dose of drug should be soluble in the GI fluid. Though GI fluid is aqueous in nature, it is composed of diverse type of chemical components viz. electrolytes, enzymes, surfactants, etc. These have direct or indirect effects on the solubility of drug in GI content. If drug has good water solubility there is less possibility of *desolvation* of drug, and then the dose of drug is not a constraint to form solution in GI fluid. But when drug is poorly soluble in water, the incomplete dissolution of dose in GI fluid, in turn incomplete bioavailability of drug is possible. For example, aqueous solubility of griseofulvin is 15 μg/ml and its dose is 500 mg. The poor bioavailability of griseofulvin may be due to incomplete dissolution of large dose. This effect is explained by *dose: solubility ratio*, which is the prime determinant of absorption of drug. The dose:solubility ratio is the volume of GI fluids necessary to dissolve the administered dose.

2. Drug Stability

The acidic or alkaline nature of GI content, presence of enzymes and bacteria are reasons of drug degradation after oral administration. For example, antibiotics are relatively stable between pH 6-8 but are rapidly destroyed at gastric pH. The longer is the gastric emptying time more likely the drug is to be degraded by acidic pH of the stomach. The enteric coating is the widely used technique to overcome this problem but it delays the drug release and hence absorption. Alternatively the drug can be given by other suitable route such as sublingual, transdermal or rectal.

Consequences of degradation of drug:

1. Incomplete bioavailability as only a fraction of the parent drug gets absorbed.

2. Degraded product may be more toxic e.g. salicylic acid is more irritant than aspirin.

3. The process may be essential for drug absorption after administration of pro-drug, which after degradation in the GI tract releases the therapeutically active molecule.

The compromise between solubility and stability of drug in GI content is a key factor determining the bioavailability of the orally administered drug. For example, Progabide is a weak base with pK_a of 3.41. It is reasonably soluble below pH 3 and poorly soluble above pH 4. At acidic pH the drug undergoes hydrolysis to release GABA and benzophenone. At pH 6.3 it has maximum solubility and it has rapid absorption from small intestine. In such cases, following critical characteristics of drug decide the design of dosage form and bioavailability.

(*i*) Micronization of drug will increase the solubility in small intestine, which is a better absorption site but at the same time because of increased surface area there will be increased rate of drug degradation in stomach.

(*ii*) Enteric coating will protect drug from acidic environment, but the insoluble drug will reach small intestine.

(*iii*) The rapid gastric emptying of micronized drug will ensure faster drug dissolution and minimum drug degradation.

3. Dissociation and Lipid Solubility

The solubility of weak acids and weak bases is dependent on their ionization constant pK_a and pH of the dissolution medium. At pH values exceeding $pK_a +1$, a linear relation between the logarithm of the solubility and the pH is observed until the limiting solubility of the ionized form is reached.

Diffusion of drug through membranes depends on lipid-water partition coefficients and thus the degree of ionization of the drug. The unionized form of the drugs has more solubility in lipoidal membrane. The ionic drug has poor absorption, which is attributed to:

(a) Poor lipid solubility.

(b) Electrostatic repulsion at membrane surface.

(c) Enlargement of molecules due to hydration.

The proportion of ionized form to unionized form of drug is affected by the pH of fluids on both sides of the membrane and pK_a of the drug. The effect of pH of fluids on trans-membrane partitioning of drug is explained by *pH-partition theory*. *The pH-partition theory states that the absorption of a weak electrolyte is a function of the extent to which the drug exists in its unionized state in aqueous solution at the site of absorption.* The passive diffusion of unionized drug takes place until equilibrium is reached. In acidic gastric content, the weak acidic drug exists almost entirely in its unionized form. After partitioning of unionized form, drug reaches blood circulation, having alkaline pH (pH 7.4). Where, a major portion of drug exists in the ionized form. Because of this, once the drug is absorbed in blood circulation it cannot pass back into the stomach. This effect is referred to as *ion-trapping*. The concentration of the ionized form on each side of the membrane may not be equal. In intestinal tract the reverse is true because the increasing pH in the intestine causes weak bases to be more completely unionized and weak acids more ionized.

The ratio of unionized to ionized molecules is important in predicting absorption in the GI tract. The *Henderson-Hasselbalch equation* can be used to calculate such ratio when pK_a of the drug and pH of the fluid are known.

For acids

$$pH = pK_a + \log \frac{[\text{Ionized acid}]}{[\text{Unionized acid}]} \qquad \text{...1.4}$$

For bases

$$pH = pK_a + \log \frac{[\text{Unonized acid}]}{[\text{Ionized acid}]} \qquad \text{...1.5}$$

Table 1.4: pK_a values for some drugs

Weak acids	pK_a	Weak bases	pK_a
Aspirin	3.5	Atropine	9.65
Ibuprofen	4.4	Codeine	7.9
Nalidixic acid	6.7	Diphenhydramine	8.3
Phenobarbital	7.41	Diazepam	3.7
Salicylic acid	3.0	Theophylline	0.7
Tolbutamide	5.4	Trimethoprim	6.4

Absorption of weakly acidic drug (pK_a 4) and weakly basic drug (pK_a 8) is explained as follows:

For acids

(*i*)
$$\log \frac{[A^-]}{[HA]} = pH - pK_a$$
$$1.2 - 4 = -2.8$$

Therefore,
$$\frac{[A^-]}{[HA]} = \text{antilog}(-2.8) = 0.06310$$

(*ii*)
$$\log \frac{[A^-]}{[HA]} = pH - pK_a$$
$$7.4 - 4 = 3.4$$

Therefore,
$$\frac{[A^-]}{[HA]} = \text{antilog}(3.4) = 251.2$$

Thus in acidic fluid of pH 1.2, the ratio of $[A^-]$ to $[HA]$ of weak acidic drug (pKa 4) is 0.06310. It indicates that the majority of drug exists in unionized form, which has better absorption. When drug enters in blood it exists almost entirely in an ionized form.

For bases

(*i*)
$$\log [BH^+]/[B] = pK_a - pH$$
$$= 8 - 1.2 = 6.8$$

Therefore,
$$\log [BH^+]/[B] = \text{antilog } (6.8) = 6.31 \times 10^6$$

(*ii*)
$$\log [BH^+]/[B] = pK_a - pH$$
$$8 - 7.4 = 0.6$$

Therefore,
$$\log[BH^+]/[B] = \text{antilog } (0.6) = 3.981$$

It indicates that majority of drug remains in ionized state in gastric fluid.

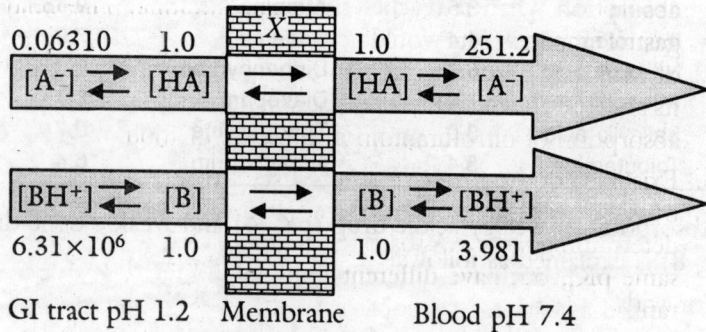

GI tract pH 1.2   Membrane   Blood pH 7.4

Fig. 1.10. pH- partition hypothesis

Limitations of pH-partition Theory

1. The pH-partition theory is based on assumption of attainment of equilibrium distribution between unionized and ionized forms of a drug. However, due to blood circulation the drug is continuously swept away maintaining *sink condition*. Therefore, it is the biggest failing of this hypothesis to calculate absorption from equilibrium distribution.

2. The hypothesis is more suitable in describing absorption of weak acids and weak bases.

3. The ionization of drug in the lumen is similar to that in the blood and little ion trapping occurs.

4. Absorption from GI tract is not only attributed to the pH at different regions or lipid solubility of drug but it also depends on other factors such as the gastric residence, surface area available for absorption, degradation of drug, etc.

5. Some weak acidic drugs may show better absorption from small intestine. It is because that poorly soluble weakly acidic drug has a high dissolution rate in an alkaline environment. Thus, the higher surface area is available for absorption of dissolved drug; secondly the weakly acidic pH (pH 5.3) at surface of the intestinal mucosa is responsible for effective absorption of weakly acidic drug that exists in unionized state. This hypothesis then raises questions regarding absorption of weak bases. The weak bases may interact with organic cations, which are secreted from blood into the lumen of the intestine.

A poorly water-soluble weakly basic drug, which highly dissociates and dissolves in stomach, may also show better absorption when it reaches the small intestine. The delayed gastric emptying rate would permit a longer time for dissolution of weak-basic drug in acidic fluid and in turn it would increase its absorption when it reaches the small intestine, e.g. enhanced absorption of nitrofurantoin in presence of food.

6. Existence of drug in its unionized state is not the sole criteria but the solubility of unionized form of drugs is the rate determining step, e.g. barbituric acid derivatives have almost same pK_a, but have different lipid solubilities, which can be ranked as barbital < apobarbital < pentobarbital.

7. Certain drugs despite of ionization, have good solubility in all the parts of GI tract e.g. tetracycline and theophylline

4. Dissolution Rate

Presence of the drug in solution state at absorption site is one of the prerequisite of absorption of drug. Therefore, factors that influence the rate of dissolution of the drug in GI fluid influence the bioavailability of drug. *Dissolution rate may be defined as the amount of substance that goes into solution per unit time under standard conditions of temperature, pressure and solvent composition.* Dissolution is a dynamic process and is considered to involve mass transfer. Following are some of the theories to explain process of dissolution of drug.

(a) **Noyes-Whitney Theory or Stagnant Film Theory:** Noyes-Whitney equation describes the process of dissolution. It states that *the rate of dissolution of drug (d_c/d_t) is directly proportional to the diffusion coefficient of the drug in solution in GI fluid (D), the effective surface area of the drug particle available for drug dissolution (A), difference in the saturation solubility of the drug in the diffusion layer (C_s) and the concentration of drug in solution in the bulk of GI fluid (C) and inversely proportional to the thickness of diffusion layer (x)* (Equation 1.6).

$$\frac{d_c}{dt} = \frac{DA(C_s - C)}{x} \qquad \ldots 1.6$$

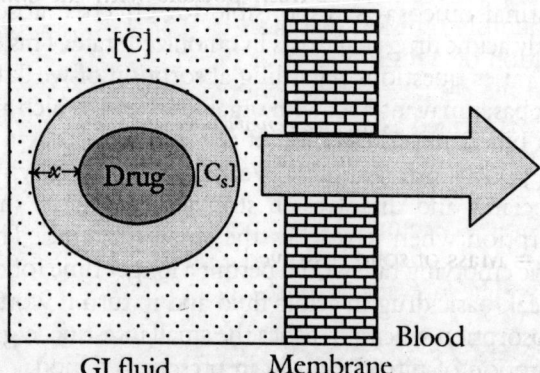

Fig. 1.11. Dissolution process of drug in GI tract

The equation is based on diffusion controlled dissolution process. The driving force for this first-order process is $(C_s - C)$. But the *in-vivo* conditions are different. GI motility affects the thickness of diffusion layer by disturbing it. Additionally the rapid and continuous absorption of drug in blood circulation increases the concentration gradient. The equation 1.6 may be expressed as:

$$\frac{d_c}{dt} = \frac{D \cdot A \cdot C_s}{x} \qquad \ldots 1.7$$

This theory assumes that the surface area of the dissolving solute remains constant during dissolution, but practically it is not possible. Hixson and Crowell modified the Noyes-Whitney to explain the effects of change in the surface area:

$$W_0^{1/3} - W^{1/3} = K \cdot t \qquad \ldots 1.8$$

where, W_0 = Initial powder weight, W = Powder weight at time t, K = Constant which is function of particle density, viscosity, diffusion coefficient, C_s and x.

Equation 1.8 is also termed as *Hixson and Crowell's Cubic Root Law.*

(b) **Danckewrt's Model:** Danckewrt's model of dissolution does not consider the formation of diffusion layer and the solid surface is continuously exposed to fresh solvent causing the mass transfer. It is assumed that the dissolution medium is under the turbulence, which extends up to surface of the solid. The agitated dissolution medium consists of a mass of eddies or pockets. These continuously get exposed to the solid surface, absorb the solute by diffusion and carry it to the bulk of the solution. The contact of fresh pockets with the solid surface continuously transfers the mass to the bulk, not allowing the formation of diffusion layer or C_s. This process of dissolution due to the contact of fresh pockets of solvent with new solid surface is termed as *surface renewal process.*

$$\frac{V d_c}{dt} = \frac{dm}{dt} = A\sqrt{\gamma\, D(C_s - C)} \qquad \dots 1.9$$

where, V = Volume of dissolution medium,

m = Mass of solid dissolved

γ = The rate of surface renewal or interfacial tension.

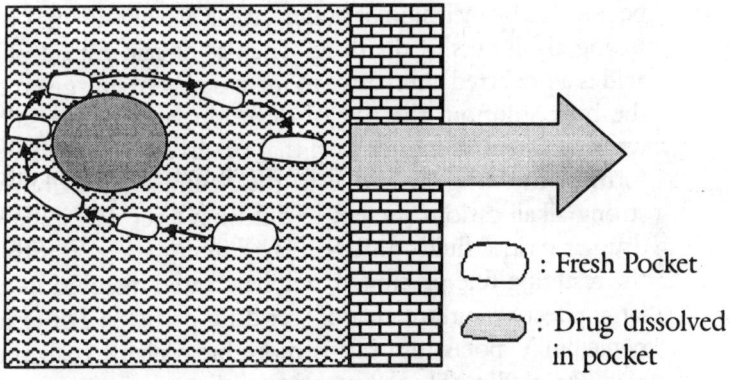

( ) : Fresh Pocket

( ) : Drug dissolved in pocket

Fig. 1.12. Surface renewal process of dissolution

(c) **Limited Salvation Theory:** It states that an intermediate concentration less than saturation exists at the interface as a result of salvation mechanism, which is the function of solubility than that of the diffusion. In the dissolution of crystals the different faces of a crystal will have different interfacial barrier. It can be explained by following equation:

$$G = K_i \cdot (C_s - C) \qquad \dots 1.10$$

where, G = The dissolution rate per unit area,

K_i = The effective interfacial transport constant.

Factors Affecting Dissolution of Drug

1. **Physiological Conditions:** Presence of food, viscosity of GI fluid and GI motility affect the thickness of diffusion layer. An increase in viscosity of GI content can decrease the ability of molecule to diffuse away from the surface. GI motility and absorption of drug in blood circulation increases the concentration gradient by disturbing the diffusion layer and maintaining sink condition, respectively.

2. **Salt Forms:** As discussed above, the solubility of unionized drug in GI fluid is important for its absorption. For the dissociation of weak acids and weak bases, the pH of the diffusion layer plays significant role. The pH of the GI fluid is not necessarily equal to the pH in the diffusion layer or microenvironment of the drug particle. Though weakly acidic drugs have poor solubility in stomach, the unionized form produced in acidic gastric content has better absorption. However, due to its insolubility it produces low C_s. Thus, raising the pH of microenvironment could increase C_s; it could be possible by inclusion of buffers, weak alkaline agents or using strong alkali salts of the drug. The use of salt instead of weak acid is a preferred alternative to increase C_s. At any given pH of the bulk solution, the pH of diffusion layer of the salt of a weak acid will be higher than that observed with the free acid form of the drug. It is due to the neutralizing action of the strong alkali cations present in diffusion layer. Precipitation of drug at gastric fluid- diffusion layer interphase is possible but the resulting fine precipitate will have rapid dissolution due to large effective surface area of wet drug particles. For example, penicillin V potassium salt is more bioavailable than the free acid. At acidic pH, tolbutamide sodium is 500 times more soluble than that of free acid. The solubility of ibuprofen and its sodium salt is as follows

Drug	pH 2	pH 6.5	pH 8
Ibuprofen	5.02	5.65	30.4
Ibuprofen Sodium	8.90	42.00	57.8

When a drug is a weak base, its maximum ionization and dissolution will occur in gastric fluid. However, due to effective absorption capacity of small intestine, state of ionization of drug will have insignificant effect on drug absorption.

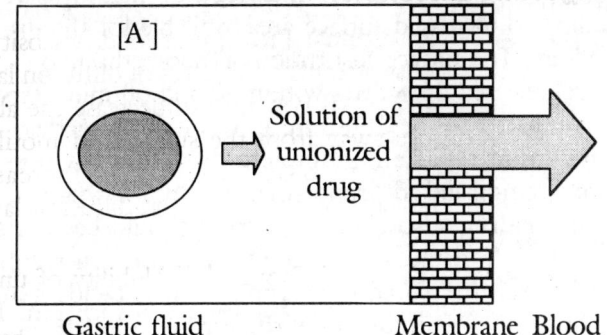

(a) Weak acidic drug

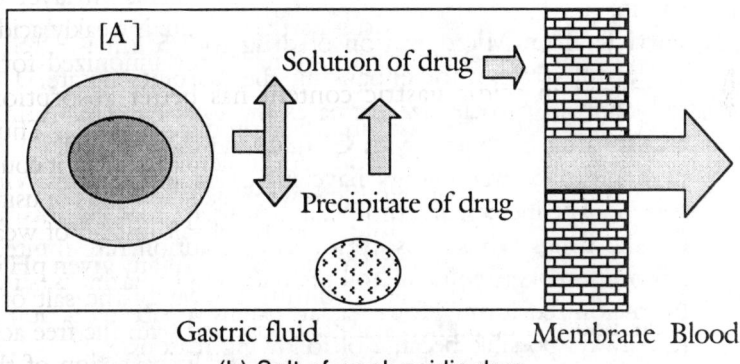

(b) Salt of weak acidic drug

Fig. 1.13. Dissolution process of weak acid and its salt in gastric fluid

3. **Complexation and Adsorption:** In this methodology drug is either complexed with sequestering agent or adsorbed on an inert substance with large surface area to increase its solubility. For example, nicotinamide is used to enhance solubility of poorly soluble drug such as diazepam and progesterone. Progesterone solubility increases by almost 600 fold. The cyclodextrins have been used as complexing agent to enhance aqueous solubility of various drugs viz. β-cyclodextrin complexed with piroxicam or ibuprofen. A complex with γ-cyclodextrin increases both rate and extent of absorption of benzodiazepines.

   The *miniscular drug form* is a recent technique to achieve enhancement in dissolution rate of drug. It involves the surface adsorption of drug on inert substances such as kaolin, microcrystalline cellulose, which reduces the drug particle size leading to increased surface area available for the dissolution medium. The surface adsorption of indomethacin on kaolin or Avicel released 25% drug within 30 and 60 min. respectively, as compared to the 140 min. in case of indomethacin alone. Thus more rapid and complete dissolution is possible by complexation and adsorption of drug. But the drug-complexing agent or drug-adsorbent interaction should be reversible to liberate free drug. For example, reduction in solubility of antibiotics due to complexation with antacids containing calcium or aluminum or with ferrous sulphate present in haematinic preparations or adsorption of drug when co-administered with antidiarrhoeial preparation containing kaolin.

4. **Particle Size:** Micronization of drug to 3-5 μm is often a successful strategy for enhancing the dissolution rate. The reduction in particle size increases the total effective surface area of drug in contact with GI fluid and these particles with higher surface free energy have increased interactions with solvent. The increase in absorption by this approach is possible for the drugs whose absorption is dissolution rate limited. Absorption of griseofulvin, tolbutamide, sulphadiazine is better in micronized form. However, an extensive size reduction is not always possible because of following reasons:

   (a) An increased surface free energy and electrostatic forces also increase agglomerating tendency.

   (b) Absorption of air on larger surface area reduces wettability of powder,

   (c) Chemical degradation due to heat generated during milling or increased reactivity of fine particles towards environmental factors, e.g. crystalline form of Penicillin G is more stable than amorphous form. Milling at low temperature or under inert gases can be attempted to overcome degradation of drug.

   (d) Rapid dissolution of drug in stomach may increase chances of drug decomposition, e.g. erythromycin.

5. **Wetting:** Reduction in particle size should go hand in hand with good wettability. The aggregation of powder and adsorption of air on powder surface can be minimized by

adding wetting agent. Surfactants and hydrophilic polymers have been included in dosage forms to enhance drug dissolution and bioavailability. When phenytoin is agglomerated by spherical crystallization, the agglomerates containing polyethylene glycol (PEG) demonstrated higher area under the blood concentration-time curve (AUC) and C_{max}. A drug, which has poor wettability in water or in conventional dissolution media, may have good wetting by GI fluid. The native surfactants in GI tract such as bile salts may assist the wetting of drug.

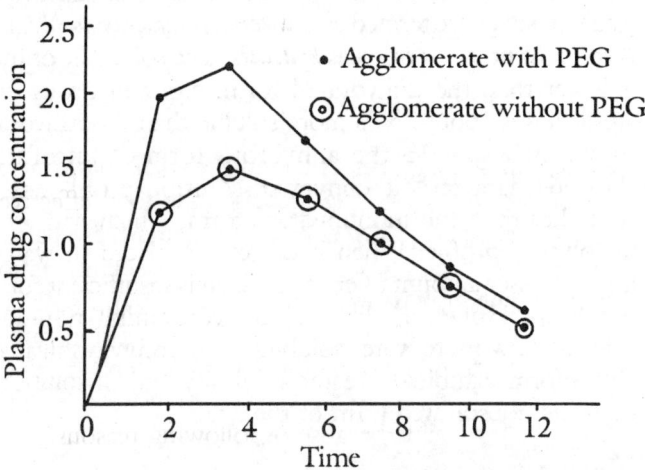

Fig. 1.14. Effect of PEG on bioavailability of the phenytoin

6. **Crystal Form:** The crystalline and amorphous are the two basic properties of solids. The crystalline form is associated with lattice energy of crystallization. As, greater energy is required for a drug molecule to transfer from the lattice of crystalline to a solvated state, their solubility and rate of dissolution are inferior than the corresponding amorphous form, e.g. the orally administered amorphous novobiocin is therapeutically effective whereas crystalline novobiocin is ineffective. *Existence of a drug in more than one crystalline form is called as polymorphism,* in which the constituent molecules are aligned in different arrangements with respect to one another in the lattice structure. Since they possess different lattice energies they show difference in solubility. The lowest energy polymorph is generally more resistant to chemical degradation, has highest melting point

and least solubility and hence it is preferred in pharmaceutical suspensions. The metastable polymorph is unstable, but it has more solubility. Metastable form has a thermodynamic tendency to convert to the stable form. Chloramphenicol palmitate exists in three polymorphs; A, B and C. Form B which is metastable produces 7 times more blood concentration than stable polymorph, A. Solubility of a stable form of diflunisal, an analgesic drug is 14 μg/ml, whereas its metastable form has comparatively more solubility, 26 μg/ml.

In addition to polymorphism, a crystalline substance may associate with solvent from which it is crystallized and the resultant solids are termed as *solvates* or *pseudopolymorphs*. If water is the solvent it is termed as *hydrates*. The solubility of hydrates is lower than the unhydrated form, e.g. anhydrous form of ampicillin is about 25 % more soluble than the trihydrate. As shown in Fig. 1.15 the anhydrous form of nitrofurantoin showed characteristic convex dissolution profile and more solubility than the monohydrate form, which had a normal dissolution profile. When hydrates are placed in water they liberate lesser amount of energy, which is insufficient for crystal break-up. However, the solvates containing non-aqueous solvent show more water solubility. Griseofulvin solvated with chloroform exhibited greater solubility and dissolution rates than the nonsolvated form of the drug.

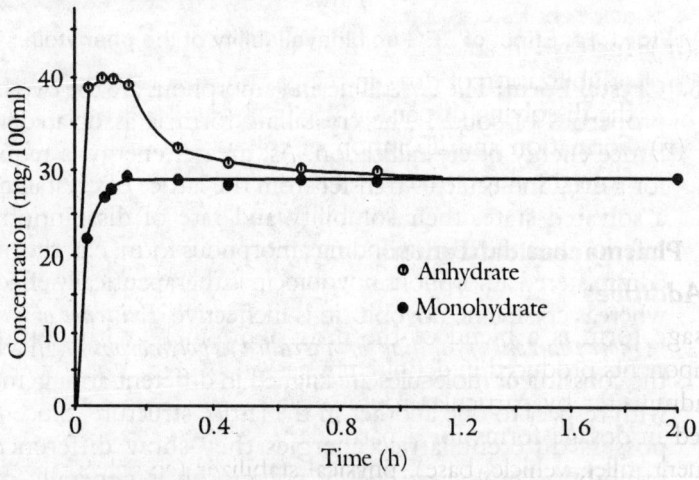

Fig. 1.15. Dissolution of nitrofurantoin

The order of dissolution of various crystal forms is:

Amorphous > metastable/anhydrous > stable

Therefore, the rate of conversion of soluble form to the less soluble form should be monitored during processing and storage of the dosage form.

7. **Solid Dispersion:** Solid dispersions are dispersion of one or more drug(s) in an inert carrier to produce solid-state molecular dispersion. It is prepared by various techniques such as solvent evaporation, fusion or combination of these. The carriers employed include, polyethylene glycol (PEG), polyvinyl pyrrolidone (PVP), citric acid and urea. The increased dissolution rate of solid dispersion is attributed to formation of molecular dispersion of the drug. The various observations are as follows:

(*i*) A solid dispersion containing highly energetic forms of the drug possess higher dissolution rates, e.g. griseofulvin-PVP dispersion.

(*ii*) The presence of amorphous form and metastable polymorphs can increase the dissolution rates, e.g. lack of crystalline structure increases dissolution rates of sulphathiazole-PVP dispersion; formation of indomethacin II, a metastable polymorph in dispersion with PEG 6000 by fusion method.

(*iii*) The increased wettability, e.g. use of bile salts such as cholic acid, cholesteryl esters.

(*iv*) Increase in aqueous solubility due to microenvironmental solubilization of drug in the gastric fluid layer surrounding the dissolving dispersion, e.g. paracetamol-urea.

(*v*) Formation and liberation of colloidal particles or crystals from the dispersion, e.g. b-carotene -PVP.

(C) Pharmaceutical Factors

1. Additives

Dosage form is a blend of the drug component with non-drug components produced in definite physical shape, which is convenient to administer by particular route of administration. Additives are added in dosage forms for a particular function, viz. to make bulk (diluent, filler, vehicle, base), physical stabilizer (co-solvent, wetting agent, suspending agent, emulsifying agent), chemical stabilizer (antioxidant, buffer) and organoleptic additives (coloring agent, flavors, sweeteners).

(a) **Additives Used in Solid Dosage Form:** Lactose, dicalcium phosphate dehydrate are the commonly used diluents in tablets and capsules. Diluent should not adsorb the drug or form complex with drug, e.g. tetracycline and phenytoin form insoluble complex with calcium-based diluents. Magnesium stearate and talc are used as lubricants during manufacturing of solid dosage forms. Its hydrophobic nature often retards penetration of liquid and thus disintegration of the dosage form. The water-soluble lubricants such as sodium lauryl sulphate, sodium oleate do not show such retarding effect. Phenothiazines are adsorbed on silicates such as talc and kaolin.

Tablet disintegration is also affected by compression pressure, aging of dosage form, type and concentrations of diluent, binder, lubricant, and disintegrating agent. Diluents such as Avicel, Starch 1500 possess direct compressibility; in addition they have good disintegration properties. Adsorption of drug on large surface area of Avicel has been exploited to improve distribution and dissolution of drug. The use of effervescent salts is one of the ways to formulate dispersible or soluble tablets of analgesics, antibiotics etc.

The presence of alkaline substance in formulation may raise the microenvironment pH, which can increase the solubility of weakly acidic drug or protect the degradation of drug in the acidic gastric pH.

Use of hydrophilic polymers as granulating agent e.g. sodium alginate, chitosan and guar gum due to their bioadhesive properties, may retain the drug in upper GI tract for prolonged period of time. Some of the additives show pH dependent effect on drug release, e.g. Eudragit polymers. These polymers are available in different varieties such as pH dependent, pH independent, swellable, erodable etc. The specific type and concentration of such polymers is used to modify the drug release. Sodium alginate is widely used polymer in manufacturing of microspheres. In acidic fluid, this polymer retards drug release due to formation of alginic acid, whereas in alkaline pH of small intestine gelling of sodium alginate followed with gel relaxation gives faster drug release.

(b) Surfactants: Inclusion of surfactants in solid dosage forms is a usual practice to increase release of poorly soluble drug. The reduction of solid/liquid interfacial tension enhances penetration of GI fluid into solid dosage form. Effects of surfactants on absorption of drug can be summarized as:

(*i*) Increased wettability and solubility of drug. Surfactants increase drug solubility by micelle formation but may have negative effects on the drug absorption if the concentration of free drug gets reduced.

(*ii*) Prevent aggregation of dispersed phase and maintain fine particles in wet form.

(*iii*) Increases contact between drug and membrane.

(*iv*) Disrupt the integrity and permeability of membrane.

(c) Viscosity Enhancing Agents: These are hydrophilic polymers used as suspending agent or as body builders in monophasic liquids. The flavor built on viscous liquid improves palatability and mouth feel effects of liquid formulations. These agents influence drug absorption in following ways:

(*i*) Complex formation with drug may reduce free drug concentration.

(*ii*) Decrease in rate of drug diffusion in the GI tract.

(*iii*) Delay in gastric emptying, in turn the time required to reach drug in small intestine.

(*iv*) Retain drug in gastric content, which is advantageous for drugs having absorption in upper GI tract e.g. ferrous sulphate.

(*v*) Enable local effect of drug, e.g. antibacterials, antiseptics and in addition also form soothing coat on inflamed membrane.

2. Dosage Forms

Drugs can be formulated in solid, liquid or semisolid dosage forms. Irrespective of physical state of dosage form and drug, the drug must be in solution state in the GI fluids for its absorption. In other words, ability of dosage form to present drug in the form of solution is rate-determining step for the absorption of drug. Hence, the bioavailability of drug after oral administration from various dosage forms can be ranked as:

Aqueous solutions > aqueous suspensions > powders > granules > capsules > uncoated tablets > coated tablets.

The possible steps involved in the drug release from various dosage forms are as follows:

(a) **Aqueous Solution:** In this case, drug is available in solution state and is ready for absorption. Since solvent and GI fluid are aqueous in nature, drug gets readily mixed and distributed in GI content. If by any means precipitation of drug occurs, the resulting precipitate remains fine and wet and readily soluble when unsaturated gastric fluid becomes available. If solution is achieved by miceller solubilization, the drug should get released in GI tract for absorption. However, drug in dissolved state is more susceptible to chemical degradation.

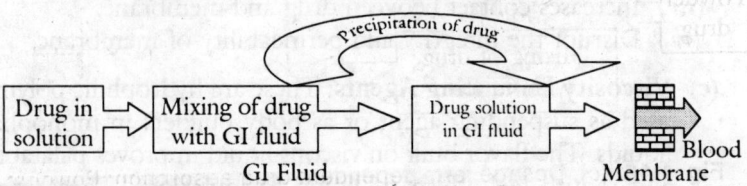

Fig. 1.16. (a). Dosage form dependent drug absorption: Aqueous solution

(b) **Aqueous Suspension:** As compared to powder dosage forms, suspensions contain fine particles with wet surfaces. Smaller is the particle size of drug more will be the surface area and faster will be the rate of dissolution of drug in GI fluid. Suspensions containing surfactants as wetting agent may have rapid absorption properties due to its surface tension lowering effect, which keeps the drug particles deagglomerated, and easy to wet by GI fluid. The crystal stability of drug, viscosity of suspension, complexation of drug with suspending agent, gastric residence and bioadhesiveness of viscous suspension are other factors which may affect absorption of suspended drug. As compared to solid dosage forms drugs in suspensions are more sensitive to chemical degradation.

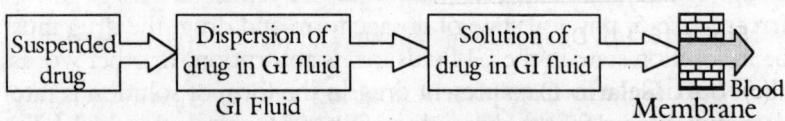

Fig. 1.16. (b). Dosage form dependent drug absorption : Aqueous suspension

(c) **Powders:** Fineness, wettability, and dissolution rate of powder are main factors, which influence the drug absorption. Powders can be formulated as granules. Then the size of granules and rate of deaggregation of granules are additional factors, which influence the drug absorption. Effervescent salts have been used for fast dispersion and taste masking. Since the effervescent granules contain acids and alkali surrounding the drug particle, different pH environment exists on the surface; it may show different dissolution characteristics than the conventional granules.

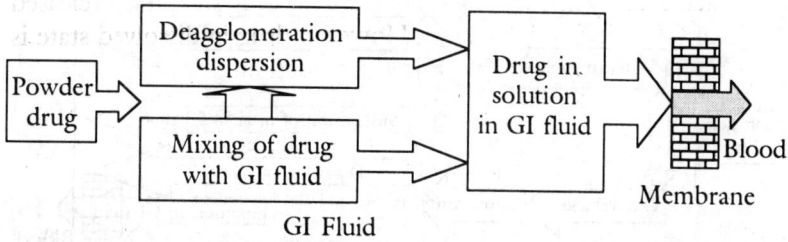

Fig. 1.16. (c). Dosage form dependent drug absorption: Powders

(d) **Hard Gelatin Capsules:** Powder, as dosage form is less convenient to administer and handle compared to tablets and capsules. In capsules, the fine particles of drugs are not normally subjected to high compression forces. The disintegration of capsule shell in GI tract releases drug in the form of powder. Disintegrating agent or surfactant can be used to enhance the deagglomeration of powder plug or to disintegrate granules that are filled in capsules.

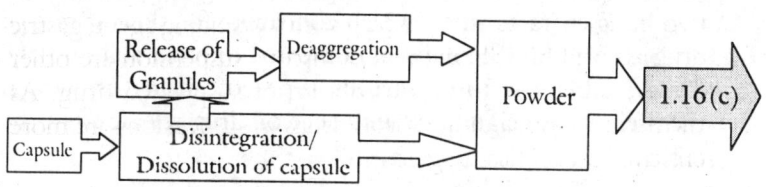

Fig. 1.16. (d). Dosage form dependent drug absorption: HGC

(e) **Soft Gelatin Capsules:** A solution or dispersion of drug in suitable vehicle, which is encapsulated in soft gelatin capsule, may give better drug absorption compared to powder filled in hard gelatin capsules. Vehicle used may be water miscible like polyethylene glycol 400 or 600, polysorbate 80, or water immiscible vehicle like vegetable oil or mineral oil. A formulation containing water miscible base rapidly disperses or dissolves drug in GI fluid. If oily base is a digestible oil, the dissolved drug shows rapid absorption than those dissolved or dispersed in non-digestible oil. Oily vehicles in presence of emulsifying agents, or due to the action of bile salts, form emulsion with aqueous GI fluids. Thus drug release from oily vehicles occurs by partitioning from oil to aqueous GI content.

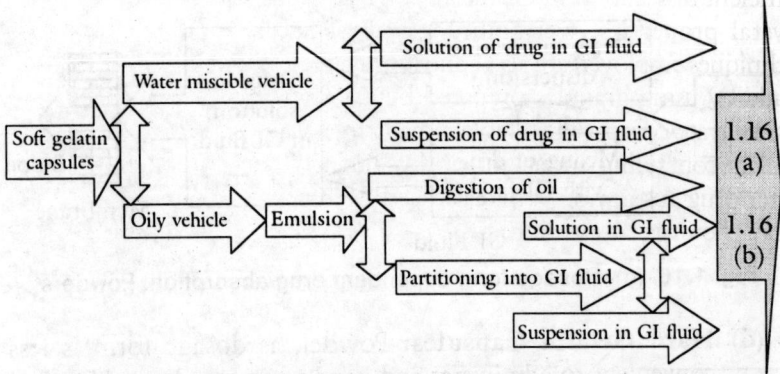

Fig. 1.16. (e). Dosage form dependent drug absorption: Soft gelatin capsules

(f) **Tablets:** The basic difference in tablets and all other dosage form is densification of drug particles. In tablets, powder particles are subjected to compression forces to bring about densification. The reduction in effective drug surface area and difficulty to regenerate well dispersed drug particles are the two basic characteristics, which contribute for slowest rate of drug absorption. Secondly, as compared to other solid dosage forms, tablets require various types of additives, which themselves have significant influence on drug release from the tablet.

After oral administration, tablets undergo disintegration into granules or directly in primary drug particles. When disintegrating agent is blended with granules (inter-granular) the disintegration product is granule and when disintegrating agent is blended with powder before granulation (intra-granular) it yields primary particles. Once primary particles are generated then drug dissolution will occur rapidly. But disintegration of intra-granular disintegrant added tablets is delayed as compared to inter-granular disintegrant added tablets.

Due to immediate interaction of GI fluids with disintegrating agent, inter-granular disintegration is a comparatively fast process. But the drug release may be slower, as the deaggregation of granules to primary particles is the rate-determining step.

The disintegration rate of tablet is not the only rate-determining step in absorption of drug from tablets. Disintegration mainly contributes in the drug release but the released drug should have sufficient dissolution in GI fluid. The factors discussed above such as crystal properties, wettability, effect of additives and tabletting techniques employed are also contributing factors. For example, tablets made by using granules prepared by dry granulation are difficult to disintegrate compared to tablets made by wet granulation technique. Tablets containing surfactant or any other wetting agent may show faster drug absorption, whereas excess of lubricant and/or binder may delay the drug absorption.

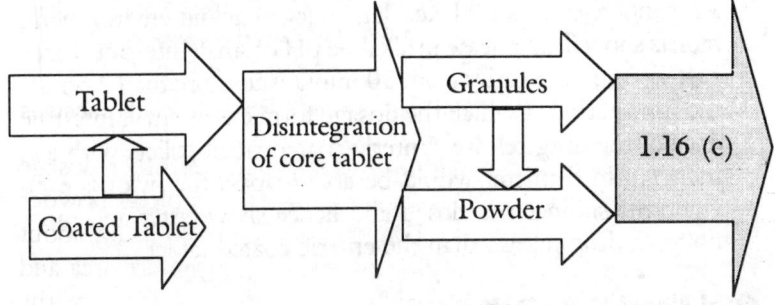

Fig. 1.16. (f). Dosage form dependent drug absorption: Tablets

(g) **Coated Tablets:** Coating of the tablets is an additional physical barrier applied on core tablet. Therefore, the coating should be removed or become permeable to drug release. The solubility of coating material, its concentration and thickness of coat are some of the important properties of coat, which determine drug release. Though sugar is soluble component used in sugar coating, sugar coating process involves use of water impermeable polymers as seal coat, insoluble powders such as talc, dicalcium phosphate and binders as subcoat and waxy materials for polishing. The concentration of additives in each coat, number of coats and thickness of coats significantly affect the drug release. Polymers like cellulose acetate phthalate, shellac are employed in minimum concentration in seal coating. Otherwise, at higher concentration these polymers may show enteric effect. Film coating involves deposition of thin polymer film on substrates including tablet, pellets, granules etc. Film coating may serve various purposes viz. delay the drug release, e.g. enteric coat, or achieve sustained release or it may be non-functional to improve handling and aesthetic properties. The polymers used have diverse properties such as hydrophilic (hydroxypropylmethyl cellulose), hydrophobic (ethyl cellulose, acrylic polymers) or polymers having pH dependent solubility such as cellulose acetate phthalate. Comparatively, the hydrophilic polymers have no significant effect on the disintegration and drug release, but the slight variation in concentration of hydrophobic polymer has significant affect on drug release. Enteric-coated tablets are based on use of pH dependent polymers. The poor insolubility and reactivity of the enteric polymer protects drug from gastric environment. After no release period i.e. 'lag time' in acidic environment, tablets show drug release in alkaline pH of small intestine. Since gastric emptying varies from 30 minutes to more than 2 hours, the time period at which the dosage form enters small intestine decides the drug release. Enteric-coated small pellets with less than 1 mm diameter would be able to pass the pylorus even when the sphincter is closed and hence show faster and more uniform drug release than the enteric coated tablet.

4. Oral Novel Drug Delivery Systems

Novel drug delivery systems (NDDS) are the dosage forms which are developed to achieve better patient compliance, modified drug release, delivery of drug at the site of action, more efficient administration of drugs by various routes, and for better therapeutic effect. The main merits of NDDS are as follows:

- ◆ Enhanced bioavailability.
- ◆ Delivery of drug at desired site at a controlled rate over an extended period of time.
- ◆ More uniform blood concentration, in turn more consistent and prolonged therapeutic effect.
- ◆ Reduced side- effects.
- ◆ Improved patient compliance due to reduced dosing frequency.

The examples of NDDS for oral administration are as follows:

(a) **Sustained Release Dosage Forms (SRDF):** In general, oral dosage forms release the drug rapidly in the stomach. Its solution into gastric fluid is produced and the drug gets absorbed in blood circulation. In conventional dosage forms, a single dose of drug is delivered at each time. The fast release of drug from conventional dosage forms leads to a initial rapid surge of the drug throughout the body followed by diminished concentration of the drug. After specific time interval next dose of drug is administered to achieve desired plasma-drug profile. Therefore, the plasma-profile time curve shows typical peak-valley pattern. The conventional dosage forms need frequent dosing to achieve therapeutic effect over a period of treatment. The frequent dosing of conventional dosage forms show fluctuation in systemic drug concentration, higher dose to regain and maintain the plasma-drug profile and in turn the toxic effects. The controlled or sustained release dosage forms (CDDS) are based on slow but constant drug release for extended period of time. CDDS provide continuous release of a drug at a predetermined rate for a predetermined time.

The improved biopharmaceutical qualities of oral sustained release dosage forms includes:

(*i*) Absence of "peaks and valleys" in blood concentrations i.e. uniform blood concentrations compared to fast release dosage forms

(*ii*) Because a constant lower concentration of the drug is released, it reduces the possibility of toxic levels of drugs.

Immediate drug release to achieve rapid therapeutic plasma concentration followed by gradual and continuous release to extend the steady state level over prolonged period of time is the main characteristic of CDDS. Most of the time polymers are used as release rate controlling system. The hydrophobic, hydrophilic, swellable polymers or polymers having pH dependent solubility are used in various concentrations. The other approaches include– increase in particle size, use of ion exchange resins, osmotic agents and development of prodrug. Therefore, GI residence, volume, viscosity and pH of the GI content have greater influence on drug release. No two CDDS show the superimposible drug release profile because of the differences in the techniques used to control drug release. Therefore bioequivalency of dosage form is of paramount importance in CDDS.

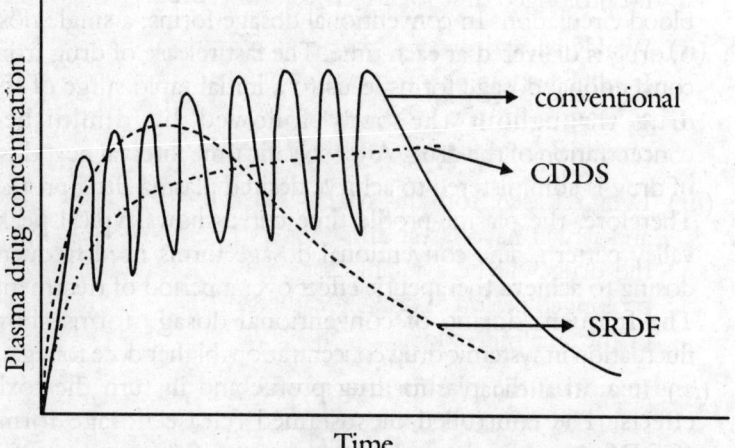

Fig. 1.17. Plasma–drug concentration profile

(b) **Gastro-retentive Dosage Forms:** The residence of the dosage forms in various regions of GI tract is usually up to 1-2 h in stomach, 3 ± 1 h in small intestine and longer, up to 35 h in large intestine. Sustained drug delivery meant for *bis in die* or o.d. administration are likely to carry the drug into an area of large intestine where drug is poorly or erratically absorbed or undergo biotransformation by colonic bacteria. The high viscosity and low fluid content of colon is not a suitable environment for swelling or erosion of polymers that are used to control the drug release from controlled drug delivery systems. Absorption from the sustained release dosage form is more questionable if it is taken on empty stomach, or after light meal, it could result in the delivery system arriving at the colon after only 3-3.5 hours.

Gastroretension of dosage form is one of the ways of prolonging the exposure of the small intestine to high concentration of drug. The gastric retention of drug has manifold effects on drug absorption. The drug released in stomach may be in dissolved, dispersed, ionized or in unionized form depending on solubility and dissociation properties of drug. The mechanisms of absorption of such drugs are as follows:

(*i*) It keeps weakly acidic drugs in unionized form in stomach for prolonged time for effective absorption from that region.

(*ii*) Weakly basic drugs will remain in ionized but soluble state. It will have low penetration through gastric membrane. But as drug is in the solution state it can rapidly reach the proximal small intestine and show better absorption.

(*iii*) Drug released from this system will be in the gastric content and it will have faster emptying into small intestine. Thus the drug will·be available for continuous, controlled and prolonged period of time in ready to absorb state over whole of the small intestine.

(*iv*) It is an alternative for drugs, which are having either low solubility or which show chemical degradation in lower GIT, e.g., diazepam, ranitidine, isradipine etc.

(*v*) Gastroretentive drug delivery system is also effective for local action, i.e. in the treatment of *H. pylori* infections.

Following are some of the approaches to design gastroretentive drug delivery systems.

(*i*) **Bio-adhesion:** It is based on the use of bioadhesive polymers such as carbopol, guar gum etc. Because of the hydrogen and electrostatic bond formation at the mucous-polymer interphase, the dosage form remains adhered to the gastric mucosa. But, the continuous mucous clearance may hinder bioadhesion. Secondly, this technique is not suitable approach for gastro-retention of irritant drugs. As higher concentrations of drug released at localized area may lead to gastric ulceration.

Albumin beads containing chlorthiazide remained bioadhesive for 6 h and increased the peak blood level from 1.0 mg/ml to ~1.8 mg/ml and showed sustained effect for 30 h after administration (Fig. 1.18)

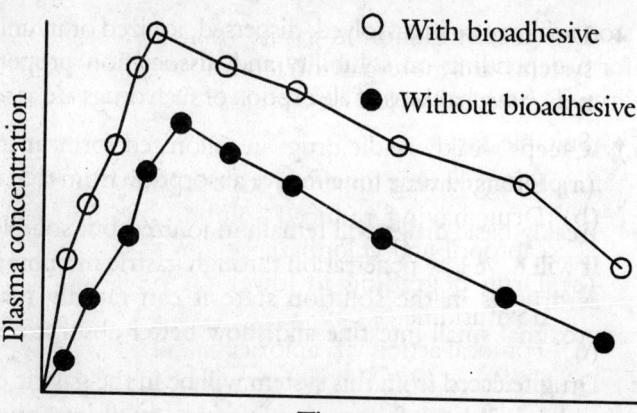

Fig. 1.18. Plasma concentration drug profile of chlorthiazide from bioadhesive and non-bioadhesive beads

(*ii*) **Floating Drug Delivery Systems (FDDS):** Floating or hydrodynamically balanced systems work on principle of floating on surface of GI fluid because of its less density (less than 1). Hydrophilic polymers such as hydroxypropyl methyl cellulose (HPMC), sodium carboxymethyl cellulose (Na-CMC) and sodium alginate have been extensively used to design floating beads, tablets and capsules. The swelling of dosage form after administration imparts buoyancy and system floats till the resulting gel retains sufficient bulk and strength. The effervescent agents such as, sodium bicarbonate or its mixture with citric acid, tartaric acid can also be combined with hydrophilic polymers. Formation and release of carbon dioxide imparts buoyancy. Because of alkaline carbonates pH may rise resulting in alkaline microenvironment, which may hasten the solubility of weak acidic drugs which otherwise have poor solubility in acid.

The characteristics of floating systems are as follows:

♦ The floating systems are not stagnant; mixing of gastric content disturbs the diffusion layer maintaining greater concentration gradient.

♦ Unlike bioadhesive system there is no possibility of localized high concentrations of drug and thus less chances of gastric irritation.

♦ Due to distribution in gastric content the multiparticulate systems are more gastroretentive than the possible 'all or non-effect' of tablets or capsules.

♦ Suitable for

(a) Drugs having upper GI tract as better absorption site.

(b) Drug having reduced solubility at higher pH viz. captopril and chlordiazepoxide.

(c) Drug degrading in lower GI tract viz. ranitidine, doxifuridine.

(d) For local action viz. amoxicillin in *H. pylori*, mesoprostol in ulcers.

The gastroretentive systems are also designed on following principles:

♦ Incorporation of caloric additives such as fats and higher free fatty acids.

♦ Use of osmotic agents, volatile substances and ion exchange resins.

♦ Bigger sized non-disintegrating tablets.

♦ Sinking beads containing heavy additives. The high-density beads retain in antrum of stomach.

The upper GI tract, especially the duodenum is the site for better absorption of iron salts. The solubility of ferrous sulfate decreases at alkaline pH of intestine. The sustained release tablets or capsules are designed to release iron gradually so that a smaller amount of iron is present in lumen at any given time. This helps to minimize the gastrointestinal irritation, nausea and other side effects that may occur at elevated localized iron concentrations. The benefits related to site-specific absorption, minimization of irritation and constant plasma-drug profile can be achieved by designing floating drug delivery systems.

(c) **Chronopharmacotherapeutic Based Drug Forms:** A number of body functions, symptoms of a disease/disorder and pharmacokinetics of drug display circadian variation. Ideally the drug release should coincide with circadian rhythm. In fact, optimum clinical outcome cannot be achieved only by maintaining constant drug plasma levels. To minimize the drawbacks of conventional and controlled drug delivery systems lot of attention has been focused on developing delivery system that is capable of releasing therapeutic agent at right site and at right time by using time controlled, pulsed triggered and programmed drug delivery devices.

Pulsatile drug delivery systems are characterized by rapid drug release after lag period of little or no drug release. The drug release from these systems is matched with the time for better pharmacokinetics and existence of disease. Press-coated tablets are suitable to release drug according to the desired time schedule. The composition and thickness of outer coat and disintegrating agent in core with enough expansion force to break outer coat, determines the pulse release after lag time (Fig. 1.19). The Pulsincap® system consists of a water-insoluble capsule filled with the drug formulation and plugged with a swellable hydrogel at the open end. The opening of capsule results in pulse release. Capsule filled with drug mixture along with osmotic agent or effervescent salts and plugged with erodable, rupturable or enzyme degradable plug are some of the techniques to achieve pulse release by physical modification of dosage forms.

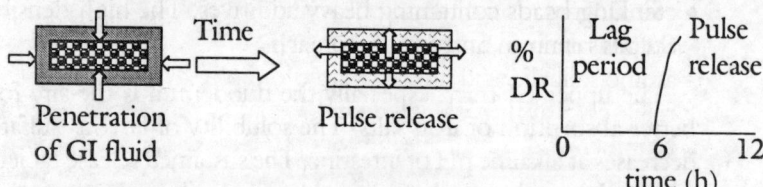

Penetration of GI fluid · Pulse release

Fig. 1.19. Press-coated pulsatile drug delivery system

Due to initial lag period, this system has limitation for the treatments needing immediate drug action. The dosage form for such treatment should contain an immediate dose and a pulse release. Three-layer tablet containing a NSAID has been developed. The immediate drug release layer releases an immediate dose of anti-inflammatory drug, which is needed for rapid relief followed by a pulse.

The success of pulsatile drug delivery system is determined by disintegration of barrier layer, gastric emptying and release of drug in GI tract where drug has best absorption.

(d) **Colon Specific Drug Delivery Systems:** Inflammatory bowel diseases such as ulcerative colitis, irritable bowel syndrome,

Crohn's disease and colon cancer are the various disease conditions that demand drug targeting to colon. Due to longer colon residence, colon has also been exploited for systemic application of drug, especially for sustained drug release. But release of drug is questionable due to low fluid content, viscosity of mass, sluggish movements, impaired swelling or erosion of the release rate-controlling polymer. By virtue of anaerobic environment of lower GI tract, colonic microflora mainly catalyzes hydrolytic and reductive reactions. For example, bioavailability of ranitidine is markedly lower from colon due to bacterial metabolism of drug.

For colon targeting, the dosage form should protect drug from exposure to upper GI tract. The two main approaches are employed, viz. pH dependent drug release and polymers with colon specific degradation. The threat of bacterial degradation is effectively utilized as an opportunity for site-specific drug release. Therefore colon specific drug delivery systems are formulated on basis of dosage forms or prodrugs based on azo polymers or polysaccharides such as pectin, chitosan, guar gum, etc. Degradation of these polymers specifically occurs in colon. Sulphasalazine, a prodrug, consists of sulphapyridine and 5-amino salicylic acid linked by azo bond. Azo reduction in colon releases 5-amino salicylic acid, an anti-inflammatory drug. Number of drugs including theophylline, ibuprofen, iosorbide dinitrate, nifedipine, metoprolol and protein and peptide drugs like calcitonin, interferon, erythropoietin, insulin have been studied for their absorption from colon.

The second approach utilizes pH dependent solubility of polymer. Here drug delivery system is coated with enteric polymer, which dissolves when the system enters the duodenum and the second polymer provides delayed release so that the system starts to deliver drug by the time it reaches the colon.

1.5 DRUG ABSORPTION FROM ROUTES OTHER THAN ORAL ROUTE

The present trends in NDDS focus on effective delivery of the drug to its site of absorption. It avoids unnecessary systemic circulation of drug, reduces degradation of drug and the associated side effects. The desired plasma concentration of drug can be obtained with the reduced dose. Drugs can be administered using variety of routes other than oral, which are discussed below.

(a) Oral Cavity

This includes drug administration through the mucosal membrane lining of the cheeks (buccal mucosa). Absorption of drug from oral cavity is one of the approaches to avoid first-pass metabolism. But due to salivary washing of the drug it is somewhat unpredictable. Buccal mucosa is considerably less permeable than the sublingual area due to which it is unable to provide the rapid absorption. The various routes of drug absorption are shown in Fig. 1.20.

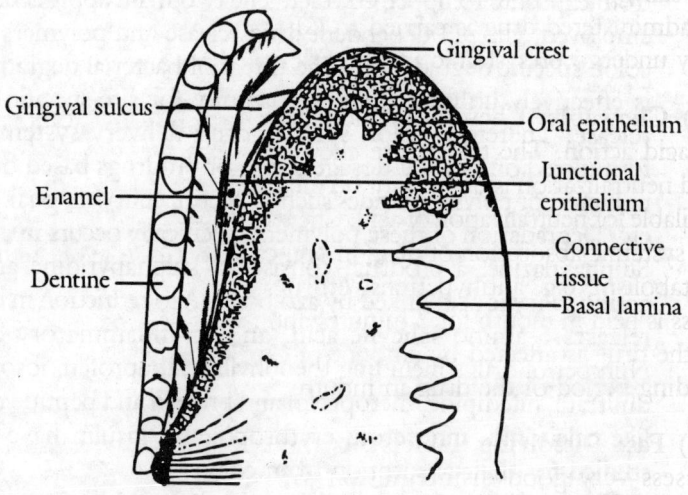

Fig. 1.20. Drug absorption sites from oral cavity

Drug absorption from the various drug delivery systems is summarized as follows.

(*i*) **Buccal and Sublingual Tablets:** Sublingual mucosa is relatively permeable, and demonstrates rapid absorption and acceptable bioavailabilities of many drugs. In addition, it is convenient, accessible, and generally well accepted. The passive diffusion of lipid soluble drug is the predominant mechanism of drug absorption from oral mucosa. Ionic drugs are poorly absorbed. Due to enriched blood and lymphatic circulation, the rapid onset of drug action is possible. The drugs absorbed through oral mucosa directly enter systemic circulation avoiding first -pass metabolism. The area of highest permeability is gingival margin. The absorption of small molecules and volatile substances is greatest from this region. The junctional epithelium in the gingival sulcus is the 'leakiest area', which allows penetration of enzymes, toxins, albumin, and histamine like substances having molecular weight up to 1 million.

Absorption of drug by sublingual route is quite quick, but is not suitable for the achievement of extended plasma concentration-time profiles. The sublingual epithelium is thinner and immersed in saliva and is more effective than the buccal mucosa. However, due to the variation in distribution of salivary glands and the water content of the saliva produced, the placement of dosage form is important. Part of administered drug is carried to GI tract via salivary drainage and may undergo presystemic and hepatic metabolism.

(*ii*) **Chewable:** Chewable tablets have been mainly designed for antacid action. The tablets are chewed and swallowed. The rate of acid neutralization is dependent on increased surface area of the tablet available for neutralization of acid. Chewable tablets are also formulated for systemic absorption of drug in oral cavity so as to avoid first pass metabolism, e.g. antihypertensive drugs. In such cases, the chewed mass is held in mouth for 2 minutes and then swallowed. Absorption of the drug is affected by amount of drug released by chewing and holding period of the drug in mouth.

(*iii*) **Fast Dissolving Tablets:** As the name indicates, these tablets possess very good disintegration capacity in oral cavity and the resulting powder mass either gets dissolved in mouth or can be easily swallowed without use of water. The drug released either gets absorbed from oral cavity or from GI tract when it is swallowed. Freeze-drying, use of sugar beads, ion exchange resins and various other super disintegrating agents are the various approaches attempted for design of fast dissolving tablets. Delivery of drugs from such formulation would not be expected to avoid first-pass metabolism since the disintegrated mass would be swallowed.

Some drugs are also administered locally in the oral cavity. Local delivery to tissues of the oral cavity has a number of applications, including the treatment of toothaches, periodontal disease, bacterial and fungal infections and dental stomatitis.

(b) Topical

Skin is the largest organ of the body. Skin is commonly employed as a site of drug administration for local as well as systemic effect. Liquid dosage forms such as liniments, lotions, sprays; semisolids like ointments, creams, pastes, gels etc are the conventional drug forms for topical drug delivery. Transdermal patch is the novel approach and has been attempted to deliver the drug in a controlled rate to the systemic circulation.

Advantages

(*i*) Protects drug from hostile GI environment and from first-pass metabolism.

(*ii*) Increased patient compliance by avoiding GI distress such as vomiting, GI irritation and reduced dosing frequency.

(*iii*) Provides constant plasma drug profile over several days without the peaks and troughs pattern and prevents hazard of dose dumping effect that is possible with oral sustained drug delivery.

(*iv*) Easy to terminate drug therapy by removing transdermal patch.

Intact skin and skin appendages are the two routes by which drug penetrates the skin. Drug transport by trans-appendageal route, which is, the eccrine sweat glands and the sebaceous glands, directly enters the dermal region where it gets absorbed in blood circulation. This route is more rapid than transepidermal drug transport. But as compared to intact skin the total area provided by this route is just a fraction of intact skin and secondly very few drugs, especially ionic drugs can enter by this route. Hence trans-appendageal route cannot be used to achieve steady -state plasma profile of the drug.

The intact skin is composed of layers of different lipophilicity and hydrophilicity. Three major layers in the skin are epidermis, dermis and subcutaneous tissue. The outer horny layer of the epithelium, the stratum corneum provides major resistance to most of the substances. The stratum corneum is dense, highly compressed lipoidal layer with hydrophilic keratinized cells. The diffusion of drug through this layer is the rate-limiting step. Lipophilic drugs show preferential penetration through this layer (intercellular route). Hydrophilic keratinized cells (intracellular route) allow penetration of polar drugs. The hydration of skin increases penetration of polar drugs. The rate of drug absorption is inversely proportional to the thickness of stratum corneum and it is low from plantar, palmar and dorsum of hand. Absorption of drug though skin is primarily by passive diffusion.

Dermis is comparatively hydrophilic in nature. It is associated with an efficient blood supply, which provides sink condition for drug absorption. Once the drug crosses the stratum corneum, it permeates rapidly and enters into blood circulation. Therefore, the drug properties such as partition coefficient of drug, pk_a, and molecular size have significant influence on transport of the drug. The other factors, which influence drug absorption, are binding of drug in stratum corneum, metabolism in epidermis and dermis.

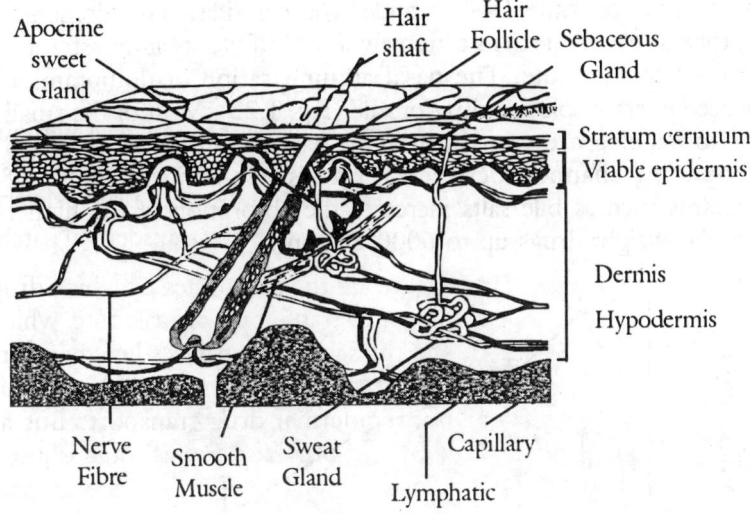

Fig. 1.21. Skin transport of drug

Use of transdermal dosage forms, in which the drug is incorporated in a stick-on patch applied to an area of thin skin is increasing e.g. glyceryl trinitrate used in angina, hyoscine to prevent motion sickness, oestrogen or hormone replacement following menopause and scopolamine to prevent motion sickness.

(c) Nasal

In recent years, nasal mucosa has been explored as drug administration route to achieve faster and higher levels of drug absorption. Extensive vascular nature of the nasal mucosa and in addition its high permeation makes the nasal route of administration beneficial for many drugs. For example, proteins and peptides e.g. dDAVP, a synthetic analogue of vasopressin, antidiuretic hormone, gonadotrophin releasing hormone and calcitonin are given as nasal sprays to avoid frequent injections. These peptides are inactive when given orally because of destruction in GIT but show enough absorption from nasal mucosa to give therapeutic effect.

Nasal cavity is employed for local action as well as for systemic effects. Like other some non-conventional route, the nasal route is also useful to avoid first-pass metabolism and GI degradation of drug. Bioavailability of some drugs after nasal administration is equivalent to the IV infusion route. Dolbutamide hydrochloride is a β_1-adrenergic receptor stimulant, due to its extremely short half-life, its administration is limited to IV route. The nasal administration of dolbutamide produced effective plasma-drug profile (Fig. 1.22). Most of the small drug molecules are transported by passive diffusion through hydrophobic channels between the cells. Co-administration of surfactants such as bile salts increases the absorption of the higher molecular weight drugs up to 6000 Daltons.

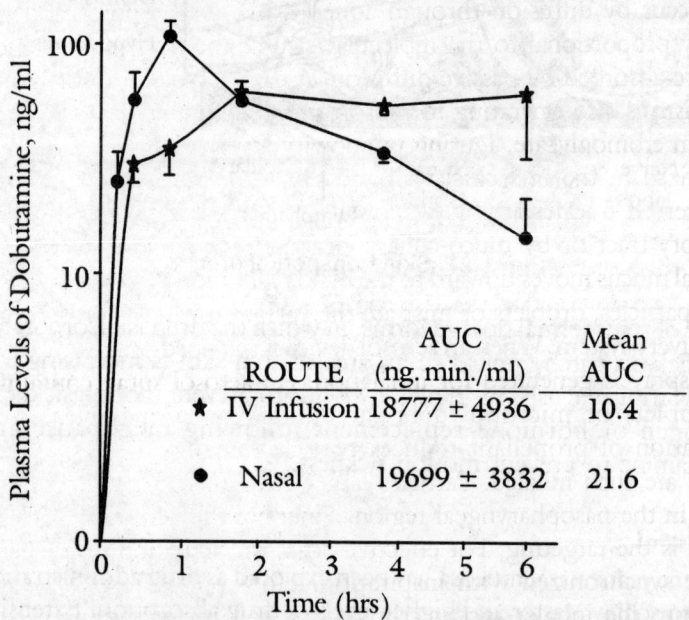

ROUTE	AUC (ng. min./ml)	Mean AUC
★ IV Infusion	18777 ± 4936	10.4
● Nasal	19699 ± 3832	21.6

Fig. 1.22. Plasma-drug profile of dobutamide after intranasal and intravenous administration

A limitation of this route is the presence of several enzymes in the nasal mucosa, which affect the stability of drugs. For example, proteins and peptides will be degraded by proteases and amino-peptidase present in the nasal mucosa. Peptides may also form complexes with immunoglobulins in the nasal cavity leading to an increase in the molecular weight and thus reduced absorption.

Absorption of drug from the olfactory region of the nose also provides a potential for many drugs to be available to the central nervous system.

(d) Inhalation

Pulmonary drug delivery is one of the examples of targeted drug delivery. Due to the direct delivery of drug to the large surface area of the tracheobronchial tree and alveoli, smaller inhaled doses can produce rapid action with reduced systemic side effects. Because of the large surface area and high blood supply, alveolus is a better site for drug absorption and is more rapid than the GI absorption. Alveolar epithelium and the capillary endothelium have high permeability to hydrophilic as well as lipophilic substances. Absorption of hydrophilic drugs occur by diffusion through aqueous membrane pores and is inversely proportional to the molecular size of the drug. Lipophilic drugs are absorbed by passive diffusion. A carrier type of absorption mechanism is also operating for absorption of fine powders such as disodium cromoglycate. During pulmonary travel of drug it may be metabolized in the bronchial wall and the lung. Secondly the drug may enter GI tract either by swallowing of drug deposited in upper respiratory tract or by muco-cilliary clearance mechanism. Tracheo-bronchial mucus moves upward to the hypopharyx and gets swallowed.

Fine particles, droplets or mist are the various forms of aerosol for drug delivery system. When an aerosol device is activated a high velocity aerosol spray is generated for inhalation. An aerosol spray contains fine droplets or micropowders surrounded by propellant. The vaporization of propellant reduces particle size and these smaller particles are then inhaled. Particles larger than 10 μ deposit almost entirely in the nasopharyngeal region. Finer are the aerosol particles effective is the targeting. For effective dose, the actuation of inhaler must be synchronized with inspiration. However, almost 50% of patient use the inhaler incorrectly. Secondly, if the inhaler is used correctly, only 10% of dose released from inhaler reaches lungs. Almost

80% is deposited in the oropharyx and remaining adheres to the devise. The deposited drug is then swallowed, the systemic absorption of which leads to side effects. The attachment of long mouthpiece (spacer) to a metered dose inhaler overcomes these problems. During the long travel distance in the tube, the resistance created by air reduces the velocity of aerosol, allows vaporization of propellant, which causes droplets to decrease in size. The mist of aerosol particles remain suspended in tube, which can be conveniently inhaled after few second of actuation. Inhalation of aerosol using spacer increases lung deposition up to 100%, and decreases throat deposition by 90%. The smaller aerosol generated after vaporization of propellant possesses good lung deposition.

In summary, pulmonary drug absorption is determined by following parameters:

♦ Physicochemical properties of drug such as partition coefficient, particle size, solubility in solvent and in propellant.

♦ Properties of propellant such as vapor pressure, toxicity and solvent action.

♦ Mechanics of device to generate fine particles with reduced velocity and with maximum removal of propellant.

♦ Effect of drug and additives on mucous viscosity, mucocilliary clearance, e.g. tetracyclines and polyvalent ions increase viscosity of mucous, β-adrenoceptor agonists increase the rate of mucocilliary clearance.

♦ Correct use of device.

(e) Intraocular

Cornea is the rate-limiting barrier for the absorption of drug into the intraocular tissues. Like skin, cornea is also composed of lipoidal and aqueous layers. The epithelial and endothelial cells are lipoidal and stroma is acellular with high water content. The unionized drug easily penetrates epithelium and endothelium, the former serves as the depot for lipophilic molecules. The stroma allows rapid passage of water-soluble and ionized drugs and also serves as a depot for them. Once the drug enters stroma it is distributed to all the internal tissues of the eye. Therefore, the drug should have balanced hydrophilicity and lipophilicity. Proteins present in tears bind with drugs and such bound drugs due to bulkiness are difficult to absorb.

The rates of tear turnover and efficient drainage system of eye affect the bioavalability of instilled drug. The instilled drug immediately gets diluted in the tear film, gets spread over the eye lid margin and the remainder is rapidly drained into the nasolacrimal duct. Among various ophthalmic preparations, suspensions and ointments provide prolonged duration of action. Newer formulations like ocular inserts provide slow continuous delivery of small amounts of drug. Side effects from such systems are very low as very little amount of drug is passed through drainage.

(f) Rectum

Although unpopular, rectum is a useful route when oral administration of a drug is not possible e.g. when patient is unconscious or when vomiting is present.

Enema and suppositories have been administered by rectal route for local actions and for systemic effects. This route is an alternative to oral route for administration of unpleasant tasting drugs, to avoid nausea, vomiting, or in case of unconscious patients. Among all applications, an avoidance of first-pass metabolism and protection from degradation in GI content are the main value adding parameters of the rectal route. The site of release of drug in the rectal canal determines possibility of occurrence of the first-pass metabolism. The drug released in the lower rectum and anal canal is transported via the haemorrhoidal plexuses and internal iliac veins, which do not drain into the liver. But the spreading of suppository or enema may carry drug in upper rectum, from where drug is transported by superior and inferior mesenteric arteries. This drug undergoes liver metabolism. The rectal absorption of drug occurs by passive diffusion of the unionized drug by apparent first order kinetics. The absorption via lymphatic is also another absorption mechanism available for absorption of rectally administered drug.

Administration by this route is convenient for long term care and can be undertaken by unskilled persons and by the patient himself/ herself. The disadvantage is that absorption is sometimes irregular and incomplete and many drugs cause irritation of rectal mucosa. Examples of drugs that can be given rectally are– indomethacin in rheumatoid arthritis, aminophylline for bronchospasm and diazepam for status epilepticus.

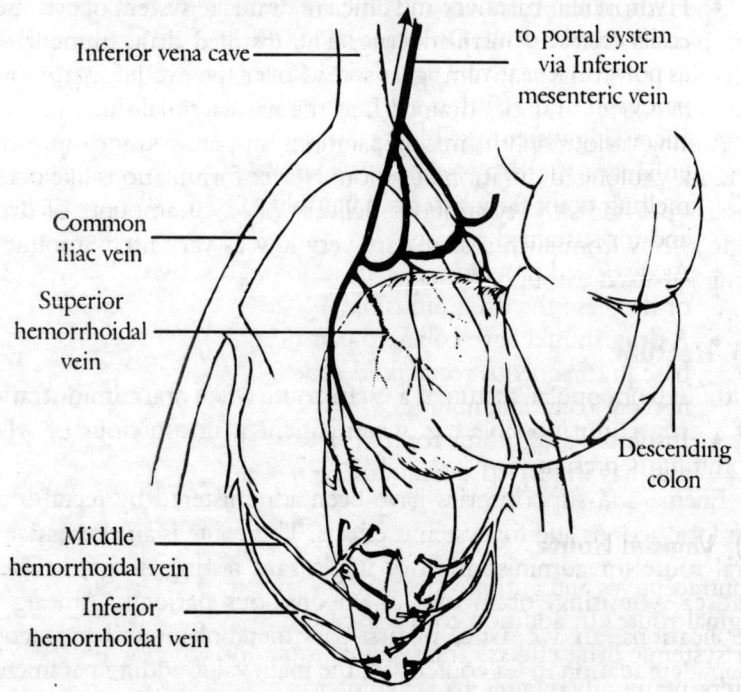

Fig. 1.23. Absorption of drug through rectum

Factors affecting the rectal absorption of drug

♦ Anorectal fluid has no effective buffer capacity; therefore, medicaments dissolved in this fluid may largely determine the pH. The co-administration of buffer can increase the rectal absorption of drug by keeping it in unionized form.

♦ Drug absorption is maximum when the colon is empty, where drug has greater contact with the mucous membrane.

♦ The volume of anorectal fluid available for the solubility of drug is very small, which may slow down the absorption of slightly soluble drug.

♦ Vehicles in formulation having more affinity toward the drug lower its release. Lipophilic drug may have somewhat slower drug release from oily bases than that from the hydrophilic bases. Hence, for rapid action water-soluble drug should be formulated in fatty base. The lipid soluble drug in oily base may provide sustained release.

♦ Hydrophilic bases are miscible with rectal fluid therefore they easily release drug. On other hand, the hydrophilic bases such as polyethylene glycol may dehydrate the mucosa. The resultant irritation and reflux evacuation may expel the dosage form. Increasing water miscibility of oily bases through emulsification enhances the drug release. The slower release from higher melting point fatty bases can be utilized to achieve local action and for sustained release.

♦ As discussed previously, the inclusion of surfactant can increase or decrease the drug diffusion and drug absorption.

♦ A drug should have balanced partitioning, first to diffuse from base in to aqueous rectal fluid and second for partitioning into lipoidal rectal membrane.

♦ Insoluble drug in micronized state causes less rectal irritation, and has improved dissolution.

(g) Vaginal Route

Contraceptives and antiinfectives are the main drugs administered by vaginal route. In addition to the local effects, vagina is also utilized for systemic drug effects. Transvaginal route for systemic medication offers many advantages like, avoidance of first pass metabolism, minimization of proteolytic degradation, etc. In spite of all these studies fluctuation in vaginal absorption resulting from variation in serum estrogen level throughout the life cycle of women is a major hindrance in the use of this route. In general the vaginal absorption is slower and more erratic than oral absorption.

(h) Injections

Injections are choice of drug administration in emergency when immediate drug action is required. Secondly, it is an alternative route of drug administration when the oral route is inappropriate. Disadvantage of injections is that the dose, once injected, cannot be withdrawn.

Intravenous (IV) injection is used to introduce drug directly into the systemic circulation, where the drug is completely bioavailable. Intravenous drip or an infusion pump is used to obtain continuous drug levels in body. Suspensions may block the capillaries therefore these should not be injected by IV route.

Intramuscular (IM) injection introduces drug in muscles. Therefore, as compared to IV route the absorption of drug is slower and incomplete. Also, unpredictable drug levels may be achieved because of metabolism of drug in muscle tissues and precipitation of drug at the injection site. Drugs, which degrade after oral route such as insulin, can be administered by IM. An aqueous suspensions or oily formulations are also administered by IM route for sustained effects. The absorption of drug is determined by vascularity at injection site, degradation of drug, solubility and molecular size of drug, volume, pH and viscosity of injection.

◆ The higher is the blood circulation, the faster is the drug cleared from the site of injection, e.g. absorption from arm muscles is faster than thigh muscles.

◆ Absorption of drug occurs by blood circulation and lymphatic system. The lipophilic drugs enter the blood circulation rapidly by passive diffusion. This absorption is independent of molecular size. Hydrophilic and ionic drugs are absorbed into blood circulation via the capillary pores and absorption is restricted to smaller molecules. The molecules with larger size are absorbed via lymphatics.

◆ Drug dissolved or dispersed in oily vehicle show slow release. The insoluble or precipitated drug also results in slower absorption. Smaller injected volumes show faster drug absorption. The slow release is also observed with slightly hypertonic IM injections.

Drug absorption from the *subcutaneous (SC) injection* is slower than the IM route. It is due to the poor blood circulation. Subcutaneous (SC) administration is used only when the drug does not cause irritation, otherwise severe pain, necrosis or tissue damage may occur. When the drug is administered in the SC tissues, drug absorption is slow but uniform. Isotonic solutions are injected to reduce pain and can be utilized for sustained effect. Following means can control the rate of absorption:

◆ Absorption of insoluble insulin is slow as compared to soluble preparation.

◆ Incorporation of vasoconstrictor substance will retard the absorption.

♦ Instead of a solution, sterile compressed pellet (subcutaneous implant) can be used which releases drug slowly and uniformly. Thus the drug effect can be prolonged. Testosterone is effectively administered by this method.

♦ Massage, exercise, application of heat or inclusion of vasodilator will increase the blood flow and hence will increase the absorption.

♦ Inclusion of *hyaluronidase* will reduce the degree of polymerization of the connective tissue and will permit a more rapid and extensive spreading of injected material. Hyaluronidase is generally used in a technique called as *hypodermoclysis*, in which large volumes are administered subcutaneously.

Intraperitoneal (IP) administration is rarely employed in human beings. But is one of the most widely used routes of administration in laboratory animals. It involves penetration of thick muscle layers and blind injection into organ filled abdominal cavity. By this route, absorption of the drug is very rapid.

The drugs can be directly administered into the subarachnoid space and thus the effects will be localized to the spinal nerves and meninges e.g. in case of spinal anaesthesia or CNS infections like tuberculous meningitis in which streptomycin may be given intrathecally.

In humans, *intraarterial* administration is only limited for the administration of radio-opaque media for diagnostic purposes or to localize the effect of drug to a particular tissue or organ e.g. treatment of liver tumors and head/neck cancers. It has wider application in experimental work. This route generally requires great care and is reserved for experts.

1.6 IN VITRO MODELS OF ABSORPTION

Various models, which are used for drug absorption studies, are discussed below.

Physicochemical Methods

(a) Partition Coefficient

Partition coefficient between an oil and water phase, **log P**, is one of the easiest property of a drug molecule that can be determined. Partition coefficient provides a measure of the lipophilicity of a molecule and can be used to predict to what extent it will cross the biological membrane. Usually octanol is selected as an oil phase as it has similar properties to biological membranes.

It is important to note that log P does not take the degree of ionization into consideration. Hence **log D** is generally used. Log D is the distribution coefficient where aqueous phase is at a particular pH and thus it takes into account the ionization of the molecule at that pH. The log D measured at intestinal pH (e.g. 6.8) will give a much better idea about extent of drug permeability across gastrointestinal membrane than log P.

(b) Artificial Membranes

Artificial membranes are very useful in studying passive membrane permeability as they are reproducible and are suitable for high throughput screening. Artificial membranes show comparable results with Caco-2 cells (see below). Membranes used in these studies are mixture of lecithin and an inert organic solvent on a hydrophobic filter support. These membranes do not give an absolute prediction but show a trend in the ability of molecules to permeate by passive diffusion.

Immobilized artificial membranes are also used. These membrane columns are better than octanol/water or other solvent/solvent partition partitioning systems. A modification of this system is immobilized liposome chromatography (ILC). On ILC many compounds with same log P have been shown to demonstrate variable membrane partitioning based on their charges.

Liposomes, lipid bilayers produced from mixture of lipids are also useful in investigating passive diffusion of drugs through lipid membranes. This system has been used to study passive absorption of many monocarboxylic acids.

PAMPA (Parallel Artificial Membrane Permeation Assay) is an *in vitro* high throughput assay for the permeability of new compounds. A modified version of this is the filter-immobilized artificial membrane (filter-IAM) permeability assay. This coupled with an instrument PSR4p (Permeability-Solubility-Retention; pION, USA) can be used for high throughput permeability screens. PAMPA helps to prioritize molecules for further studies. It also provides information on solubility, lipophilicity and ionization status of a drug.

(c) Chromatographic Retention Indices

Immobilized artificial membranes (IAM) chromatography along with physicochemical parameters is used for evaluation of passive intestinal absorption. IAM packings are prepared by covalently immobilizing monolayers of membrane phospholipids to silica particles.

Micellar Liquid Chromatography (MLC) is also used for the prediction of passive drug absorption. In this system retention of drugs depends on hydrophobic, electronic and steric interactions.

In general chromatographic techniques are easy in operation and have high analytical sensitivity.

(d) Cell Culture Techniques

There are now well-accepted cell culture models for drug absorption studies. These models are based on the assumption that passage of drugs across the intestinal epithelium is the main barrier for drugs to reach the circulation.

Primary cultures of enterocytes (these constitute 90% of the cells in the intestinal epithelium and are responsible for the majority of the absorptive functions) are unable to form an organized epithelium and hence do not display an apical and basolateral surface.

Human intestinal cell lines are generally divided in to four different groups:

◆ **Type I:** These cells differentiate spontaneously under normal culure conditions and hence are polarized (i.e. apical and basolateral surface), form domes, have tight junctions and brush border e.g. Caco-2 cells.

◆ **Type II:** These cells differentiate into enterocytes-type cells only under specific culture conditions e.g. HT29 in presence of glucose; HT29 clone can differentiate into mucus cells.

◆ **Type III:** These cells form domes but do not express any biochemical or morphological markers of differentiated cells e.g. T84, SW1116 and Col115 cell lines.

◆ **Type IV:** These cells do not differentiate e.g. HCA7 and SE480 cell lines.

Caco-2 is the most widely used cell line. *Caco-2 cells are a human colon carcinoma cell line.*

In culture, Caco-2 cells differentiate to form a monolayer of enterocytes, which resemble those in the small intestine e.g. they contain microvilli and many transport systems such as for sugars, amino acids, vitamins, peptides and P-glycoprotein efflux transporters. They exhibit morphological and functional similarities to intestinal enterocytes. The monolayer of Caco-2 cells adhere through tight junctions more like those of the colons than those of the leakier small intestine. These cells also express some Cytochrome P450 enzymes and Phase II enzymes e.g. glutathione S-transferases and sulphotransferases

In general Caco-2 cells are grown on porus membrane (supports) for a period of 15-21 days in culture medium, typically, it is Dulbecco's Modified Eagle Medium supplemented with 20 % fetal bovine serum, 1 % non essential amino acids and 2 mM l-glutamine.

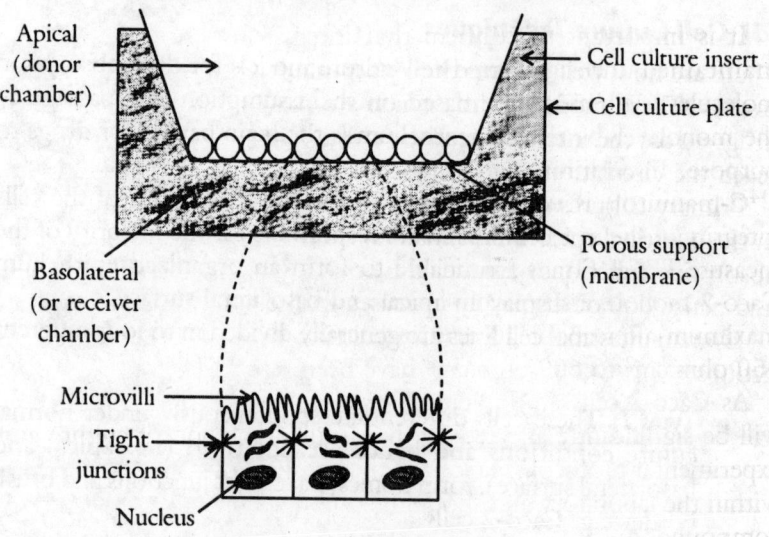

Fig. 1.24. Caco-2 cell culture

The cells are grown at 37°C in 10 % CO_2 at relative humidity 95%. The culture medium is replaced twice a week.

Transport experiments are carried out in Hank's Balanced Salt Solution (pH 6.5) on the apical surface and Hank's Balanced Salt Solution (pH 7.4) on basolateral surface. After a brief incubation period (30 min) at 37°C in shaking water bath, buffers are replaced with fresh buffers with dilute solution of drug in the apical chamber. At regular intervals the concentration of the drug in the basolateral chamber is determined. Note that, in relation to *in vivo* situation, the apical surface faces the intestinal lumen and the basolateral surface faces the blood stream. Thus,

$$P_{app} = \frac{d\theta}{dt}\left(\frac{1}{C_oA}\right) \qquad ...1.11$$

where,

P_{app}	:	Apparent permeability coefficient (cm/S)
C_o	:	Initial concentration in apical chamber (μg/ml or ng/ml)
A	:	Surface area of the monolayer (cm^2)
$\dfrac{d\theta}{dt}$	:	Rate of drug transport (μg/S or ng/S)

It is important to confirm that integrity of the monolayer is maintained through out the experiment. Hydrophilic marker molecules, such as mannitol, which are passively transported across the monolayer by the paracellular route, are generally used for this purpose. In addition, for simplicity usually radiolabelled mannitol (^{14}C-mannitol) is used. If it shows less than 2 % transport then integrity of the monolayer is maintained. An alternative method is to measure TEER (Trans Epithelial Electrical Resistance). TEER across Caco-2 monolayers typically increases with culture time and reaches maximum after about 10 days in culture. Resistances ranging from 150 ohm.cm^2 to 600 ohm.cm^2 have been reported.

As Caco-2 cells are biological systems the apparent permeability will be significantly affected by their source, method of culture and experimental protocol. Hence the procedure should be standardized within the laboratory and should be calibrated with a set of standard compounds.

Caco-2 cells can also be used to identify mechanisms of permeability. For example:

1. If P_{app} increases with increasing concentration i.e. transport is not saturated, is independent of pH, is same in both directions, meaning apical to basolateral or basolateral to apical, then it can be concluded that it is passive and not active transport.

2. If basolateral to apical transport is significantly greater than apical to basolateral then drug must be actively effluxed from the cells by a P-glycoprotein like system. This can be further confirmed by the inhibitors of P-glycoproteins such as verapamil.

3. It is possible to use the competitive inhibitors of a particular transporter to check its involvement in the transport of a particular drug.

4. It enables to check if drug follows paracellular or transcellular transport. Calcium is involved in keeping tight junctions together. So by using chelators such as EDTA the tight junctions can be opened which can be assessed by mannitol. If opening of tight junctions does not affect drug permeability then drug transport is considered to occur via transcellular pathway.

5. If mass balance on both sides of the membrane does not account for 100% of the drug, then the drug could be binding to porous membrane, it needs to be investigated in detail or drug could be metabolized by the enzymes secreted by the cells or even biotransformation by CYP450 within the cells.

Thus Caco-2 cells can evaluate the permeability and in addition can provide information regarding stability and presystemic biotransformation and how they are likely to affect rate and extent of absorption.

Advantages of Caco-2 Cells:

➤ Understanding of mechanisms of absorption of drug.
➤ They are non-animal models.
➤ Require only small amount of drug.
➤ Rapid screening tool to assess permeability of large number of drugs.
➤ Evaluate potential toxicity of drugs to cells.
➤ Investigate impact of excipients in drug absorption and mechanisms of enhancement of permeability.
➤ Can be used as an experimental tool for drug-drug interaction studies at the level of transporters.

Disadvantage of Caco-2 cells:

➤ Culture time is longer of about 20 days.
➤ Handling of the cells is labor-intensive.
➤ Because of tight junctions they are reflective of the permeability of the colon rather than small intestine.
➤ They lack mucus layer.
➤ Require analysis of large number of samples.

To overcome these bottlenecks, many pharmaceutical industries are using automated "high-throughput" permeability screens e.g.

automated cell feeding techniques, 96-well format. Use of LC-MS instead of HPLC with UV or fluorescence detection also increases throughput. In spite of all these things inter-laboratory variation is a major concern and is mainly because of polyclonal nature of Caco-2 cells and sensitivity to minor variation in culture conditions e.g. serum content and composition.

HT-29-18C1, a subclone of human intestinal adenocarcinoma cell line, can differentiate into absorptive cells having microvillus structure and mucus secreting goblet cells. Also has resistance similar to small intestine. So it could provide better information about transcellular and paracellular absorption. In order to mimic small intestinal mucosa *in vivo*, co-cultures of Caco-2 cells and mucus secreting HT29-MTX cells have been used.

Another cell line derived from dog kidney is the MDCK (Madin-Darby Canine Kidney) cell line. MDCK share many common characteristics with Caco-2 cells. The major advantage is that it requires only 3 days in culture to reach membrane integrity (Caco-2 cells require 15-21 days). Hence MDCK is becoming more and more popular.

Another cell line of interest is LLC-PK. This cell line can be used to express CYP3A4 and thus metabolism and drug permeation can be studied in one cell line, but more research is needed as this cell line is yet to be well characterized as an absorption model.

Absorption models have also been investigated for other routes such as skin and pulmonary administration. For example use of skin models using full-thickness human skin mounted in diffusion cell; Calu-3 epithelial cell monolayers for predicting pulmonary drug absorption; 16HBE14o human bronchial epithelial cells.

Thus irrespective of various limitations, cell culture techniques, especially Caco-2 cell models is widely used to predict the intestinal absorption potential of new drugs.

(e) Tissue Techniques

The various tissue techniques, which have been used as an absorption model, are as follows:

Model	Details
Everted sacs	Measures uptake into intestinal segments
Everted intestinal rings	Studies the kinetics of uptake into the intestinal mucosa
Isolated sheets	Measures the transport across sheets of intestine

Isolated sheets and everted (inside out) intestinal rings are the most popular models.

Isolated sheets of intestinal mucosa are generally obtained by cutting the intestine into strips. After removal of musculature the sheet is mounted in diffusion chamber or an *Ussing chamber* filled with buffers (Fig. 1.25). Ussing Chamber technique was originally developed to study transepithelial ion transport.

In this technique small intestinal sheets are mounted between two compartments (Ussing chambers). The mucosal (i.e. luminal) and serosal (i.e. basolateral) compartments are usually supplied with Krebs-Ringer bicarbonate buffer. The integrity of the tissue is confirmed by transepithelial resistance measurement. The system is maintained at 37°C with constant stirring and supply of oxygen and carbon dioxide mixture ($O_2 : CO_2 \equiv 95 : 5$).

The permeability can be measured by adding drug to the donor chamber and checking appearance of drug in receiving chamber. Fluxes in both the directions i.e. mucosal to serosal and serosal to mucosal can be studied. Effect of pH can be studied simply by altering the pH of the buffer in appropriate chamber.

For this technique mostly rat intestine is preferred as its permeability correlates well with that of human intestine.

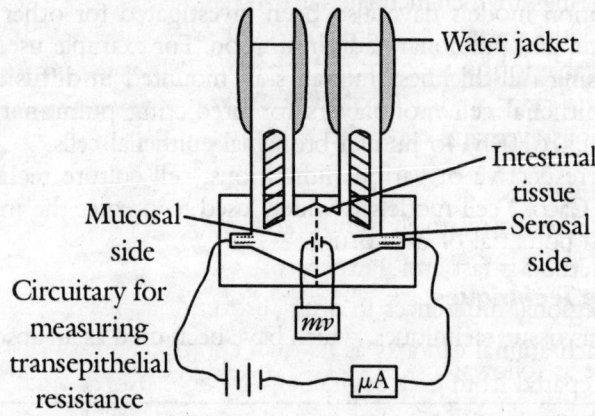

Fig. 1.25. Diffusion chamber for isolated intestinal sheets

Advantages:

➢ Permeability across different regions can be determined and thus resgional differences in intestinal absorption can be studied.

➤ Determination of permeability in different animal models can be done by using different animal tissue. Thus species differences with respect to intestinal absorption characteristics can be determined.

➤ Transepithelial drug transport can be investigated in combination with intestinal metabolism.

➤ Amount of drug needed is relatively small (mg quantities).

➤ Samples are analytically clean/pure.

Disadvantages:

❖ The viability of intestinal tissue mounted in Ussing Chamber is quite controversial

❖ Dissection of epithelial tissue is quite difficult and serosal muscle layer can only be partially removed

Everted intestinal rings (everted gut sacs) were first introduced by Wilson and Wiseman in 1954. In *everted intestinal rings* the musculature is intact as whole intestinal segments are used. Briefly, intestinal segments are quickly excised, usually from rats, and flushed with saline solution. The segment is tied at one end and by placing on glass rod it is carefully everted and cut into small rings. The everted intestinal rings are then incubated in drug containing buffer maintained at 37°C with constant oxygenation. Under optimal conditions, rings remain viable for up to 2 hours. The transport of drug is stopped by rinsing the rings with ice-cold buffer and drying them. The drug content is assayed and expressed as mol/gm/time.

Advantages:

➤ Method is relatively simple and quick

➤ Method is fast and inexpensive

➤ Regional differences in drug absorption can be studied

➤ Each animal can acts as its own control as many rings can be prepared from each segment of the intestine isolated

➤ Mechanism of drug absorption can be studied by changing the experimental conditions

Disadvantages:

❖ Extreme care is needed to maintain the viability of the tissue throughout the experiment.

❖ Tissue needs to be disrupted completely for the determination of drug contents, which complicates the assay procedure.

❖ Polarity of the absorption cannot be assayed.

❖ A compound has to cross all the layers including muscle of the small intestine instead of just the intestinal mucosa

These methods are also first calibrated with standard drugs as in case of Caco-2 cells.

(f) Perfusion Models (In situ Models)

For perfusion studies, most popular is the rat model. Some of the *in situ* models are as follows:

Model	Details
In situ perfusion	Measurement of drug disappearance from either closed or open loop perfusate of segments of intestine
Vascularly perfused intestine	Measurement of drug disappearance from perfusate and its appearance in blood

The main advantage is that whole animal is used and hence normal physiology is maintained such as, nerves, lymphatic and blood supply, all the transport mechanisms are present and are functional. Also viability of the tissue is not an issue here because of intact blood supply and innervation with minimal interference of the intestinal function and architecture. *In situ* model also enables the study of intestinal events in isolation without complication of billiary excretion and enterohepatic circulation. Among various absorption models, *in situ* perfusion of intestinal segments in anesthetized rats most closely mimics *in vivo* rat absorption.

Several modifications of the *in situ* approach have been developed. In case of open loop method, dilute drug solution will be passed slowly through the intestine. Drug concentration of the solution at the inlet and outlet is determined. Thus permeability coefficient can be calculated as follows:

$$P_{eff} = \frac{Q \cdot \ln(C_i - C_o)}{2 \cdot \pi \cdot r \cdot l} \qquad \ldots 1.12$$

where, P_{eff} = Effective permeability coefficient; cm/s

Q = Flow rate; ml/s

$$C_i \quad = \text{Initial drug concentration}$$
$$C_o \quad = \text{Final drug concentration}$$
$$r \quad = \text{Radius of intestinal loop; cm}$$
$$l \quad = \text{Length of intestinal loop, cm}$$

In case of closed loop method, dilute drug solution is added to the section of intestine (10-20 cm long) and the intestine is closed. The intestine is then excised and drug content in luminal solution is analyzed at specified intervals. This method has the same disadvantage as everted intestinal rings as the drug content measurement requires tissue disruption. Also by this approach it is not always practical to determine the steady state disappearance rate of drug from the lumen. As the disappearance of the drug from the lumen is used for the calculation of 'absorption rate', it is important to confirm that there is not degradation of the drug.

In situ models are based on the assumption that disappearance of drug from the intestinal lumen correctly reflects drug absorption i.e. appearance of drug into the portal circulation. Thus this approach may overestimate the absorption in case of drugs undergoing extensive intestinal metabolism or drugs having significant accumulation in the intestine. This shortcoming can be overcome by collecting the samples from mesenteric vein, which is draining the blood from the perfused intestinal segment.

These models are also first calibrated with standard drugs.

(g) Human Models

Some of the human models are as follows:

Model	Details
Loc-I-Gut	Measures drug disappearance from perfusate of human intestine
High frequency capsule	Measures drug in systemic circulation; non-invasive method

The Loc-I-Gut is a multichannel tube system with a proximal and a distal balloon. It is a perfusate technique, which gives insight into human permeability (Fig. 1.26).

The balloons are 100 mm apart. Thus isolates a 100 mm long intestinal segment to be perfused. As soon as proximal balloon passes the ligament of Treitz, both balloons are filled with air. This separates the luminal contents of the isolated segment of intestine from rest of the luminal contents of the intestine. The proper working of the balloons is checked by using the non-absorbable markers. The passage of distal balloon down the GI tract is enhanced by attaching tungsten weights.

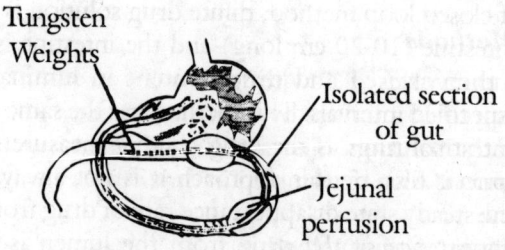

Tungsten Weights

Isolated section of gut

Jejunal perfusion

Fig. 1.26. Loc-I-Gut model

The use of high frequency capsule has also been tried to study absorption. The transit of high frequency capsule through gastro intestinal tract is followed by X-ray fluoroscopy. As soon as capsule reaches its intended release site, drug release is initiated by high frequency signal, which leads to rupturing of latex balloon, which is loaded with drug.

This technique is limited as loading of drug in balloon is difficult and also exposure to X-ray makes it a somewhat harmful model.

(h) Models for Buccal Permeation Studies

These studies involve methods that would examine *in vitro* and/or *in vivo* buccal permeation profile and absorption kinetics of the drug.

A. In vitro Methods

Most of the *in vitro* studies of drug transport across buccal mucosa have used buccal tissues from animal models. Animals are sacrificed immediately before the start of an experiment. Buccal mucosa with underlying connective tissue is removed from the oral cavity. Connective tissue is carefully removed and the buccal mucosal membrane is isolated. The membranes are placed and stored in ice-cold (4°C) buffers (usually Krebs buffer). Membranes are mounted between side-by-side diffusion cells for the *in vitro* permeation experiments. Membrane viability is always a major concern in this technique.

Buccal cell cultures have also been suggested as useful *in vitro* models for buccal drug permeation and metabolism. However, to utilize these culture cells for buccal drug transport, the number of differentiated cell layers and the lipid composition of the barrier layers must be well characterized and controlled. This has not yet been achieved with the buccal cell cultures used thus far.

B. *In vivo Methods*

The technique involves the swirling of a 25 ml sample of the test solution for up to 15 minutes by human volunteers followed by the expulsion of the solution. The amount of drug remaining in the expelled solution is then determined in order to assess the amount of drug absorbed.

The drawbacks of this method include:

> ➤ salivary dilution of the drug,
> ➤ accidental swallowing of a portion of the drug solution,
> ➤ inability to localize the drug solution within a specific site (buccal, sublingual, or gingival).

Various modifications of the buccal absorption test have been reported correcting for salivary dilution and accidental swallowing, but these modifications also suffer from the inability of site localization. Absorption site localization can be achieved by using a bioadhesive system. Bioavailability can then be calculated from the plasma concentration vs. time profile.

Another *in vivo* method includes use of a small perfusion chamber attached to the upper lip of anesthetized dogs. The perfusion chamber is attached to the tissue by cyanoacrylate cement. The drug solution is circulated through the device for a predetermined period of time and sample fractions are then collected from the perfusion chamber to determine the amount of drug remaining in the chamber. Blood samples are drawn after 0 and 30 minutes to determine amount of drug absorbed across the mucosa.

1.7 IN SILICO METHODS OF DRUG ABSORPTION

In silico (computational) methods are the most recent advances. These are used to predict intestinal absorption based on chemical structure and hence are quite useful before the synthesis of compounds. In general, *in silico* models involve approaches ranging from simple QSAR (quantitative structure activity relationship) to complex physiologically based pharmacokinetic and pharmacodynamic models.

One of the first and best-known computational models to predict drug absorption was established in 1997 by Lipinski and co-workers and is known as 'Rule-of-Five'. Some of the simplest models are based on a single descriptor e.g. log P or log D or polar surface area which is a descriptor of hydrogen-bonding potential. Now more sophisticated and accurate *in silico* models are commercially available. For example, QMPRPlus™ (Quatitative Molecular Permeability Relationships), GastroPlus™ (both developed by Simulations Plus Inc., USA: **www.simulations-plus.com**) and iDEA™ (*in vitro* Determination for the Estimation of ADME; Lion Bioscience Inc., USA: **www.lionbioscience.com**).

In silico models can be used to rank compound analogues for permeability and absorption characteristics based on chemical structure. But much more research is needed in this area as *in silico* models are not as reliable as experimental models.

QUESTIONS

1. Explain in detail various mechanisms of drug absorption.
2. What are various factors affecting drug absorption.
3. Explain *in situ* models for drug absorption studies.
4. Explain cell culture techniques used for drug absorption studies.
5. Explain buccal route of drug administration. Add a note on models used for buccal absorption.
6. Explain isolated tissue techniques used in drug absorption studies.
7. Explain structure of cell membrane in detail.
8. Write note on:
   (a) Passive diffusion
   (b) Carrier mediated transport
   (c) pH partition hypothesis
   (d) Floating drug delivery system
   (e) Gastroretentive dosage forms
   (f) Intranasal drug administration
   (g) Loc-I-Gut model of drug absorption
   (h) Topical application of drug
   (i) Rectal application of drug.

2 Distribution of Drugs

2.1 INTRODUCTION

Distribution of drug refers to the reversible transfer of drug from one location to another or one compartment to another within the body. After absorption, as the drug is in the blood and as the distribution process is carried out by the circulation of blood, one compartment (location) is always blood. Whereas, the other can be extra vascular fluids and/or various body tissues. Thus, distribution can be rephrased as reversible transfer of drug from blood to extra vascular fluids and / or various body tissues. Distribution is a passive process and continues till the net flux between blood and extra vascular fluids and/or various body tissues is zero i.e. till equilibrium is achieved. In other words, till amount of drug entering and leaving the extra vascular fluid and/ or tissues is same.

As the drug flow differs from tissue to tissue, the rate and extent at which tissues receive the drug will also be different. Hence distribution will also be different from tissue to tissue. i.e. distribution will not be uniform throughout the body. Thus, in liver, which is highly perfused, the distribution rate will be very high and equilibrium will be reached rapidly. The concentration of drug at the site of action will decide the pharmacological effect and it depends on distribution. Hence distribution plays a vital role in the onset of action, intensity of the effect and duration of the drug action.

2.2 FACTORS AFFECTING DRUG DISTRIBUTION

Various factors will affect the rate of distribution of drug and are as follows:

(1) Body perfusion
(2) Permeability of the drug
(3) Permeability barriers

1. Body Perfusion

The differences in the blood perfusion will affect the rate of drug distribution, as well as concentration of drug in the various organs. Organs which are highly perfused e.g. liver, heart, kidney, lungs, will show rapid drug distribution whereas, organs which are poorly perfused e.g. fat tissue, bones, will show slow/poor distribution of the drug. Organs which are highly perfused will rapidly attain drug concentration that of blood but organs which are poorly perfused will take longer time to attain such concentration. Thus there is a direct correlation between tissue perfusion rate and the time required to distribute a drug to a tissue. *Perfusion rate* is defined as the volume of blood that flows per unit time per unit volume of tissue (Table 2.1).

Table 2.1: Blood flow, perfusion rate, percent body volume and percent cardiac output received by different organs

Organ	% of body volume	Blood flow (ml/min)	% of cardiac output received	Perfusion rate (ml/min/ml of tissue)
Highly Perfused				
Lungs	1.6	5000	100	10
Kidneys	0.5	1100	22	4.0
Liver	2.3	1350	27	0.8
Adrenal glands	0.03	25	0.2	1.2
Heart	0.4	200	4	0.6
Brain	2.0	700	14	0.5
Thyroid gland	0.03	50	1	2.4
Spleen	0.3	77	1.5	0.4
Moderately Perfused				
Muscle (inactive)	43	750	15	0.025
Skin (cool weather)	11	300	6	0.04
Poorly Perfused				
Fat	20	200	4	0.03
Bone	16	250	5	0.02

Imagine a situation where drug is presented to a tissue at an arterial blood concentration of C_A and at a rate equal to the product of blood flow, Q, and C_A.

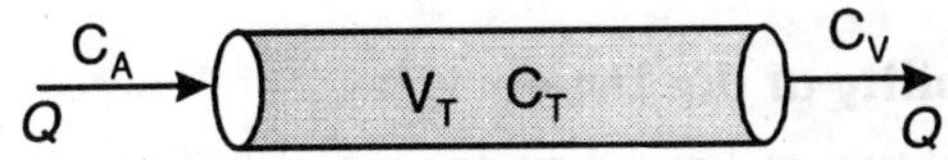

Thus,

$$\text{Rate of presentation} = Q \cdot C_A \qquad ...2.1$$

The drug leaves the tissue at a venous concentration of C_V and considering there is no elimination, then

$$\text{Net rate of uptake} = Q \cdot (C_A - C_V) \qquad ...2.2$$

Blood and tissue can be considered as one compartment if we consider there is no resistance to movement. At equilibrium between concentration of venous·blood (C_V) and tissue (C_T);

$$\text{Amount of drug in tissue} = V_T \cdot K_P \cdot C_V \qquad ...2.3$$

Where,

V_T = Tissue volume

$K_P = C_T/C_V$; equilibrium distribution ratio

Hence,

$$\text{Fractional rate of exit } (K_T) = \frac{\text{Rate of exit}}{\text{Amount of drug in tissue}}$$

$$= \frac{Q \cdot C_V}{V_T \cdot K_P \cdot C_V} \qquad ...2.4$$

or

$$K_T = \frac{\left(\dfrac{Q}{V_T}\right)}{K_P} \qquad ...2.5$$

where,

$\dfrac{Q}{V_T}$ = Tissue perfusion rate

K_T = distribution rate constant (with units of reciprocal time) is a measure of how rapidly drug would leave the tissue if the arterial drug concentration becomes zero.

Thus it is analogues to elimination rate constant. Hence,

$$\text{Distribution half-life} = \frac{0.693}{K_T}$$

or

$$= \frac{0.693 \cdot K_P}{(Q / V_T)} \qquad ...2.6$$

Thus if the drug has high affinity (K_P) and if tissue is poorly perfused (low Q/V_T) then distribution half life will be large i.e. drug will leave slowly from the tissue.

(2) Permeability of the Drug

The permeability-rate limitation for the distribution is particularly important for polar drugs. The drug distribution is influenced by various physicochemical factors such as molecular size, degree of ionization and partition coefficient. Only small, water soluble molecules and ions of size below 50 Daltons can enter the cells through water filled pores. However, entry is restricted for larger size molecules except when specialized transport systems exist for them.

The degree of ionization in plasma or extracellular fluid (ECF), which is dependent on pK_a of the drug, also plays important role in drug permeability. As pH of plasma or ECF essentially remains constant at pH 7.4, except under pathological conditions such as systemic acidosis or alkalosis, it plays less role in the diffusion of the drug. Thus drug which remains unionized at physiological pH will easily permeate the cells, whereas polar, hydrophilic drug which remains ionized at physiological pH can not penetrate the cell. Besides drug pK_a and ionization, partition coefficient ($K_{O/W}$) also plays important role in drug permeability. It is possible that drug may have same $K_{O/W}$ but may have different ionization at physiological pH. In this condition the drug which is more unionized at physiological pH will show better penetration. For example, pentobarbital and salicylic acid have almost same $K_{O/W}$, partition coefficient of unionized form [n-heptane/water] is 0.05 and 0.12 for pentobarbital and salicylic acid respectively, but at physiological pH pentobarbital is more unionized. The fraction unionized at pH 7.4 for pentobarbital and salicylic acid is 0.8 and 0.004 respectively. Thus as pentobarbital is more unionized at physiological pH it penetrates and distributes more rapidly than salicylic acid.

Thiopental, a weak acid (pK_a 7.6), a nonpolar and lipophilic drug is only partially ionized at plasma pH. Its penetration is perfusion-rate limited and because perfusion of brain is greater than that of muscle, entry of thiopental is more rapid in brain. Consider another drug, penicillin, which is a large polar and water soluble compound. It is ionized at plasma pH and hence does not readily pass through the membranes. Thus, entry of penicillin is better in muscles than brain because of greater porosity of muscle capillaries.

Some pathological or drug induced conditions may alter the plasma pH. It may affect the ionization of the drug, hence drug penetration and ultimately its actions. Acidic drugs will be present in more unionized form in acidosis than alkalosis, and will be present in higher concentrations intracellularly and hence will show enhanced pharmacological actions in acidosis. Advantage of this phenomenon has been taken therapeutically very intelligently. For example, in pentobarbital poisoning, high doses of sodium bicarbonate are administered. Sodium bicarbonate will produce systemic alkalosis because of which pentobarbital, being an acidic drug, will be present in ionized form and hence will demonstrate much less penetration in CNS and instead will have enhanced excretion.

(3) Physiological Barriers to Distribution

Variety of membranes in the body act as permeability barriers for distribution of drugs and many of these membranes have specialized structural features.

- Simple capillary barrier
- Simple cell membrane
- Blood-brain barrier
- Cerebrospinal fluid barrier
- Placental barrier
- Blood-testis barrier

Simple Capillary Barrier

Protein free plasma is filtered from the capillaries into the tissue spaces. Any drug dissolved in the plasma but not bound to proteins will leave the capillaries with the tissue fluid. In reality, membranes of capillaries do not act as barriers to drug molecules and drugs in their free from with molecular size less than 600 Daltons, irrespective of being ionized or unionized, will diffuse through the capillary membrane into tissue fluid. Once in tissue fluid (interstitial fluid), molecules of many drugs are readily taken up by the cells.

Simple Cell Membrane

Movement of drug from interstitial fluid or extracellular fluid into the cell is restricted by cell membrane (Fig. 2.1).

The details of cell membrane and movement of solutes across the cell membrane have already been discussed before (Refer to Chapter 1).

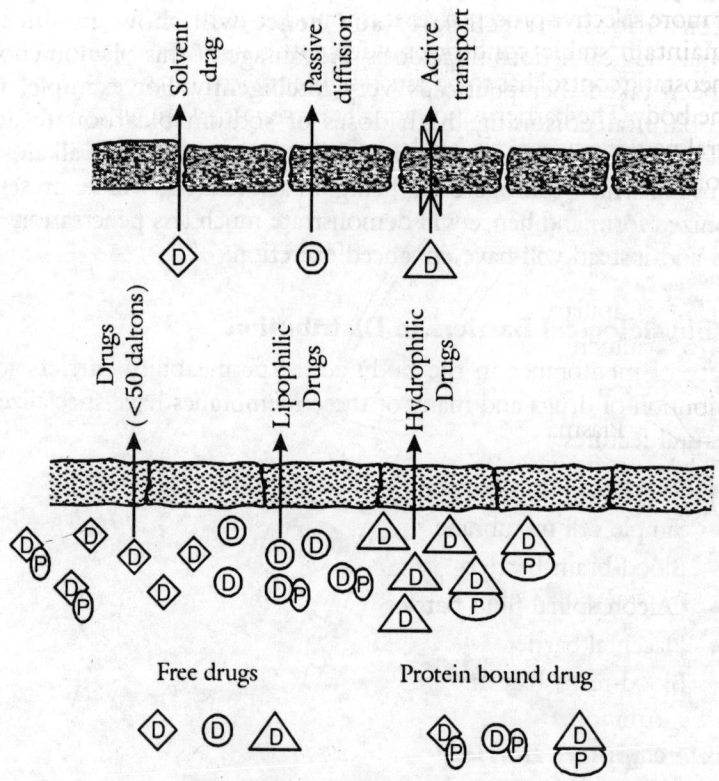

Fig. 2.1. Cell membrane barrier

Blood-Brain Barrier

Although small molecules generally pass with ease from the blood to the tissues, many blood borne substances do not pass readily into the brain. This is because of the operation of metabolic and physical barriers, collectively known as *blood-brain barrier*. It is best to think of the brain capillaries as having no pores, where endothelial cells are joined to one another by tight junctions. In addition, *astrocytes* form a solid envelop around the brain capillaries. Hence any material that leaves the vessel must do so by passing through the endothelial cells and not between them (Fig. 2.2).

Thus, substances that dissolve readily in the lipid components of the plasma membranes enter the brain quickly.

The consequence of this partial impermeability of the cerebral capillary endothelium is that the transfer of material into the brain is a far more selective process than it is for other tissues. This is necessary to maintain stable conditions within the nervous system where homeostatic control has to be much tighter than it is needed elsewhere in the body. The barrier is not equally impenetrable in all parts of the central nervous system. It is relatively permeable in the hypothalamic region.

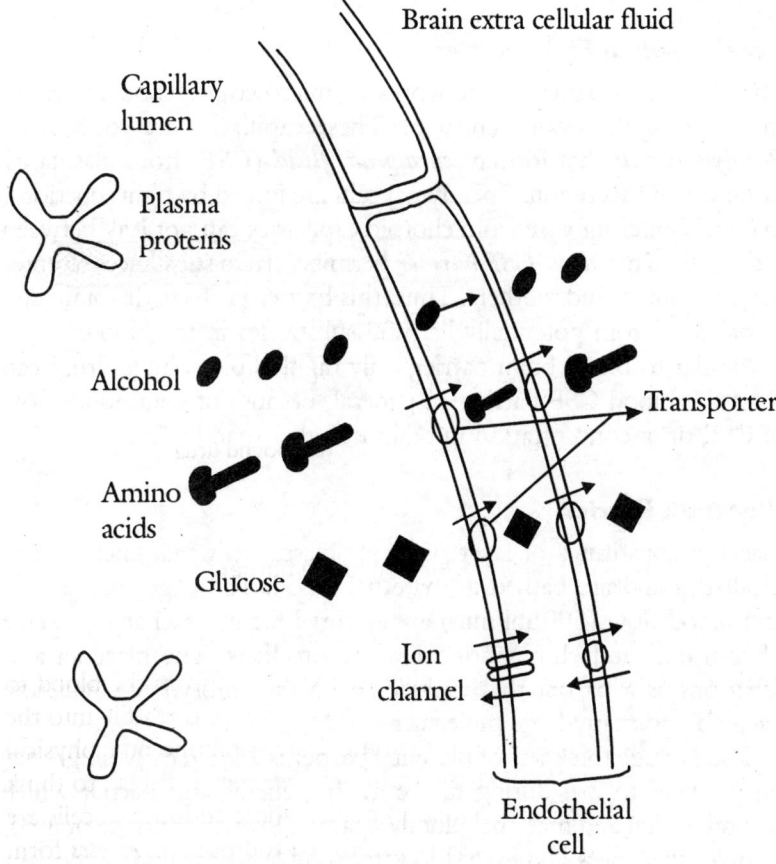

Fig. 2.1. Blood brain barrier

The blood-brain barrier accounts for some drug actions too e.g. morphine differs chemically from heroin only in that morphine has two hydroxyl groups whereas heroin has two acetyl groups. This small difference renders morphine highly lipid insoluble and heroine highly lipid soluble. Thus, heroin crosses the blood-brain barrier more readily than morphine. Other drugs that have rapid effects in the central nervous system because of their high lipid solubility are the barbiturates, nicotine, caffeine and alcohol.

For the treatment of parkinsonism, instead of dopamine levodopa is used, as later can easily cross the blood brain barrier. Polar, water-soluble drugs e.g. penicillins, which are ionized at plasma pH do not cross blood brain barrier under normal circumstances.

Cerebrospinal Fluid barrier

The choroid plexuses are networks of microscopic blood vessels in the walls of the brain ventricles. These capillaries are covered by *ependymal cells* that form *cerebrospinal fluid (CSF)* from plasma by filtration and secretion. Ependymal cells are joined by tight junctions, materials entering CSF from choroid capillaries can not leak between these cells. This *blood-CSF barrier* permits certain substances to enter the CSF but excludes others. Thus, this barrier protects the brain and spinal cord from potentially harmful substances in the blood.

Similar to blood brain barrier, only highly lipid soluble drugs can cross the blood-CSF barrier. In general, because of continuous flow of CSF, drug concentration in brain is higher than in CSF.

Placental Barrier

Placenta constitutes of layer of trophoblastic cells that enclose fetal capillaries and are bathed in maternal blood. The large surface area and blood flow (500 ml/min) are essential for gas exchange, uptake of nutrients and elimination of waste products. The placenta also functions as a barrier that excludes from the embryonic circulation bacteria and many large molecules.

The average thickness of placental barrier is 25 μ in early pregnancy but reduces to 2 μ during full term. In general, this barrier which separates fetal and maternal blood streams allows the passage of lipid-soluble substances and excludes water soluble compounds, especially those with molecular weight larger than 600. For example, drugs used as muscle relaxant during Caesarian section e.g. tubocurarine (MW 772) or gallamine (MW 891) do not affect the infant.

Other Factors Affecting Drug Distribution

1. **Plasma Protein and Tissue Binding**
   This topic will be discussed separately

2. **Age**
   The reasons for differences in drug distribution based on age are as follows:
   - *Total body water*: Much larger in infants compared to older children. In neonates amount is ~ 80 % as compared to 65 % in older children.
   - *Fat content*: Much larger in infants and elderly.
   - *Skeletal muscle*: Lesser in infants and elderly.
   - *Organ composition*: In infants, blood brain barrier is poorly developed. So much higher drug penetration in the brain is seen.
   - *Plasma protein content*: Infants have low levels of plasma albumin.

3. **Pregnancy**
   Fetus represents a separate compartment for drug distribution and because of growth of uterus, placenta and fetus, larger volume is available for distribution. In pregnancy, total body water increases up to eight litres. As a result of haemodilution, plasma albumin declines to ~10 g/L (normal levels 35-55 g/L). The renal plasma flow also almost doubles and there is more rapid loss of drugs that are excreted by kidney e.g. amoxicillin, whose dose should be doubled for systemic infections.

4. **Obesity**
   In obese individuals the high content of adipose tissue may take up large proportion of lipid soluble drugs.

5. **Diet**
   High levels of free fatty acids in blood because of high fat diet will affect binding of acidic drugs e.g. NSAIDs binding to albumin.

6. **Disease State**
   A number of physiological changes are involved in the disease states e.g. hypoalbuminaemia from any cause viz. burns, malnutrition, sepsis, allows a higher proportion of free

(unbound) drug in plasma. Thus, there is a risk of enhanced or adverse responses especially with initial doses of drugs that are highly protein bound e.g. phenytoin.

In inflammation, there is an increase in the concentration of α_1-acid glycoprotein, which binds to number of basic drugs e.g. lignocaine, disopyramide etc.

In meningitis or encephalitis, blood brain barrier becomes more permeable. So many polar antibiotics which generally would not cross, will now cross blood brain barrier e.g. penicillin G.

2.3 VOLUME OF DISTRIBUTION

The drug concentrations in plasma achieved after its distribution completely depend on the dose of the drug administered and the extent of organ and tissue distribution. This extent of distribution can be determined by relating the concentration obtained with a known amount of drug in the body.

Volume of distribution or more correctly ***apparent volume of distribution*** of a drug is not literally a volume and it should not be considered as a particular physiological space/volume within the body. Thus, apparent volume of distribution is the apparent volume into which a drug distributes in the body at equilibrium. Hence, (apparent) volume of distribution, V_d, is the volume of plasma (as plasma rather than blood is usually measured) at drug concentration C, required to account for the entire drug in the body, X.

$$V_d = \frac{X}{C} \qquad \qquad ...2.7a$$

i.e.

$$\frac{\text{Apparent Volume of}}{\text{distribution}} = \frac{\text{(Amount in body)}}{\text{(Plasma drug concentration)}} \qquad ...2.7b$$

Volume of distribution is useful in estimating plasma concentration when a known amount of drug is in the body or in estimating the dose required to achieve a given plasma concentration.

One can also estimate the fraction of drug in and outside plasma. The drug amount in plasma $= V_P \cdot C$

where,

$\qquad V_P$ = Plasma volume
$\qquad C$ = Plasma drug concentration

According to equation 2.7a

The amount of drug in the body is $V_d \cdot C$

Hence,

$$\text{Fraction of drug in the body plasma} = \frac{V_P \cdot C}{V_d \cdot C}$$

$$= \frac{V_P}{V_d} \qquad \qquad ...2.8$$

or   Fraction of drug in body outside plasma $= \dfrac{(V_d - V_P)}{V_d}$ ...2.9

It is clear from equation 2.8 that the larger the volume of distribution, the smaller fraction of drug is in the body plasma.

As evans blue or indocyanine green are high molecular weight substances, they are essentially confined to the circulating plasma when administered intravenously. Hence they can be used to estimate plasma volume or even blood volume if the hematocrit is determined (Hematocrit value is the ratio of red blood corpuscles to plasma). Whereas, ions such as chloride or bromide which rapidly distribute throughout the extracellular fluid but do not readily cross cell membranes can be used to estimate extracellular water or extracellular fluid volume. The volume of total body water or fluid may be estimated by using heavy water (D_2O) or certain lipid soluble substances e.g. antipyrine, which distributes rapidly throughout the total body water or fluid.

The average volumes for body water compartments are approximately as follows (in percent volume/body weight):

Plasma– 5%

Extracellular fluid– 20%

Total body water– 70%

OR

Plasma– 3 litre

Vascular fluid/blood– 6 litre

Extracellular fluid– 12 litre

Intercellular fluid– 24 litre

Hence total body water– 42 litre.

The apparent volume of distribution of each of tracers explained above approximates its true volume of distribution as plasma protein or tissue binding is negligible. In reality most drugs are significantly bound to vascular or extravascular components or both. Drugs which are mainly bound to plasma proteins have apparent volumes of distribution that are smaller than their real volume of distribution. The V_d of such drugs lies between blood volume and total body water volume (i.e. between 6 to 42 litre) e.g. warfarin has V_d of about 7 litre. Drugs that are mainly bound to extra vascular tissues have apparent volume of distributions which are larger than their real distribution space. For example, V_d for amitriptyline is 1400 litre indicating that amount of drug in plasma is small in relation to the amount in extravascular compartments and implies that tissue concentrations of drug are probably very high.

V_d is a characteristic of drug and may range from 0.04 to more than 20 litre/Kg.

2.4 PROTEIN BINDING

Protein binding is one of the major determinants of drug distribution. When drug is present in the blood it can bind to many components including blood cells and plasma proteins. The various blood proteins to which drugs bind are—human serum albumin, α_1-acid glycoprotein and lipoproteins. It is important to note that pharmacological effects are related closely to the free concentration of drug at its site of action rather than the total plasma concentration. Only unbound drug can pass through most cell membranes. The protein bound drug being too large, can not pass through cell membranes. Generally, because of ease of detection, total drug concentration in plasma rather than free drug concentration is determined. For the same reason, recommended therapeutic concentrations are also expressed as the total drug concentration in plasma. The methods employed to measure free drug concentrations are often too tedious, costly and lack accuracy and precision compared to determination of total drug concentration in plasma.

Besides being a determinant of drug distribution, protein binding sometimes serves a particular physiological function e.g. transferrin, a β-globulin, acts as a vehicle for the transport of ferrous ions to bone marrow. Ferrous ions are essential for hemoglobin formation, but if they are not bound to proteins, they can produce toxic effects.

For the purpose of present discussion, drugs can be classified either as acidic or basic (Table 2.2). Acidic drugs commonly bind to plasma albumin and simultaneous administration of acidic drugs may displace one another from their binding sites. Basic drugs may bind to either albumin or α_1-acid glycoprotein.

Table 2.2: Representative acidic and basic drugs, demonstrating more than 90% binding to plasma proteins

Acidic Drugs	Basic Drugs
Aspirin	Alfentanil
Cloxacillin	Amitriptyline
Naproxen	Desipramine
Penicillin	Diazepam
Phenylbutazone	Lidocaine
Phenytoin	Lorazepam
Probenecid	Nifedipine
Sulfinpyrazone	Propranolol
Tolbutamide	Qunidine
Warfarin	Verapamil

One of the important aspects of protein binding is that it is quite variable within and among patients in various therapeutic settings. Diseases can alter drug-protein binding by decreasing the amount of proteins available for binding (Table 2.3).

Table 2.3: Plasma protein altering conditions

	Decreased plasma protein	Increased plasma protein
Albumin	Burns, chronic liver disease, pregnancy, chronic renal failure, trauma	Hypothyroidism,
α_1-acid glycoprotein	Nephritic syndrome	Celiac disease, Crohn's disease, myocardial infarction, rheumatoid arthritis, renal failure, trauma

The degree of protein binding is frequently expressed as the bound drug to total drug concentration ratio. The ratio values range from

0 to 1 and drugs with values greater than 0.9 are said to be highly protein bound drugs. The drug protein binding will depend on molar concentrations of both drug and protein. Assume that protein has a single binding site, then—

$$\text{Drug} + \text{Protein} \underset{}{\overset{K_a}{\rightleftharpoons}} \text{Drug} - \text{Protein complex} \quad ...2.10$$

where,

K_a is association constant i.e. affinity of the protein for a drug

High affinity means that equilibrium lies far to the right. Also, greater the protein concentration for a given drug concentration, the greater the bound drug concentration or vice versa.

Equation 2.10 can be written as:

$$C_U + P \rightleftharpoons C_b d$$

Where, C_U = Concentration of unbound drug

$\qquad\quad$ P = Unoccupied protein

$\qquad\quad$ $C_b d$ = Bound drug

Hence from mass law consideration:

$$K_a = \frac{C_b d}{C_U \cdot P}$$

The drug-protein binding can be specific or non-specific. Some ionized substances become loosely and non-specifically bound to plasma proteins. Because, at the pH of blood, the proteins carry net positive or negative charges which allow binding with oppositely charged ions. This represents a very less important binding as coulombic forces provide only weak bonds, which can be easily disrupted.

Another, and more important type of binding involves chemical groups of drugs and specific binding sites on proteins e.g. plasma albumin. The specific binding sites are in every way analogues to drug receptor sites in the tissues. *Plasma albumin has four different binding sites* viz. Site I (warfarin binding site); Site II (diazepam binding site); Site III (digoxin binding site), Site IV (tamoxifen binding site) (Fig. 2.3).

Site I and Site II are responsible for most of the drug binding. This type of binding mainly involves hydrophobic bonds.

A drug binds to *lipoproteins* by dissolving in the lipid core of lipoprotein. The capacity of lipoproteins to bind drugs depends upon their lipid content. Also, drug binding to lipoprotein is noncompetitive. The examples of drug binding to lipoproteins are– diclofenac (acidic), cyclosporine A (neutral) and chlorpromazine (basic).

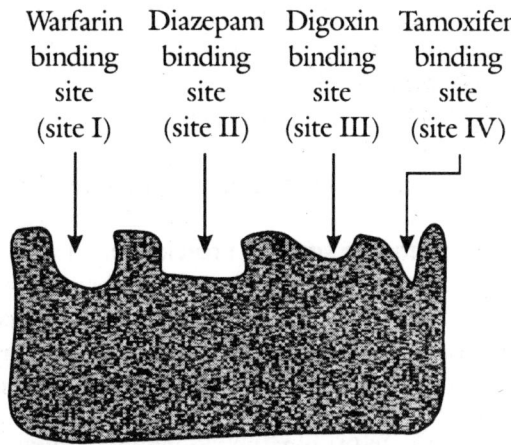

| Warfarin binding site (site I) | Diazepam binding site (site II) | Digoxin binding site (site III) | Tamoxifen binding site (site IV) |

Fig. 2.3. Plasma albumin has four binding sites

Binding of drug to plasma protein may be advantageous and it may cause facilitation of drug absorption. Because once the drug crosses the intestinal membrane and if it is highly protein bound, then concentration of 'unbound' drug in the plasma is kept low. Thus, high concentration gradient between intestine and blood is maintained, increasing drug absorption, e.g. coumarin type anticoagulant drugs. According to their physicochemical properties it could be predicted that they should be absorbed with difficulty from gastrointestinal tract but this difficulty is overcome by their high degree of protein binding.

Drug-protein binding is also clinically important. Because drug-protein complex may act as depot of drug. When plasma containing protein bound drug is exposed to another agent that has higher affinity for the binding site than the original drug, then the invader agent by simple competition displaces the original drug. This provides the basis of an important class of drug interaction.

2.5 FACTORS AFFECTING PROTEIN BINDING

Protein binding is affected mainly because of drug related and patient related factors. Lipophilicity plays important role in drug-protein binding e.g. highly lipophilic drug tends to localize in adipose tissues. Neutral, unionized drugs bind more to lipoproteins. Acidic and basic characteristics of drugs also influence the protein binding. The concentration of drug in the body also plays important role e.g. as concentration of α_1-acid glycoprotein is much less, lidocaine at therapeutic concentration will saturate the binding. Some drugs will demonstrate high affinity for a particular site e.g. digoxin has high affinity for cardiac muscle protein.

Also lipoproteins tend to bind lipophilic drugs by dissolving them in their lipid core.

Also number of binding sites on proteins play important role in protein binding e.g. albumin has more number of binding sites compared to α_1-acid glycoprotein which has limited number of binding sites. Thus, because of multiple binding sites, drug binding to albumin will require more concentration compared to drugs binding to α_1-acid glycoproteins.

Also as discussed in Table 2.3, many pathological conditions will increase or decrease amount of plasma proteins and thus will affect drug-protein binding.

2.6 KINETICS OF PROTEIN BINDING

Drug-protein binding is a reversible reaction and can be expressed as:

$$P + D \underset{K_d}{\overset{K_a}{\rightleftharpoons}} PD \qquad \ldots 2.11$$

Thus according to law of mass action

$$K_a = \frac{[PD]}{[P]\cdot[D]} \qquad \ldots 2.12$$

$$[PD] = K_a \cdot [P] \cdot [D] \qquad \ldots 2.13$$

where,

$\qquad$ [P] = concentration of free protein
$\qquad$ [D] = concentration of free drug
$\qquad$ [PD] = concentration protein bound drug
$\qquad$ K_a = association rate constant
$\qquad$ K_d = dissociation rate constant

$$P_T = [PD] + [P] \qquad \ldots 2.14$$

where,

$\qquad$ P_T = Total concentration of protein

Thus,

$$r = \frac{[PD]}{[P_T]} \text{ or } \frac{[PD]}{[PD]+[P]} \qquad \ldots 2.15$$

Where, r = moles of drug bound to total protein

Substituting equation 2.13 in 2.15

$$r = \frac{K_a \cdot [P] \cdot [D]}{K_a \cdot [P] \cdot [D] + [P]}$$

or
$$r = \frac{K_a[D]}{K_a[D]+1} \qquad \ldots 2.16$$

Equation 2.16 is valid only when protein has one binding site. But if protein has more than one binding sites (n) per mole of protein, then—

$$r = \frac{n \cdot K_a \cdot [D]}{K_a \cdot [D]+1} \qquad \ldots 2.17$$

Equation 2.17 can be used to calculate K_a and n as discussed below.

1. *Direct plot* is plot of [D] versus r as shown in Fig. 2.4.

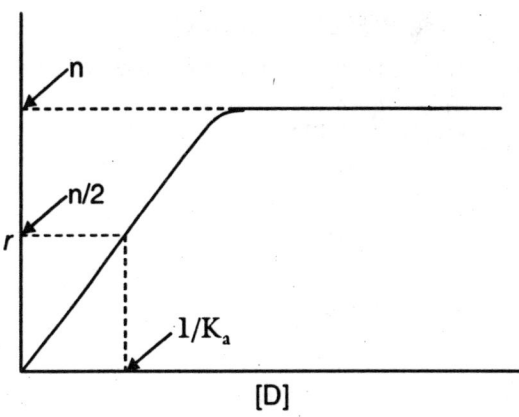

Fig. 2.4. Direct plot of [D] versus r

At saturation i.e. plateau, r = n.

2. *Sctachard plot* is obtained by rearranging the equation 2.17.

$$r + r \cdot K_a \cdot [D] = n \cdot K_a \cdot [D]$$
$$r = n \cdot K_a \cdot [D] - r \cdot K_a \cdot [D]$$

$$\frac{r}{[D]} = n \cdot K_a - r \cdot K_a \qquad \qquad ...2.18$$

Plot r versus (r/[D]) (Fig. 2.5).

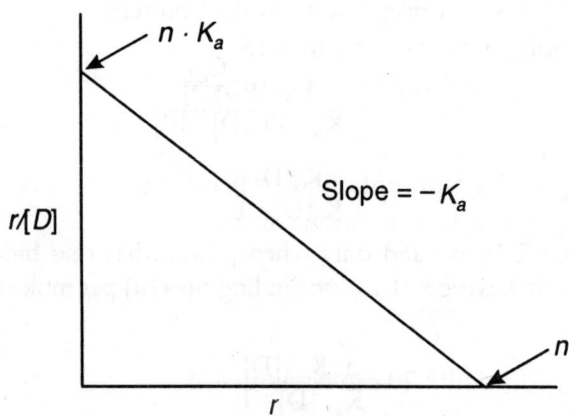

Fig. 2.5. Scatchard plot

Slope of the line is $= -K_a$, Y–intercept is $= nK_a$ and X-intercept is $= n$.

2.7 TISSUE BINDING

The total body tissue comprises 40% of the body hence drug tissue binding is quite significant. But unlike plasma binding, tissue binding can not be measured directly, as tissue will have to be disrupted resulting in the loss of tissue integrity.

Consider following equation;

Amount in body = Amount in plasma + Amount outside plasma

$$V \cdot C = V_P \cdot C + V_{TW} \cdot C_{TW} \qquad \qquad ...2.19$$

Where,

V_{TW} = Volume of plasma into which the drug distributes

C_{TW} = Corresponding total drug concentration

Divide equation 2.19 by C;

$$V \qquad = \qquad V_P + \qquad V_{TW} \cdot \left(\frac{C_{TW}}{C}\right) \qquad ...2.20$$

| Apparent volume of distribution | Volume of plasma | Apparent volume of tissue |

At equilibrium; $C_u = C_{uT}$

where,

C_u = Unbound drug in plasma

C_{uT} = Unbound drug in tissue

Also,

$$f_u = \frac{C_u}{C} \text{ and for tissues } f_{uT} = \frac{C_{uT}}{C_{TW}}$$

where,

f_u = Fraction unbound in plasma

f_{uT} = Fraction unbound in tissue

Thus,

$$\frac{C_{TW}}{C} = \frac{f_u}{f_{uT}} \qquad ...2.21$$

And hence equation 2.20 can be written as:

$$V = V_P + V_{TW} \cdot \left(\frac{f_u}{f_{uT}}\right) \qquad ...2.22$$

Thus, apparent volume of distribution increases when f_u increases and decreases when f_{uT} increases.

Binding of drugs in both plasma and tissues complicates the situation and often prevents making any conclusion about the actual volume into which the drug distributes.

2.6 DRUG INTERACTIONS

Drugs can compete for protein binding sites and thereby one drug may act as a displacer of the second, this is called as *displacement interaction*.

The clinical impact of displacement depends on:

♦ The total amount of drug in the body that is bound
♦ The extent of displacement
♦ Whether the drug is tissue bound
♦ Whether the drug is high-clearance or low clearance.

Effects of displacement are usually of clinical significance only when binding exceeds 85 to 90%. Even then, when a drug is displaced it does not necessarily mean that drug concentration in plasma will also increase proportionally because free drug can diffuse into the tissues.

Thus, if apparent volume of distribution is large, the increase in plasma concentration is minimal. If the apparent volume of distribution is small, the concentration at the receptor sites may rise significantly and show an increase in intensity of drug action and in some cases toxic effects.

As discussed in Table 2.3 many conditions are capable of altering plasma proteins. Thus, in disorders or situations in which free fatty acid levels are increased, acidic drugs are displaced from albumin binding sites. It is because the free fatty acids bind to albumin. Quantitatively, when the free fatty acids/albumin ratio exceeds 3.5, the binding of acidic drugs is reduced significantly.

Several orally active anticoagulants demonstrate serious drug interactions as a result of displacement from plasma protein because of:

➤ High percentage bound
➤ Small volume of distribution

For example, concomitant administration of warfarin and phenylbutazone will lead to displacement of bound warfarin to form free warfarin. This will lead to increased rate of loss but also an increased pharmacological activity and hence prothrombin time will almost double.

2.7 *IN VITRO* MODELS OF DRUG DISTRIBUTION

As described in previous sections, drug distribution is an important process and plays a vital part in various aspects of pharmacokinetics. Very little work has been carried out so far involving *in vitro* methods for drug distribution.

Plasma protein binding was one of the earliest *in vitro* measurements. Traditionally plasma protein binding was studied *in vitro* using ultra-filtration and equilibrium dialysis. But now a kind of high throughput approach has been developed i.e. use of 96-well format. Use of 96-well format increases number of compounds which can be screened in a single experiment. Thus, it decreases the time required for screening the compound and hence increases the output. Few attempts have also been made to develop *in silico* predictive models.

Distribution of drug to brain is one of the important distribution characteristics studied during drug development. Blood brain barrier (BBB) plays an important role in distribution of drugs into brain. Most of the *in vitro* models of BBB are based on either primary bovine, rat or mouse cells. Immortalized cells (cell lines) have also been used but because of their animal origin they do not express human transporters. Various other methods using immobilized artificial membranes, reverse-phase chromatography and capillary electrophoresis have also been used to investigate and predict drug permeability in CNS. Till todate no validated method for measuring human BBB function has been reported to provide a predictive model of drug distribution in brain *in vivo*.

There are few methods that have been tried for predicting volume of distribution based on *in vitro* data such as, human plasma protein binding, experimentally determined log D values and pK$_a$. For example scatter plot of volume of distribution against log D does not reveal any correlation but when correction for plasma protein binding is incorporated it gives a clear linear trend.

QUESTIONS

1. Explain various permeability barriers which affect distribution of drugs.
2. Explain the concept of "volume of distribution". Add a note on different tracers used to estimate volume of distribution.
3. Explain the role of different proteins involved in drug-protein binding.
4. Explain the importance of drug-protein binding in drug interactions.
5. Write a note on drug tissue binding.
6. What are various factors affecting distribution of a drug?
7. Explain kinetics of drug-protein binding.
8. Explain the changes in drug-protein binding in pathological conditions.

3

Drug Metabolism
(Biotransformation)

3.1 INTRODUCTION

The duration and intensity of drug action primarily depends upon the rate at which drug is removed from the body and/or site of action i.e. rate of elimination. *Elimination* can be defined as irreversible loss of drug from the body. Drugs are eliminated from the body either unchanged by the process of excretion or converted to metabolites and then excreted.

Metabolism, also called as *biotransformation,* is defined as the conversion from one chemical form to another. Biotransformation includes enzymatically driven chemical conversions and does not include conversions due to chemical instability. Xenobiotics, which are substances foreign to the body, are metabolized or biotransformed to more water-soluble compounds, because water soluble compounds are more readily excreted. Hence, lipid soluble drugs which are not readily eliminated are metabolized to more polar compounds. Without biotransformation, excretion of lipophilic xenobiotics would be extremely slow and they will eventually accumulate in the body and kill the organism.

The metabolic conversion of drugs mainly occurs in the liver, although every tissue has some metabolic activity. Other organs with significant metabolic capacity include the gastrointestinal tract, kidneys and lungs. Metabolism by organs other than the liver is called as *extrahepatic metabolism*.

3.2 INTRODUCTION TO PHASE I AND PHASE II REACTIONS

The enzymatic reactions in drug biotransformation are generally divided into two groups, called Phase I and Phase II (See Table 3.1).

Phase I reactions include hydrolysis, reduction and oxidation. Phase I reactions usually result in only a small increase in hydrophilicity. Phase II reactions include glucuronidation, sulfonation (also called as sulfation), acetylation, and methylation, conjugation with glutathione and conjugation with amino acids. Generally phase II reactions result in large increase in hydrophilicity. Phase I reactions may or may not precede Phase II reactions. For example, heroin first undergoes hydrolysis (Phase I) followed by conjugation with glucuronic acid (Phase II) to form morphine-3-glucuronide. But in case of morphine there is direct conjugation with glucuronic acid (Phase II) to form morphine-3-glucuronide.

3.3 PHASE I REACTIONS

Phase I reactions include hydrolysis, reduction and oxidation. Phase I reactions expose or introduce functional groups viz –OH, –NH, –SH or –COOH and slightly increase the hydrophilicity of drugs. These functional groups are often the sites for Phase II reactions.

Table 3.1: Reactions involved in drug metabolism and their subcellular location

Type of Reaction	Phase I	
	Enzyme Involved	Subcellular Location
Hydrolysis	Esterase	Microsomes, cytosol, lysosomes, blood
	Peptidase	Blood, lysosomes
	Epoxidase, hydrolase	Microsomes, cytosol
Reduction	-Azo & -nitro reduction	Microsomes, microflora, cytosol
	Carbonyl reduction	Cytosol, microsomes, blood
	Disulfide reduction	Cytosol
	Sulfoxide reduction	Cytosol
	Quinone reduction	Cytosol, microsomes
	Reductive dehalogenation	Microsomes
Oxidation	Alcohol dehydrogenase	Cytosol
	Aldehyde dehydrogenase	Cytosol, mitochondria
	Aldehyde oxidase	Cytosol
	Xanthine oxidase	Cytosol
	Monoamine oxidase	Mitochondria
	Diamine oxidase	Cytosol
	Prostaglandins H Synthase	Microsomes
	Flavin monooxygenases	Microsomes
	Cytochrome P450	Microsomes

| Type of | Phase II | |
Reaction	Enzyme Involved	Subcellular Location
	Glucuronide conjugation	Microsomes
	Sulfate conjugation	Cytosol
	Glutathione conjugation	Cytosol, microsomes
	Amino acid conjugation	Mitochondria, microsomes
	Acylation	Mitochondria, cytosol
	Methylation	Cytosol, microsomes, blood

3.3.1 Hydrolysis

Drugs containing functional groups such as carboxylic acid ester—procaine; amide—procainamide; thioesters—spironolactone; phosphoric acid ester—paraxon and acid anhydride—diisopropylfluorophosphate, undergo hydrolysis.

The hydrolysis of carboxylic acid esters, amides and thioesters is mostly carried out by carboxylesterases. Carboxylesterases are located in various tissues and serum. Phosphoric acid esters are hydrolyzed by paraoxonase. Paraoxonase is a serum enzyme and is also called as organophosphatase. Phosphoric acid anhydrides are hydrolyzed by diisopropylflurophosphatase.

In presence of alcohol, the carboxylesterases can catalyze the transesterification of drugs e.g. conversion of cocaine to ethylcocaine.

Carboxylic acid esters

$$CH_2 - COOCH_2CH_2N^+(CH_3)_2 \qquad CH_2 - COOH$$
$$| \qquad\qquad\qquad\qquad\quad \rightarrow \quad |$$
$$CH_2 - COOCH_2CH_2N^+(CH_3)_2 \qquad CH_2 - COOH$$

Sunccinyl choline   Succinic acid

$$+ 2HOCH_2CH_2N^+(CH_3)_2$$

choline

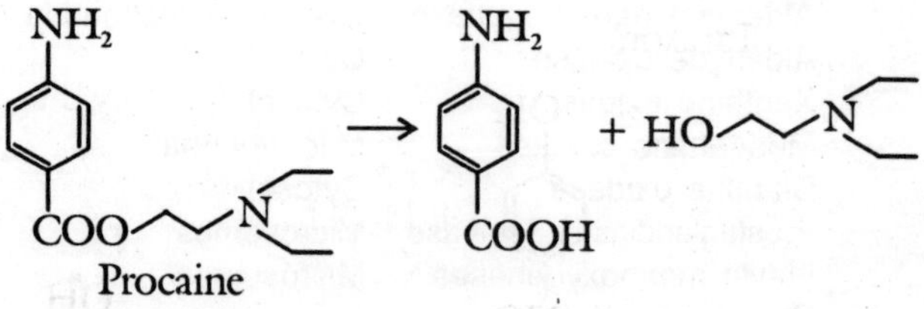

Procaine

Amides

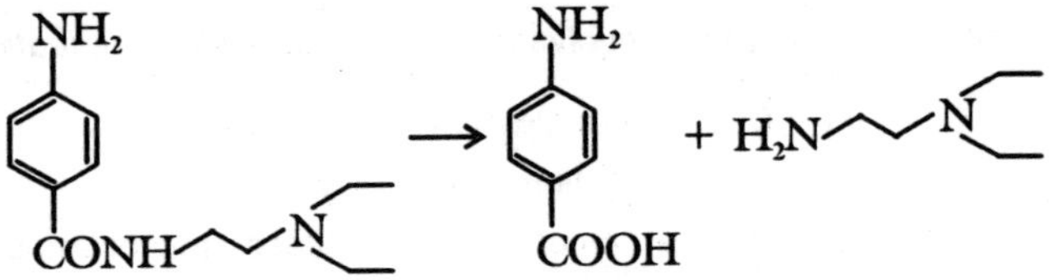

Procainamide

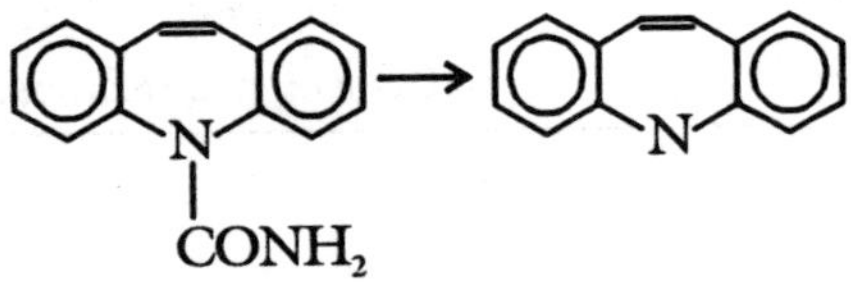

Carbamazepine

Thioesters

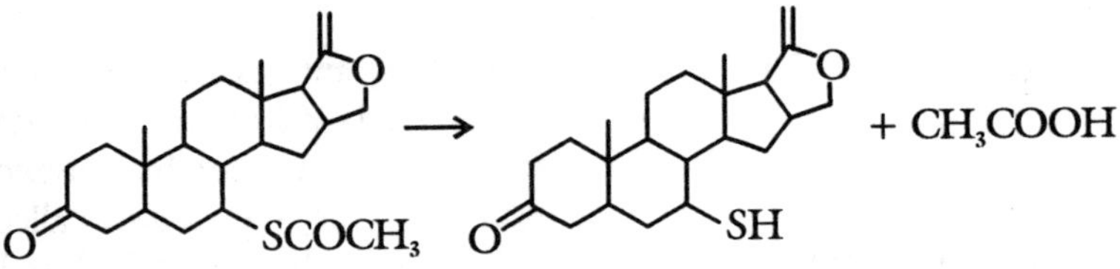

Spironolactone

Phosphoric acid esters

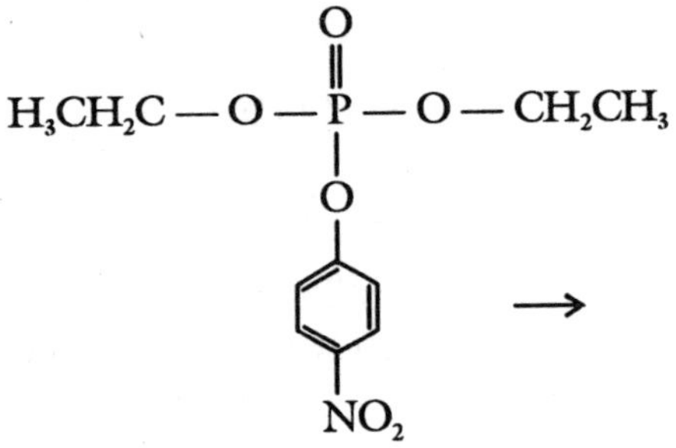

Paraxon

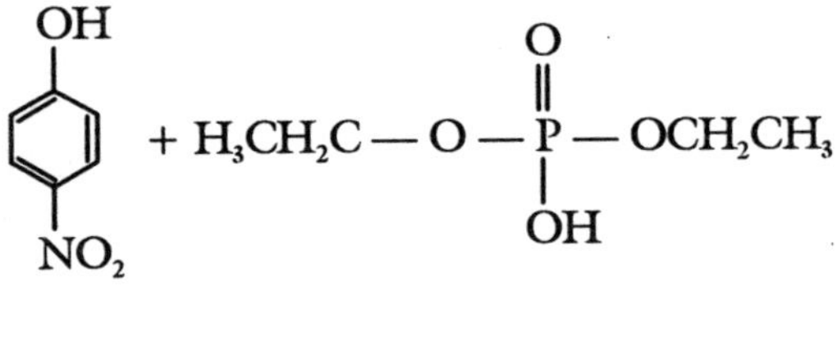

Acid anhydride

$$H_3C \diagdown \atop H_3C \diagup CH - O - \overset{\overset{\displaystyle O}{\|}}{\underset{\underset{\displaystyle F}{|}}{P}} - O - CH \overset{\diagup CH_3}{\diagdown CH_3}$$

Diisopropylfluorophosphate

$$\longrightarrow \quad H_3C \diagdown \atop H_3C \diagup CH - O - \overset{\overset{\displaystyle O}{\|}}{\underset{\underset{\displaystyle OH}{|}}{P}} - O - CH \overset{\diagup CH_3}{\diagdown CH_3} \; + \; HF$$

Metabolism of drugs by carboxylesterases is not always a detoxification process. Carboxylesterases may convert some drugs to toxic and tumerigenic metabolites.

$$H_3C - \overset{\overset{\displaystyle O}{\|}}{C} - O - CH - CH_3 \quad \xrightarrow{\text{Carboxylesterase}}$$

Vinyl acetate

$$H_3C - \overset{\overset{\displaystyle O}{\|}}{C} - OH + H_3C - \overset{\overset{\displaystyle O}{\|}}{C} - H$$

Acetate   Acetaldehyde

$\downarrow$

– can bind covalently to
DNA and Proteins
– can cause nasal tumors

$$\text{Ph} - \overset{\underset{\underset{\displaystyle NH_3}{|}}{N}} - \overset{\overset{\displaystyle O}{\|}}{C} - \overset{\underset{\underset{\displaystyle NO}{|}}{N}} - CH_3 \quad \xrightarrow{\text{Carboxylesterase}}$$

1, 3 -dimethyl -3-phenyl-
1- nitrosourea

$$\text{Ph} - \overset{\underset{\underset{\displaystyle NH_3}{|}}{N}} - \overset{\overset{\displaystyle O}{\|}}{C} - OH + HO - N = N - CH_3$$

Methyldiazonium
hydroxide

N- methyl -N- phenyl
-1- nitro formic acid

$\downarrow$

– can bind covalently to
DNA and proteins
– can cause skin cancers

Epoxides are hydrolyzed by epoxide hydrolase

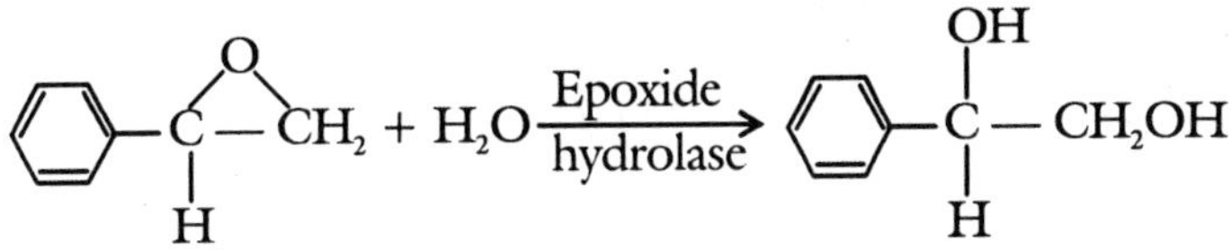

$$\text{Styrene 7, 8-epoxide} + H_2O \xrightarrow[\text{hydrolase}]{\text{Epoxide}} \text{Styrene 7, 8-glycol}$$

Styrene 7, 8-epoxide   Styrene 7, 8-glycol

Conversion of leukotriene A_4 to leukotriene B_4 is also an example of epoxide hydrolysis.

Peptidases which cleave amide linkage between adjacent amino acids function as amidases (hydrolysis reaction).

Following are few more hydrolysis reactions.

Organic acid esters

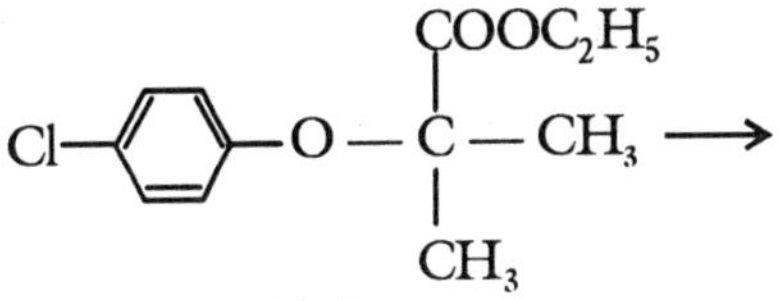

Clofibrate $\longrightarrow$

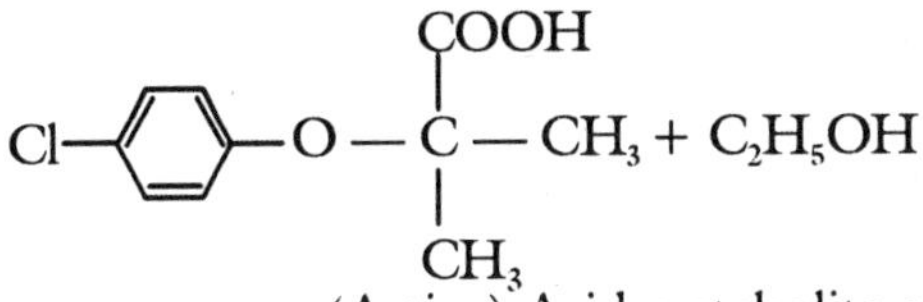

(Active) Acid metabolite of clofibrate

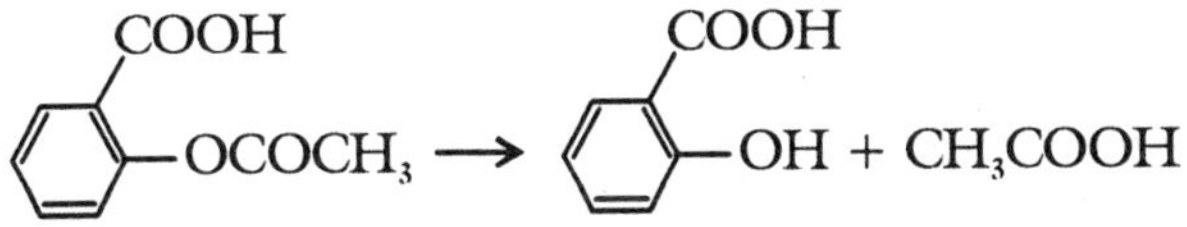

Aspirin $\longrightarrow$ Salicylic acid $+ CH_3COOH$

Inorganic acid esters

$$CH_3-\overset{H}{\underset{CH_3}{C}}-O-\overset{O}{\underset{O}{S}}-CH_3 \rightarrow CH_3-\overset{H}{\underset{CH_3}{C}}-OH + HO-\overset{O}{\underset{O}{S}}-CH_3$$

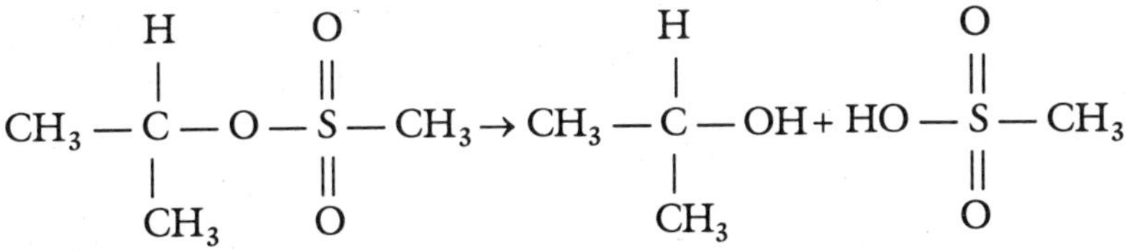

Isopropyl methanesulfonate   Isopropanol   Methanesulfonic acid

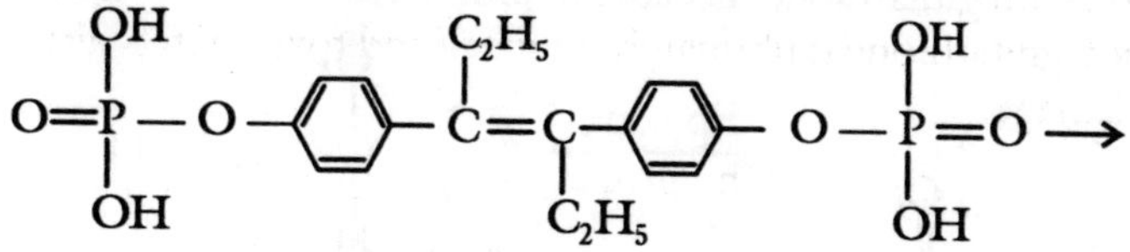

Stilbesterol diphosphate

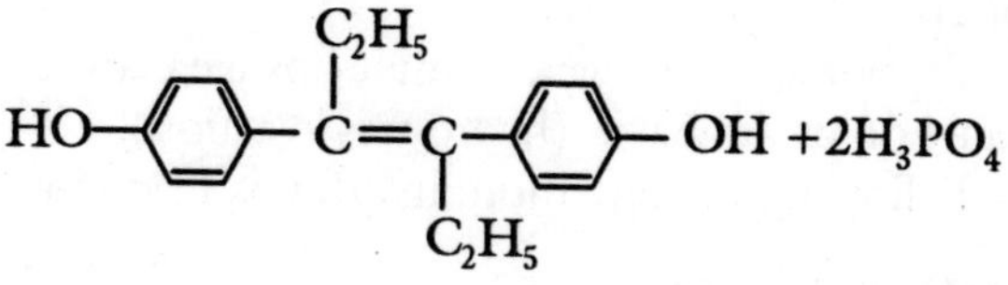

Stibesterol

N-hydroxylation

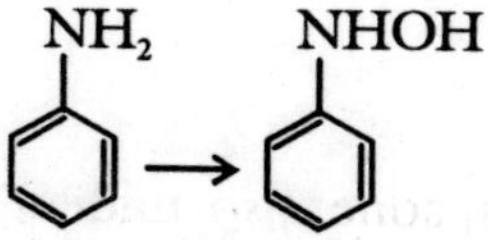

Aniline

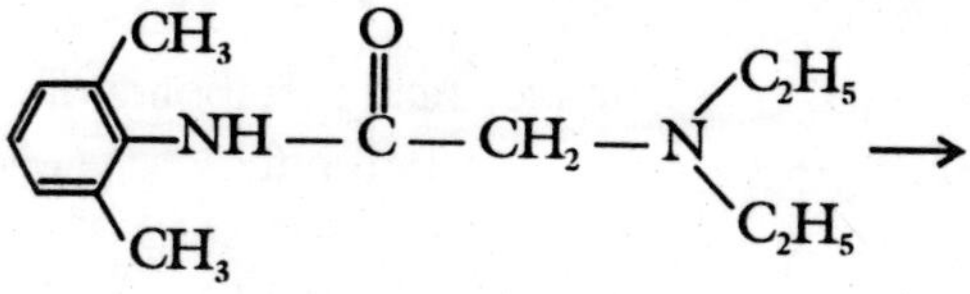

Lidocaine

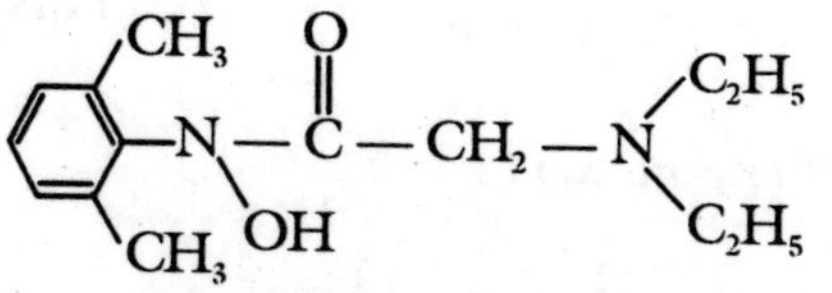

N-hydroxy lidocaine

N-hydroxylation of amides may generate reactive intermediates, which may produce toxicity by covalently binding with macromolecules e.g. paracetamol. Paracetamol on prolonged usage or overdosage causes liverdamage. Hepatotoxicity is caused by metabolite, N-acetyl-p-benzoquinone, which is generally inactivated by conjugation with glutathione. Because of prolonged use or overdose of paracetamol, glutathione is ultimately depleted and toxic metabolite causes liver damage.

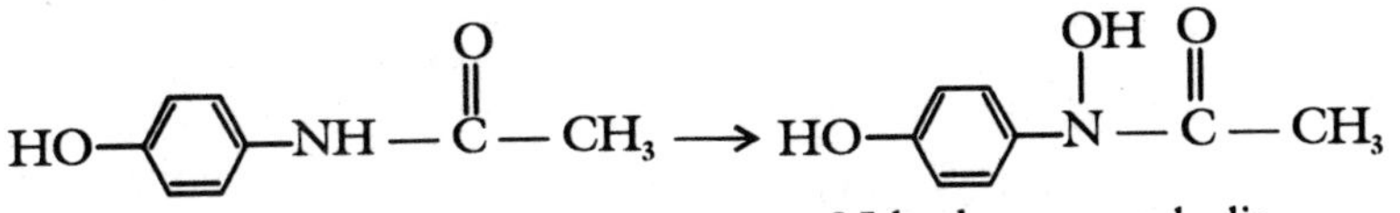

$$HO-\underset{\text{Paracetamol}}{\bigcirc}-NH-\overset{\overset{O}{\|}}{C}-CH_3 \longrightarrow HO-\bigcirc-\underset{\underset{\substack{\text{N-hydroxy metabolite} \\ \text{of paracetamol}}}{}}{\overset{\overset{OH}{|}}{N}}-\overset{\overset{O}{\|}}{C}-CH_3$$

$$\longrightarrow O=\bigcirc=N-\overset{\overset{O}{\|}}{C}-CH_3$$

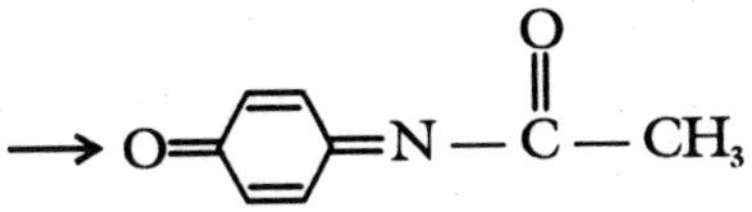

N-acetyl-P-benzoquinone

↓

covalent binding to
macromolecules

↓

Hepatotoxicity

Antileprosy drug dapsone also undergoes N-hydroxylation producing N-hydroxy dapsone. This metabolite can cause methemoglobinemia by oxidizing ferrous form to ferric form of hemoglobin.

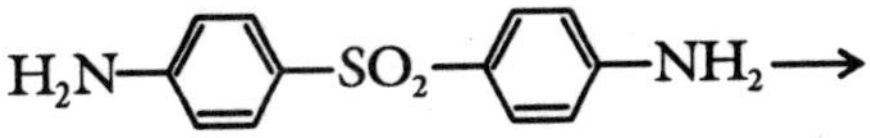

$$H_2N-\bigcirc-SO_2-\bigcirc-NH_2 \longrightarrow$$

Dapsone

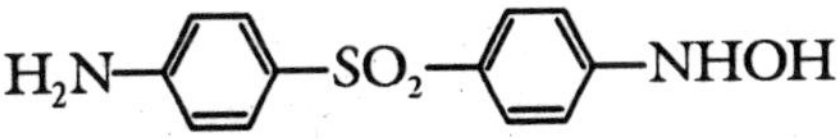

$$H_2N-\bigcirc-SO_2-\bigcirc-NHOH$$

N-hydroxy dapsone

↓

$$H_2N-\bigcirc-SO_2-\bigcirc-N=O$$

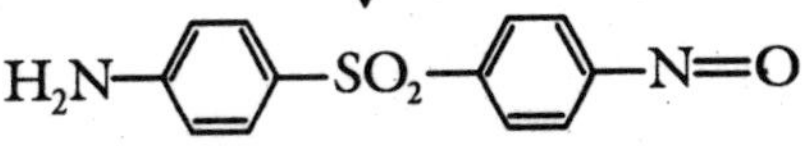

Nitroso metabolite of dapsone

Oxidation of alcohol, carbonyl and carboxylic acids

These reactions are generally catalyzed by dehydrogenases. Oxidation of ethanol to acetaldehyde and ultimately to acetic acid involves multiple organelles (microsomes, cytosol and peroxisomes).

$$C_2H_5OH \underset{\text{dehydrogenase}}{\overset{\text{Alchohol}}{\rightleftharpoons}} CH_3CHO \underset{\text{dehydrogenase}}{\overset{\text{Aldehyde}}{\longrightarrow}} CH_3COOH$$

Alcohol dehydrogenase is a zinc-containing cytosolic enzyme. Aldehyde dehydrogenase requires NAD^+ as the cofactor and different subtypes have different distribution.

N-dealkylation

Compounds such as hydrazines, N-substituted amides, secondary and tertiary amines may undergo N-dealkylation. Generally this reaction takes place without any change in oxidation state, but alkyl group which is removed generally gets oxidized.

Nonaromatic heterocyclics-hydrolytic cleavage

Phensuximide → Phenyl succinamic acid

Thalidomide → Thalidomide metabolite

Hydrolytic dehalogenation

Dichloro diphenyl trichloro ethane (DDT) → Dichloro diphenyl dichloro ethylene (DDE)

3.3.2 Reduction

Drugs containing an aldehyde, ketone, disulfide, sulfoxide, quinine, N-oxide, alkene, azo or nitro group are often reduced *in vivo* e.g. aldehyde can be reduced to alcohol or sulfoxides can be reduced to sulfide. Aldehyde oxidase is one of the enzymes involved in bioreductions.

Azo and Nitro Reduction

Generally azo– and nitro-reduction is carried out by intestinal microflora, cytochrome P450 and NAD(P)H-quinone oxidoreductase.

Azo reduction

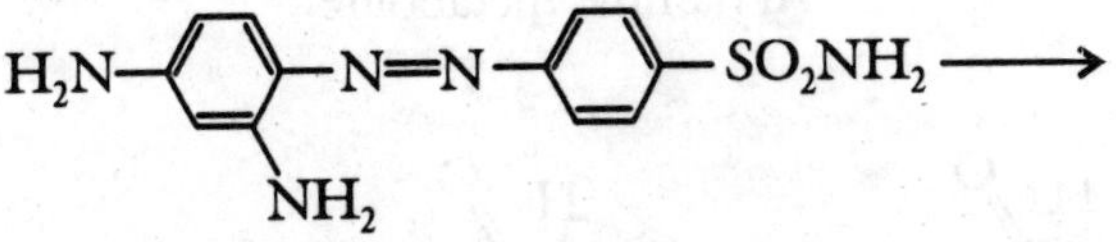

$$H_2N-\bigcirc\underset{NH_2}{-}N=N-\bigcirc-SO_2NH_2 \longrightarrow$$

Prontosil

$$H_2N-\bigcirc\underset{NH_2}{-}NH_2 + H_2N-\bigcirc-SO_2NH_2$$

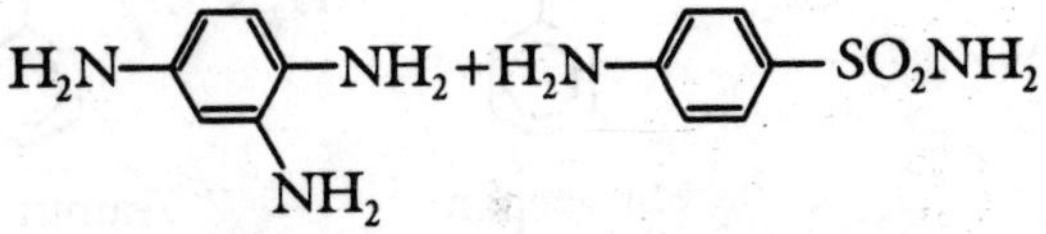

1, 2, 4-triamino benzene   Sulfanilamide

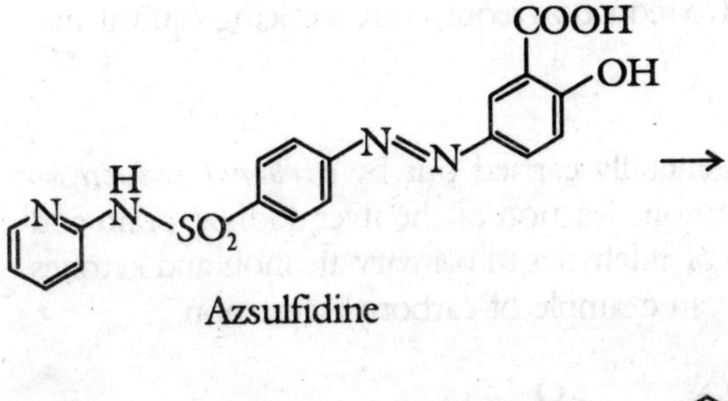

Azsulfidine

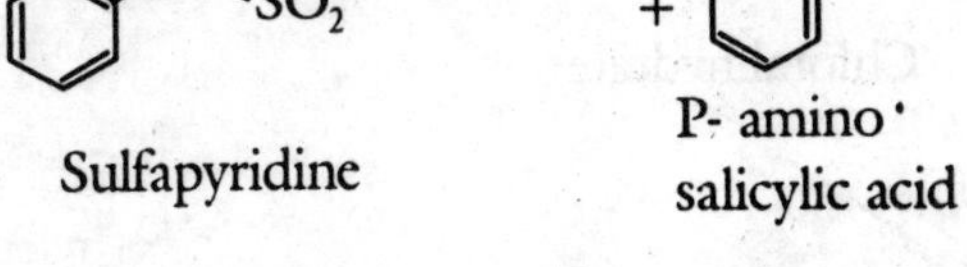

Sulfapyridine   P- amino salicylic acid

Nitro reduction

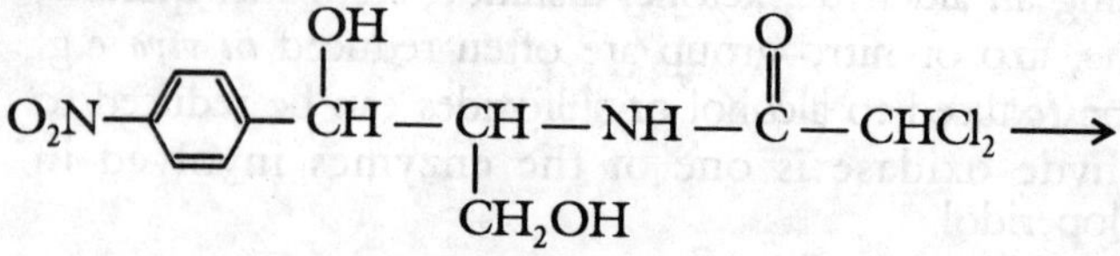

$$O_2N-\text{(ring)}-CH-CH-NH-\overset{\overset{O}{\|}}{C}-CHCl_2 \longrightarrow$$

with OH on the CH and CH_2OH below.

Chloramphenicol

$$H_2N-\text{(ring)}-CH-CH-NH-\overset{\overset{O}{\|}}{C}-CHCl_2$$

with OH on the CH and CH_2OH below.

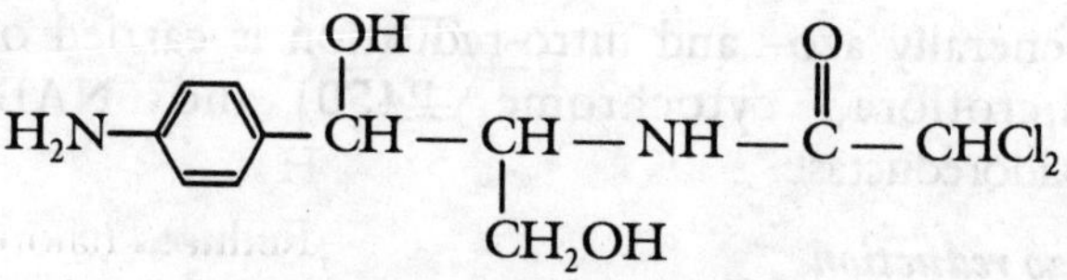

Arylamine metabolite

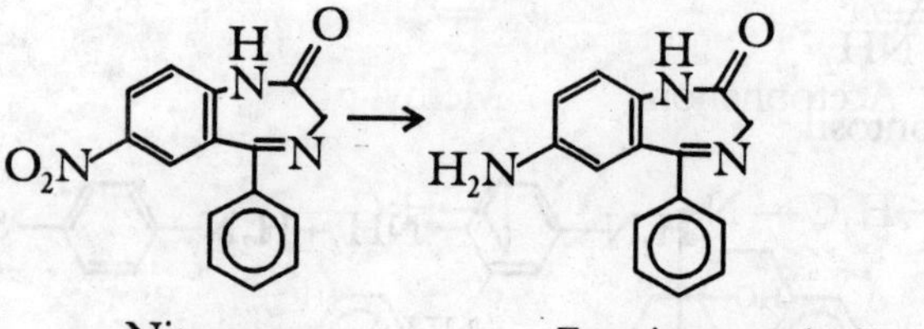

Nitrazepam   →   7-aminometabolite

During azo-reduction, $N = N$ is sequentially reduced and cleaved to produce two primary amines. This reaction requires four reducing equivalents. Whereas, nitro reduction requires six reducing equivalents.

Carbonyl Reduction

Carbonyl reduction is generally carried out by *carbonyl reductases* present in blood and cytosolic fraction of the liver, kidney, brain and other tissues. Reduction of aldehydes to primary alcohols and ketones to secondary alcohol are an example of carbonyl reduction.

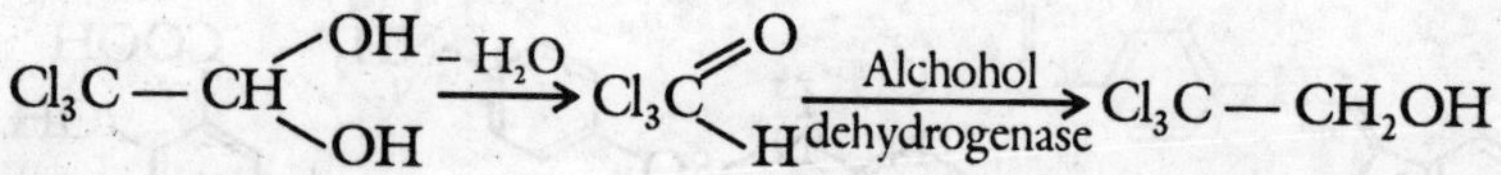

$$Cl_3C-CH\overset{OH}{\underset{OH}{\diagup}} \xrightarrow{-H_2O} Cl_3C\overset{O}{\underset{H}{\diagdown}} \xrightarrow[\text{dehydrogenase}]{\text{Alchohol}} Cl_3C-CH_2OH$$

Chloral hydrate   Trichloro ethanol

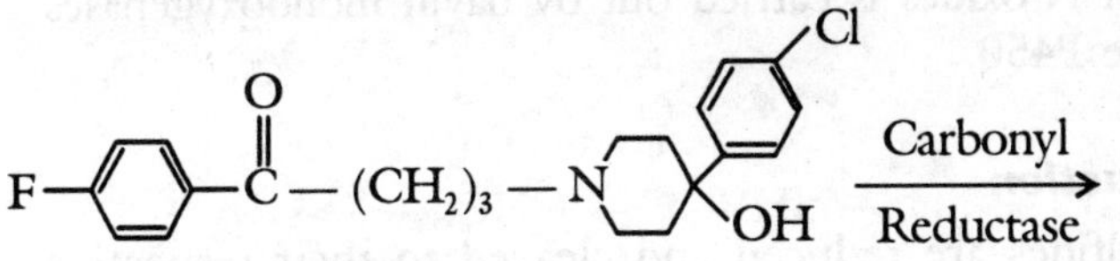

Haloperidol

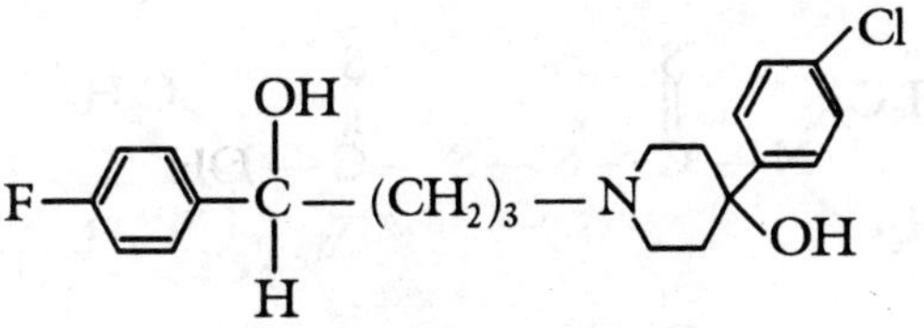

Reduced haloperidol

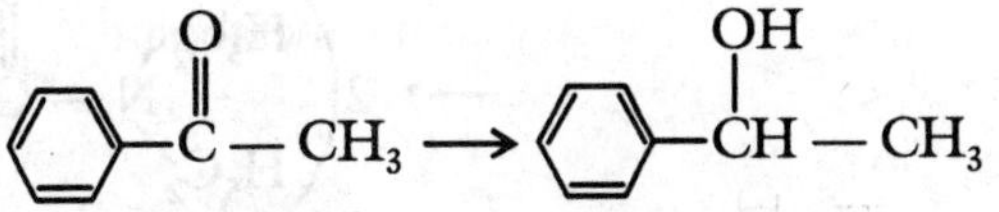

Acetophenone   Methyl phenyl carbinol

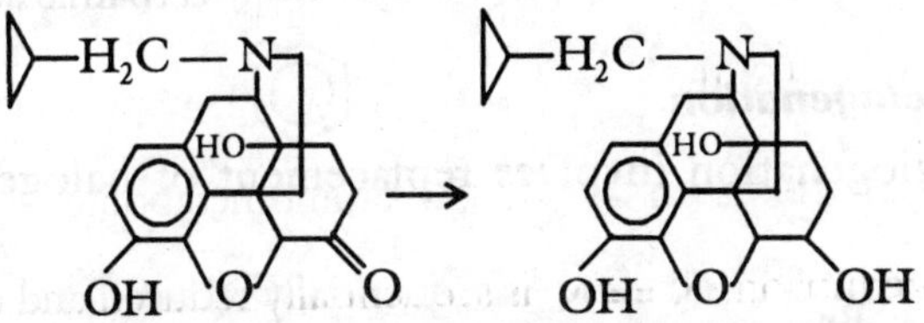

Naltrexone   Isomorphine derivative

Other drugs, which are also reduced by carbonyl reductase, include acetohexamide, daunorubicin, ethacrynic acid, warfarin and menadione.

Sulfoxide and N-oxide Reduction

Sulfoxides are reduced by thioredoxin-dependent enzymes found in liver and kidney cytosol.

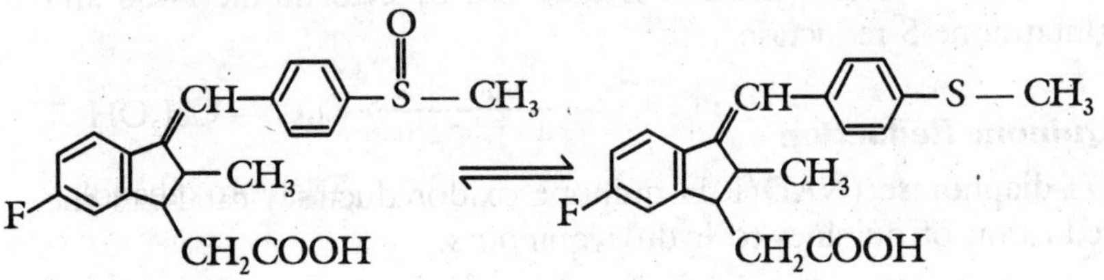

Sulindac   Sulindac sulfide

Reduction of N-oxides is carried out by flavin monooxygenases and cytochrome P450.

Disulfide Reduction

Generally disulfides are reduced and cleaved to their respective sulfhydryl components.

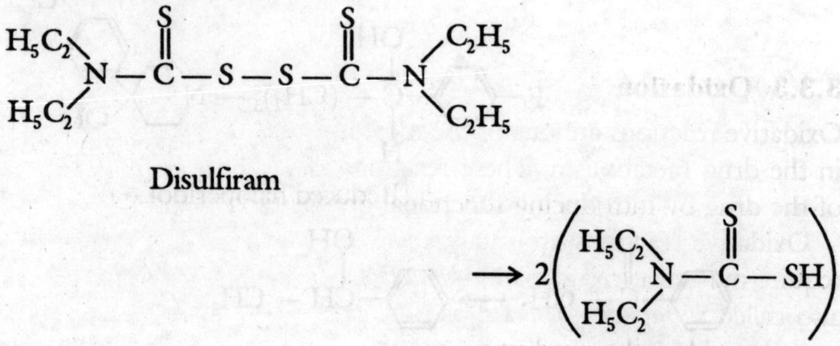

$$H_5C_2 \diagdown N-\overset{\overset{\displaystyle S}{\|}}{C}-S-S-\overset{\overset{\displaystyle S}{\|}}{C}-N \diagup^{C_2H_5}_{C_2H_5}$$
$$H_5C_2 \diagup$$

Disulfiram

$$\rightarrow 2\left(H_5C_2 \diagdown N-\overset{\overset{\displaystyle S}{\|}}{C}-SH\right)$$
$$H_5C_2 \diagup$$

Diethyldithio carbamic acid

Reductive Halogenation

Reductive halogenation involves replacement of halogen with hydrogen.

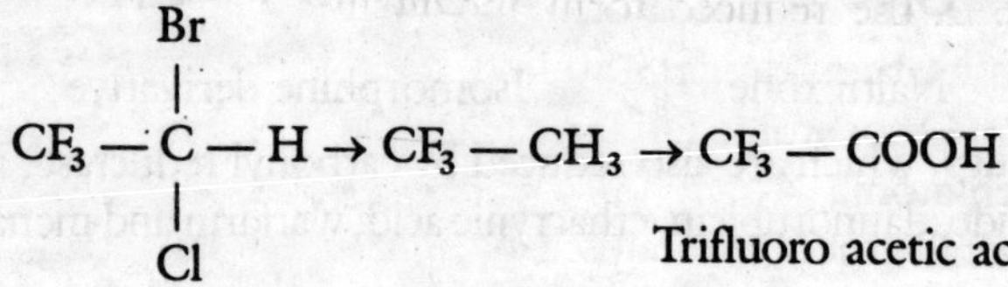

$$\underset{Cl}{\overset{Br}{\underset{|}{\overset{|}{CF_3-C-H}}}} \rightarrow CF_3-CH_3 \rightarrow CF_3-COOH$$

Trifluoro acetic acid

Halothane

The C-F bond is resistant to reduction.

Reductive dehalogenation is catalyzed by cytochrome P450 and glutathione-S-reductase.

Quinone Reduction

DT-diaphorase (NAD(P)H-quinone oxidoreductase) catalyzes the reduction of quinines to hydroxyquinones.

Menadione   DT-diaphorase   Hydroquinone

3.3.3 Oxidation

Oxidative reactions are one of the most important reactions involved in the drug metabolism. These reactions increase the hydrophilicity of the drug by introducing functional groups such as —OH.

Oxidative reactions are catalyzed by *mixed function oxidases* and require molecular oxygen and NADPH. Mixed function oxidases are also called as *monooxygenases*, as only one oxygen atom from O_2 is incorporated in the product.

The system comprises of a number of components—cytochrome P450 occupies a key function. In addition, it has two flavoproteins, which play a role in providing reducing equivalents donated by NADPH and NADH. Cytochrome b5 is also involved.

Cytochrome P450 is a heme protein (the name of the protein cytochrome P450, is derived from its ability to bind with carbon monoxide in the reduced form and form a complex which has a characteristic absorption at 450 nm). The iron atom can be divalent or trivalent. Cytochrome P450 is the site of binding for both, substrate and oxygen atom.

The overall reaction catalyzed by mixed function oxidase can be written as follows:

$$SH + NADPH + H^+ + O_2 \rightarrow SOH + NADP^+ + H_2O$$

Where SH is substrate.

A schematic representation of the functioning of the mixed function oxidase system is shown in Fig. 3.1.

Following steps are involved in the oxidation of drugs:

- A substrate (SH) binds to the oxidized form (Fe^{3+}) form of the cytochrome P450 (CYP450)
- An electron transfer from NADPH to enzyme-substrate complex via a flavoprotein (FP1) called as NADPH cytochrome

P450 reductase. Reduced (Fe^{3+}) CYP450-substrate complex is formed. This is considered as the rate limiting step.

♦ Molecular oxygen is incorporated into the reduced enzyme-substrate complex to form a ternary complex.

♦ The ternary complex accepts a second electron, which is donated by NADH via second flavoprotein (FP_2) called as NADH cytochrome b_5 reductase) and cytochrome b_5 ($CYPb_5$) and activated oxygen-CYP450-substrate complex is formed.

♦ The activated oxygen-CYP450-substrate complex splits into water molecule, oxidized form of substrate (SOH) and oxidized cytochrome P450 (Fe^{3+}). The free oxidized form of the enzyme is once again available to attach another molecule of the substrate and start a new cycle.

Thus there are *mixed functions*, i.e.

(a) Reduction of one atom from molecular oxygen to water and
(b) Incorporation of second oxygen atom into the substrate (sometimes also referred as oxygenation)

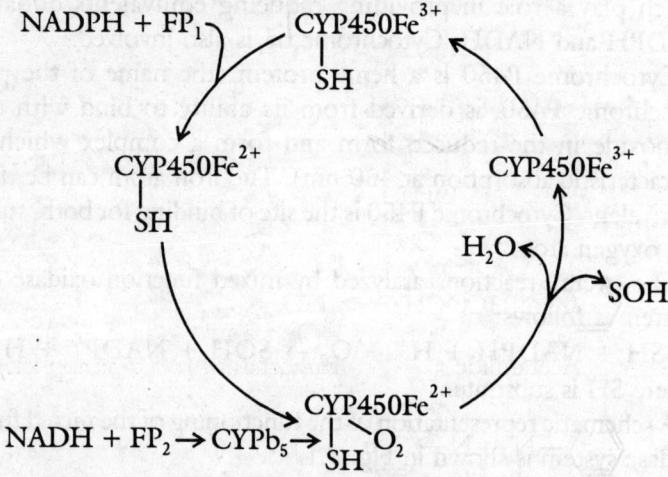

Fig. 3.1. Schematic representation of cytochrome P-450 oxidation-reduction cycle

It is important to remember that there are isozymes of cytochrome P450. Each isozyme has its own substrate for which it is to certain extent specific. Some of the important isozymes of cytochrome P450 will be discussed at the end of this section.

Following are few examples of oxidative reactions.

Oxidation of Aromatic Atoms

Oxidation of aromatic carbon atoms also called as aromatic hydroxylation proceeds via formation of an intermediate called as arene oxide. Arene oxide is highly reactive and can cause tissue damage. The oxidation of aromatic carbon atoms leads to phenolic products. The type of substitution influences the position of hydroxylation.

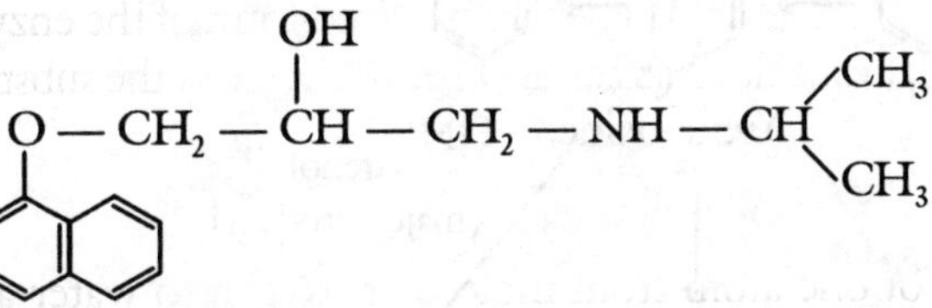

Propranolol

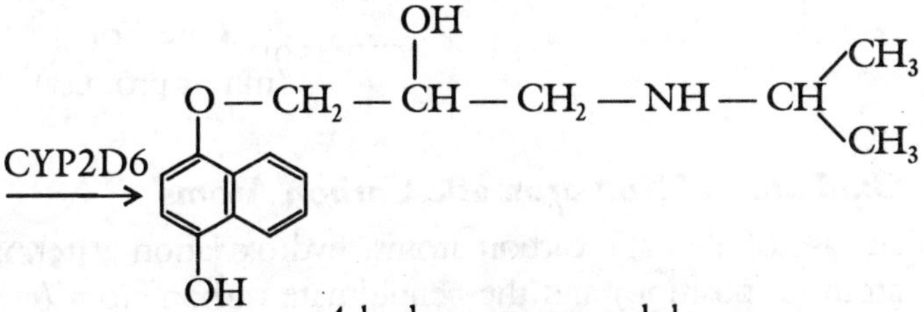

4-hydroxy propranolol

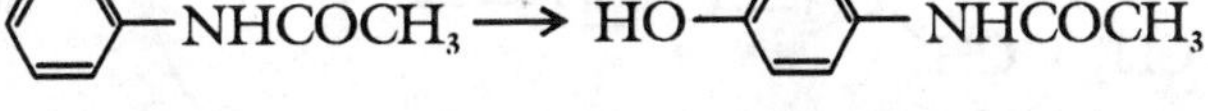

Acetanilide   Paracetamol (Acetaminophen)

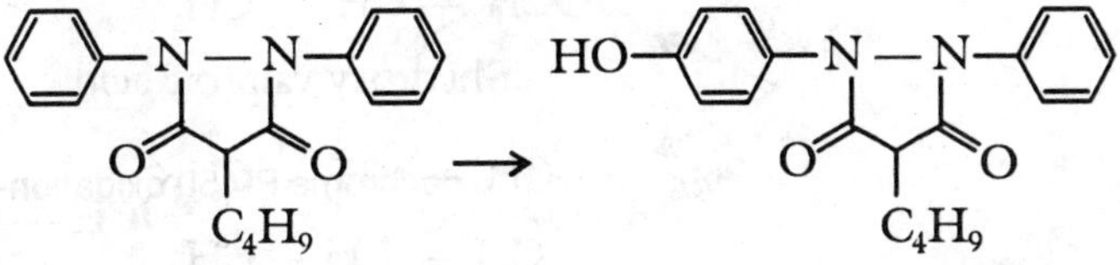

Phenylbutazone   Oxyphenbutazone

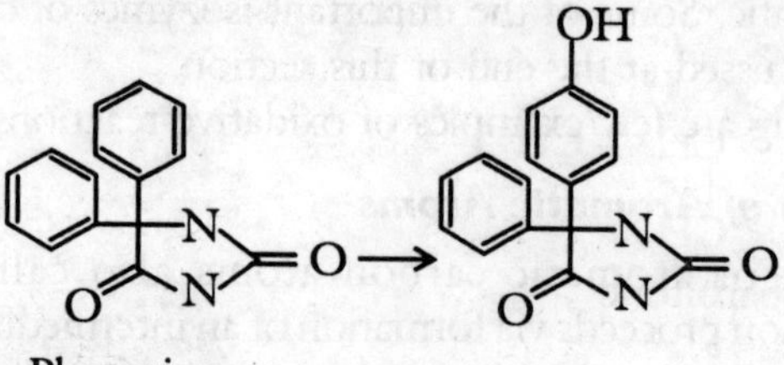

Phenytion

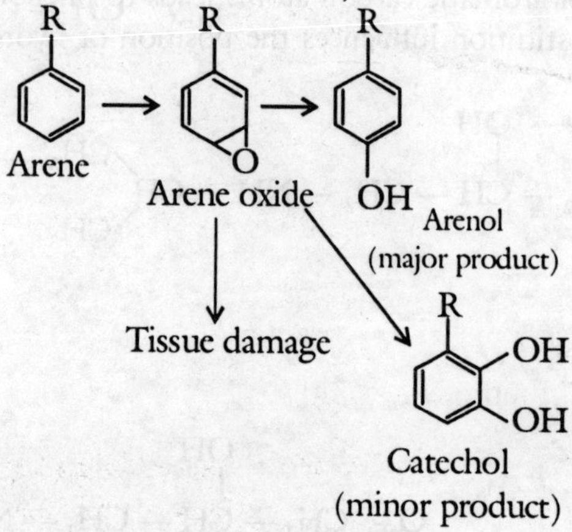

Arene → Arene oxide → Arenol (major product)

Tissue damage

Catechol (minor product)

Oxidation of Non-aromatic Carbon Atoms

In case of aliphatic carbon atoms, hydroxylation at terminal carbon atom (ω position) and the penultimate carbon atom (ω-1 position) is common.

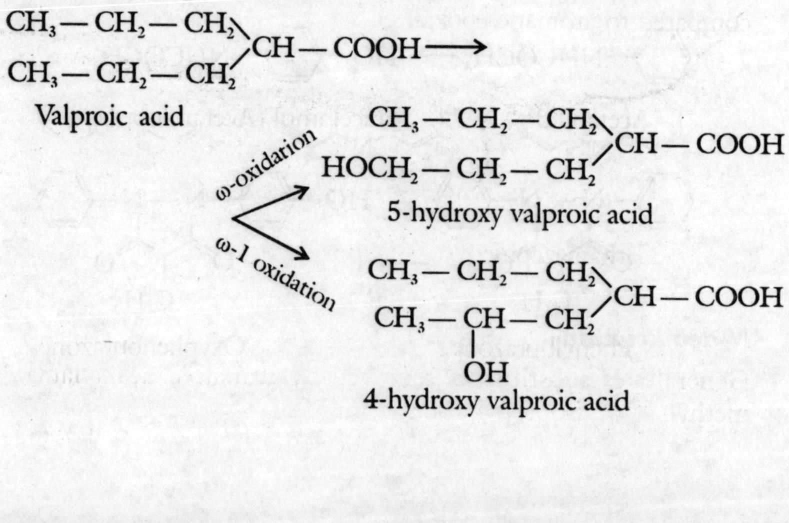

$$CH_3 - CH_2 - CH_2 \diagdown$$
$$CH_3 - CH_2 - CH_2 \diagup CH - COOH \longrightarrow$$

Valproic acid

ω-oxidation

$$CH_3 - CH_2 - CH_2 \diagdown$$
$$HOCH_2 - CH_2 - CH_2 \diagup CH - COOH$$
5-hydroxy valproic acid

ω-1 oxidation

$$CH_3 - CH_2 - CH_2 \diagdown$$
$$CH_3 - CH - CH_2 \diagup CH - COOH$$
$$\quad\quad\quad | $$
$$\quad\quad OH$$
4-hydroxy valproic acid

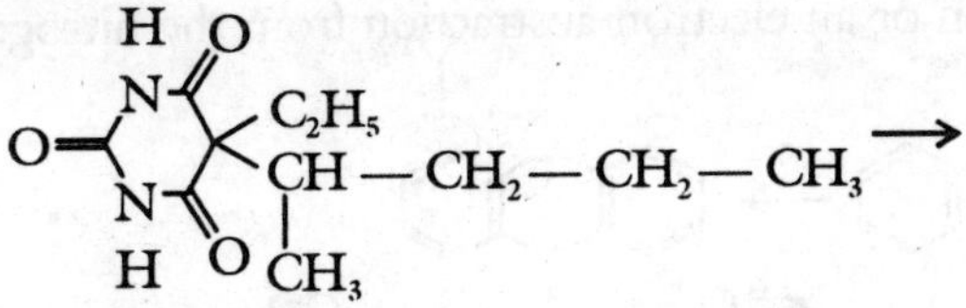

Pentobarbitone

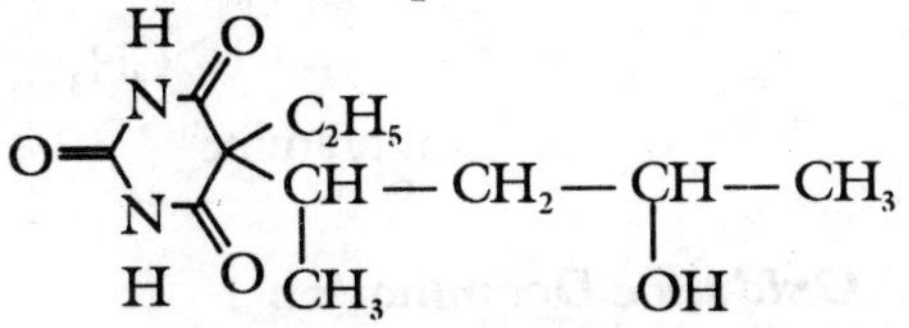

5- ethyl-5 (3-hydroxy-1-methyl butyl) barbituric acid

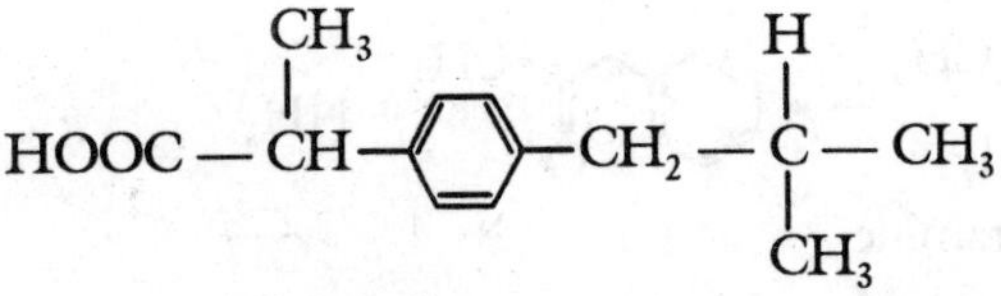

Ibuprofen

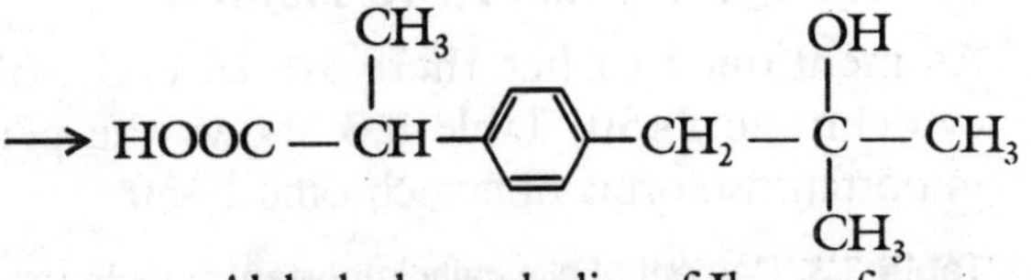

Alchohol metabolite of Ibuprofen

Similar to aromatic hydroxylation, oxidation of olefins also proceeds via epoxide formation. These epoxide intermediates are less reactive compared to aromatic epoxides.

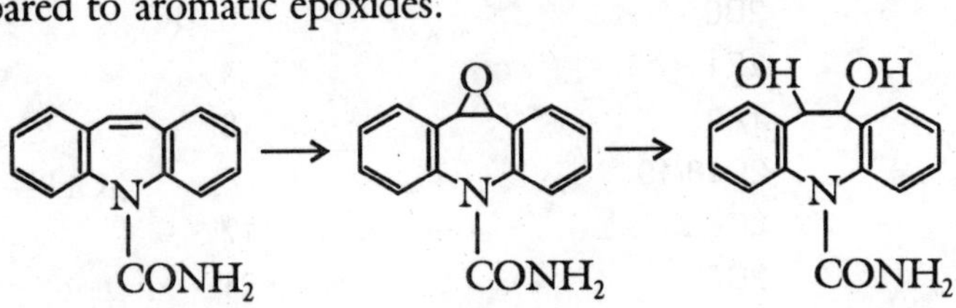

Carbamazepine

Epoxide intermediate

Dihydroxy metabolite

N-dealkylation

Generally N-substituents removed by oxidative dealkylation are methyl, ethyl, isopropyl, n-butyl and benzyl. N-dealkylation involves α-hydrogen abstraction or an electron abstraction from the nitrogen by oxygen.

Imipramine   Desipramine

Oxidative Deamination

This involves initial oxidation to imminium ion followed by decomposition to the carbonyl metabolite and ammonia.

Amphetamine

3.3.3.1 Cytochrome P450 Isoforms

As mentioned earlier there are several isoforms (isozymes) of cytochrome P450. Table 3.3 shows the percentage of clinically important isoforms of cytochrome P450.

Table 3.3: Percent of clinically important cytochrome P450 isoforms

Isoform	Percentage (%)
1A1	3
2B6	3
2E1	4
1A2	8
2C18/19	8
2C8/9	17
2D6	21
3A4/5	36

Some of the isoforms are described below.

CYP1A1: It is also called as aromatic hydrocarbon hydroxylase. CYP1A1 metabolizes a range of polycyclic aromatic hydrocarbons (mainly found in cigarette smoke), diethylstilbesterol and catechoestrogens. It is mainly expressed in small intestine, placenta, skin, lung and also in the liver (inducible).

CYP1A2: It is also called as caffeine demethylase or antipyrine N-demethylase. CYP1A2 catalyzes the oxidation of aryl amines, nitrosamines, aromatic hydrocarbons, caffeine, aflatoxin B1 etc. CYP1A2 is expressed in liver, intestine and stomach and is induced by smoking.

CYP2D6: It is involved in many drug oxidations. It is expressed in liver and to some extent in intestine and is not inducible. Polymorphism of CYP2D6 exists and has been extensively studied. Quinidine is a known inhibitor of CYP2D6.

CYP2E1: CYP2E1 plays a major role in the metabolism of halogenated hydrocarbons, acetone, ethanol, benzene, acetaminophen etc. It is expressed in liver, kidney, intestine and lung and is inducible.

CYP2C: CYP2C is a subfamily and includes CYP2C8, CYP2C9 and CYP2C19. Some of the members of this family are expressed in kidney, adrenals, brain, uterus, breast, ovary and intestine. These enzymes are involved in the metabolism of many drugs including warfarin, mehenytoin and tolbutamide. Significant degree of polymorphism exists in the expression of CYP2C isoforms.

CYP3A4: It is expressed in liver, intestine, lung, placenta, kidney, uterus and brain and is induced by glucocorticoids. Erythromycin is a known inhibitor of this enzyme. Because of the induction of CYP3A4 interindividual differences are seen in the metabolism of many drugs e.g. nifedipine, cyclosporine, triazolam and midazolam.

3.4 PHASE II REACTIONS

In Phase II reactions, drugs (or their metabolites) are combined with hydrophilic endogenous compounds resulting in the formation of complex with sufficient hydrophilic character to allow rapid excretion. These *conjugation reactions* include glucuronidation, sulfonation (also known as sulfation), acetylation, methylation, conjugation with glutathione and conjugation with amino acids such as glycine, glutamic acid and taurine (Table 3.2). Phase II reactions are generally much faster than Phase I reactions.

Table 3.2: Conjugation reactions and respective functional groups

Functional Groups	Conjugation Reactions
—OH, —COOH, —NH2, —NH, —SH, —CH	Glucuronidation
Aromatic —OH, aromatic —NH$_2$, alcohols	Sulfonation (sulfation)
Aromatic —NH$_2$, aliphatic NH$_2$, hydrazines, —SO$_2$NH$_2$	Acetylation
Aromatic —OH, —NH$_2$, —NH, —SH	Methylation
Epoxides, organic halides	Glutathione conjugation
Aromatic —NH$_2$, —COOH	Glycine conjugation

Although exceptions are there, great majority of Phase II reactions are bioinactivations. Most Phase II biotransforming enzymes are mainly located in cytosol, except UDP-glucuronosyltransferases, which are microsomal enzymes (refer Table 3.1)

3.4.1 Glucuronidation

Glucuronidation is quantitatively the most important among the Phase II reactions. Conjugation with glucoronic acid can only take place after glucoronic acid has been activated. Glucuronidation requires the cofactor uridine diphosphate-glucoronic acid (UDP-glucuronic acid) and the reaction is catalyzed by UDP-glucuronyl transferases (UGTs). UGTs are located in the endoplasmic reticulum of liver and other tissues viz. kidney, intestine, skin, brain, spleen and nasal mucosa (Fig. 3.2)

Note that UDPGA has α-linkage at C$_1$ but phenylglucuronide has β-linkage at C$_1$.

In general, site of glucuronidation is an electron rich nucleophilic heteroatom i.e. O, N or S. Thus, aliphatic alcohols, phenols and carboxylic acids form O-glucuronidation, primary and secondary amines form N-glucuronides and free sulfhydryl groups form S-glucuronides Following are some of the examples, arrow indicates the site of glucuronidation.

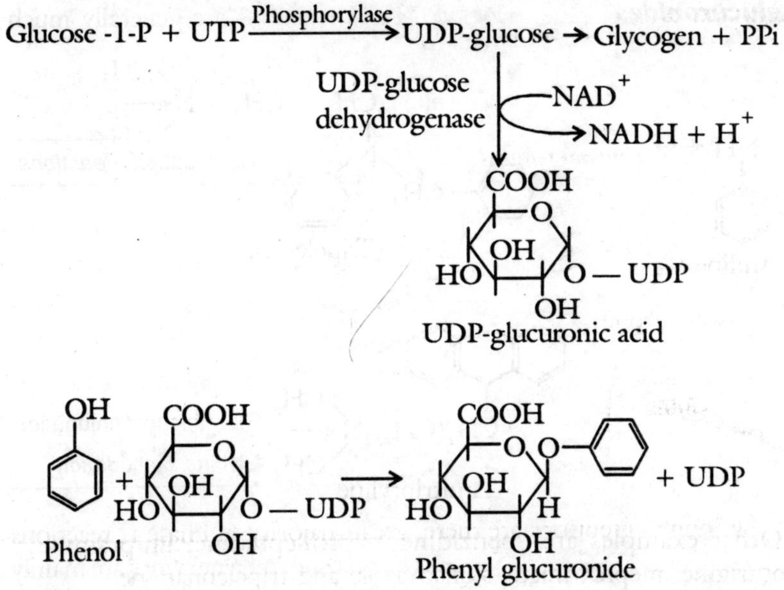

$$\text{Glucose -1-P + UTP} \xrightarrow{\text{Phosphorylase}} \text{UDP-glucose} \rightarrow \text{Glycogen + PPi}$$

UDP-glucose
dehydrogenase

NAD^+

NADH + H^+

COOH

HO — O — UDP

OH

UDP-glucuronic acid

OH

Phenol + COOH — O — UDP ⟶ COOH — O — O + UDP

Phenyl glucuronide

Fig. 3.2. Synthesis of UDP-glucuronic acid

O-glucuronides

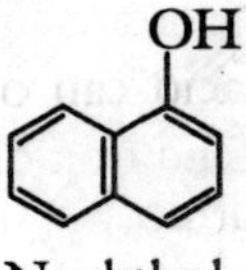

OH ←

Naphthol

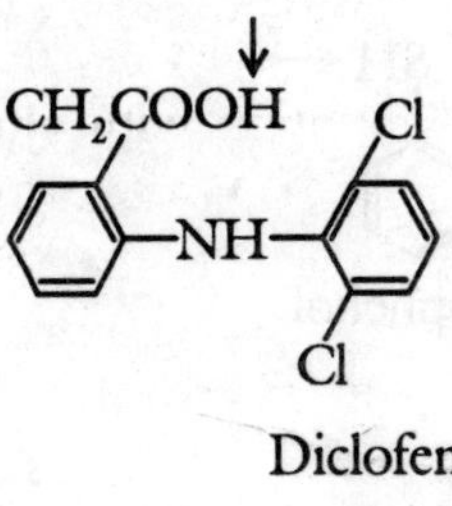

CH_2COOH

—NH—

Cl

Cl

Diclofenac

OH

O_2H— —CH — CH — CH_2OH ←

NH — CO — CHCl_2

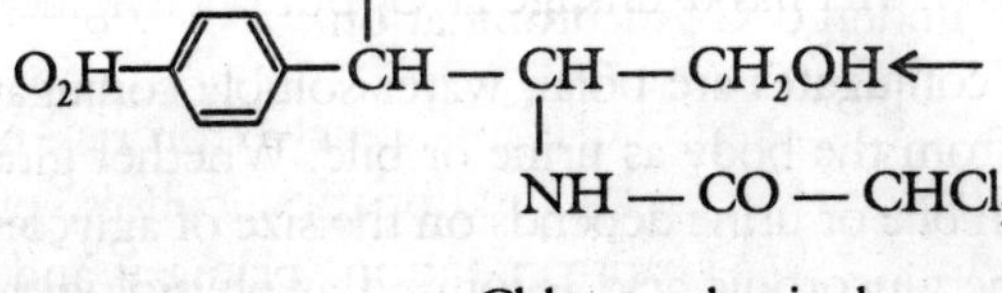

Chloramphenicol

Other examples are– acetaminophen, codeine, morphine, naloxone, oxazepam, propofol, propranolol, ketoprofen, naproxen, valproic acid, fenoprofen, chloraphenicol, and trichloroethanol.

N-glucuronides

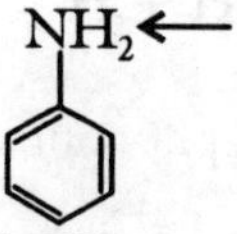

$NH_2 \leftarrow$

Aniline

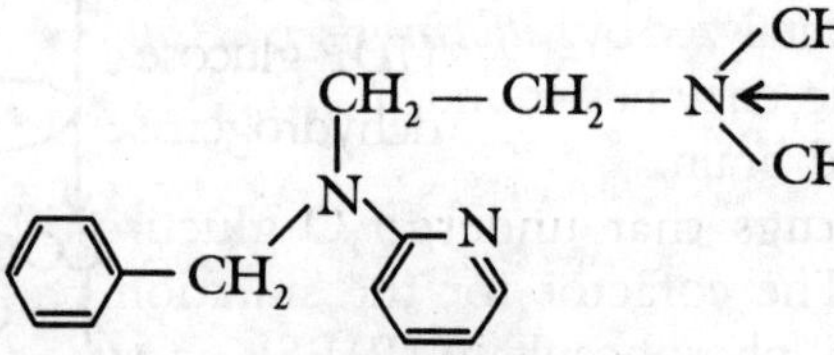

$CH_2 - CH_2 - N \underset{CH_3}{\overset{CH_3}{\leftarrow}}$

(benzyl)CH_2—N—(pyridinyl)

Tripelennamine

$CH_2(CH_2)_2 N \underset{CH_3}{\overset{CH_3}{\leftarrow}}$

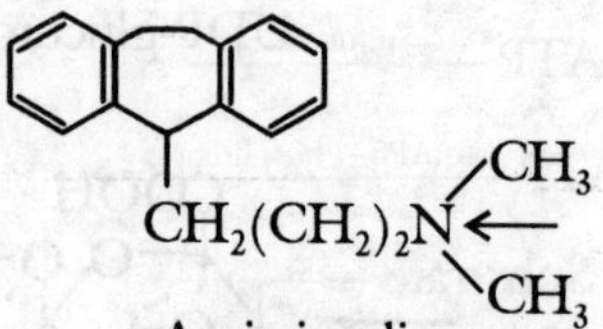

Amitriptyline

Other examples are– benzidine, cyproheptadine, imipramine, lamotrigine, meprobamate, sulfisoxazole and tripelennamine.

S-glucuronides

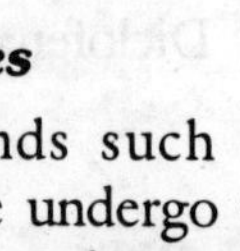

$SH \leftarrow$

Thiophenol

$\underset{C_2H_5}{\overset{C_2H_5}{N}} - C \overset{SH \leftarrow}{\underset{S}{}}$

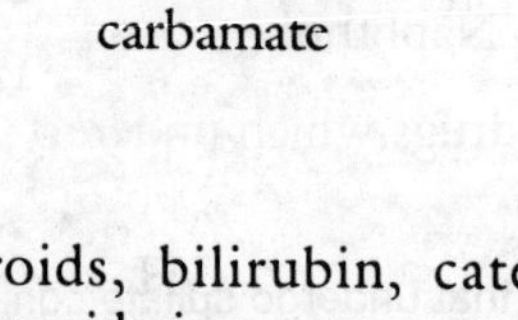

Diethyldithio carbamate

C-glucuronides

Few compounds such as steroids, bilirubin, catechols and phenylbutazone undergo C-glucuronidation.

Glucuronide conjugates are polar, water soluble conjugates which are eliminated from the body as urine or bile. Whether glucuronides are eliminated in bile or urine depends on the size of aglycone (parent compound). The glucoronic acid is ionized at physiological pH and enhances the elimination because:

1. It increases the aqueous solubility of drug or drug metabolites
2. It is recognized by the biliary and renal organic transport system thus glucuronides are secreted into urine and bile.

3.4.2 Sulfation

Sulfate conjugation produces a highly water soluble sulfuric acid ester. Sulfation is catalyzed by *sulfotransferases (sulfokinases)*. Sulfotransferases are cytosolic enzymes found in liver, kidney, intestinal tract, lung, platelets and brain.

Many drugs that undergo O-glucuronidation also undergo sulfation. The cofactor for the sulfation reaction is 3'-phospho-adenosine-5'-phosphosulfate (PAPS)

Like in glucuronidation, the sulfate needs to be activated first before the reaction with substrate.

$$SO_4^{2-} + ATP \xrightarrow{\text{Sulfurylase}} APS + PPi$$

$$APS + ATP \xrightarrow{\text{APS-Phosphokinase}} PAPS + ADP$$

$$PAPS + Substrate \longrightarrow PAP^+ + Sulfate$$

Sulfate is first converted into adenosine-5'-phosphosulfate (APS). APS is then metabolized to 3'-phosphoadenosine-5'-phosphosulfate (PAPS). A substrate then reacts with this activated sulfate.

Some of the drugs which undergo sulfate conjugation are listed in Table 3.4

Table 3.4: Drugs that undergo sulfate conjugation

Functional Group	Examples
Primary alcohol	Chloramphenicol, ethanol, polyethylene glycol
Secondary alcohol	2-butanol, cholesterol, dosaminol
Phenol	Acetaminophen, phenol, trimetrexate
Catechol	Dopamine, α-methyl-DOPA
N-oxide	Minoxidil
Aliphatic amine	Desipramine
Aromatic amine	Aniline, 2-aminonaphthalene

Phenols and aliphatic alcohols represent the largest group of substrate for sulfotransferases.

Sulfate conjugates of drugs are excreted mainly in urine.

3.4.3 Acetylation

N-acetylation is a major route of biotransformation for drugs containing an aromatic amine or a hydrazine group. N-acetylation reaction is catalyzed by N-acetyltransferases and requires cofactor acetyl-coenzyme A (acetyl CoA).

N-acetylation reaction occurs in following two steps:

1. Acetyl group from acetyl-CoA is transferred to an active site cysteine residue within an N-acetyltransferase with release of coenzyme A.
2. Acetyl group is transferred from the acylated enzyme to the amino group of the substrate. The enzyme is regenerated.

N-acetyltransferases are cytosolic enzymes and are mainly found in liver.

$$HOOC\text{—}\underset{\substack{\text{Para amino}\\\text{salicylic acid}}}{\overset{\overset{\displaystyle OH}{|}}{\bigcirc}}\text{—}NH_2 + \underset{\text{Acetyl CoA}}{CH_3CO\text{—}SCoA} \xrightarrow{\substack{\text{N-acetyl}\\\text{transferase}}}$$

$$HOOC\text{—}\underset{\substack{\text{N-acetylated para}\\\text{amino salicylic acid}}}{\overset{\overset{\displaystyle OH}{|}}{\bigcirc}}\text{—}NHCOCH_3$$

Some of the drugs which undergo acetylation reaction are listed in Table 3.5.

Table 3.5: Drugs that undergo acetylation

Functional group	Examples
Primary amines	Histamine, procainamide, dapsone
Hydrazines/hydrazides	Hydralazine, isoniazid
Sulfonamide	Sulfanilamide, sulfapyridine

3.4.4 Methylation

In general, metabolites formed by methylation reaction are not more polar or more water soluble and have equal or higher pharmacological activity than parent drug.

Methylation reaction occurs in following steps:

1. Synthesis of an activated coenzyme S-adenosyl methioine (SAM) from L-methioine and ATP. SAM is the donor of methyl group.
2. Transfer of methyl group to substrate. This reaction is catalyzed by methyl transferase.

Examples of *methyl transferases* are: Catechol-O-methyl transferase (COMT), phenyl ethanolamine-N-methyl transferase (PNMT) etc.

Some of the drugs which undergo methylation reaction are listed in Table 3.6

Table 3.6: Drugs that undergo methylation

Functional groups	Examples
Phenols	Morphine
Catechols	L-DOPA, isoproterenol
Amines	Norephedrine
Aromatic heterocyclics	Nicotine
Thiols	6-mercaptopurine

3.4.5 Glutathione Conjugation

Glutathione (GSH) is a tripeptide comprised of glycine, cysteine and glutamic acid. The formation of glutathione is catalyzed by γ-glutamylcysteine synthetase.

$$HOOC-CH-CH_2-CH_2-\overset{\overset{\displaystyle O}{\|}}{C}-NH-CH-\overset{\overset{\displaystyle CH_2}{|}\ \overset{\displaystyle SH}{|}}{\ }\overset{\overset{\displaystyle O}{\|}}{C}-NH-CH_2-COOH$$

Glutamic acid   Cysteine   Glycine

Glutathione

Substrates for glutathione conjugation include wide variety of electrophilic drugs or drugs that can be biotransformed to electrophiles. The conjugation of drugs with glutathione is catalyzed by glutathione-S-transferases. These transferases are mainly localized in cytoplasm and to a lesser extent in endoplasmic reticulum and are present in the liver, intestine, kidney, adrenal and lung.

Glutathione conjugates are thioesters formed by nucleophilic attack of glutathione thiolate anion (GS-) on electrophilic carbon atom or even electrophilic heteroatoms (O, N or S).

Glutathione conjugation reactions can be divided into two general types:

1. Displacement reactions: In these, glutathione displaces an electron withdrawing group
2. Addition reactions: In these, glutathione is added to an activated double bond.

Displacement Reaction

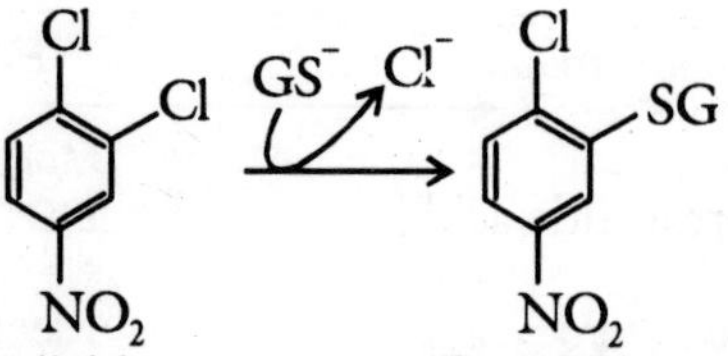

1,2 dichloro
4-nitro benzene

Glutathione
conjugate

Addition Reaction

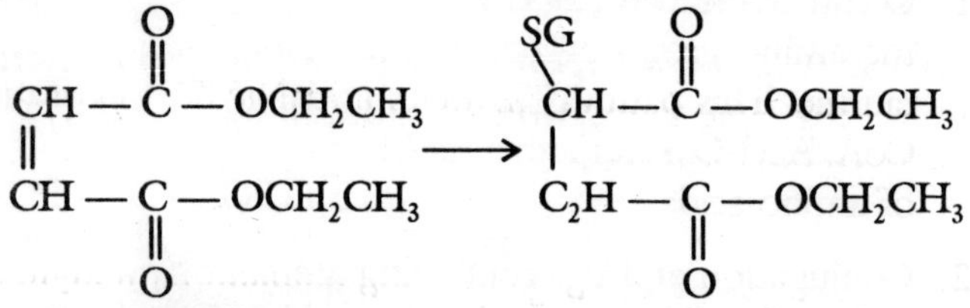

Diethyle maleate

Glutathione conjugate

Conjugation of Heteroatom

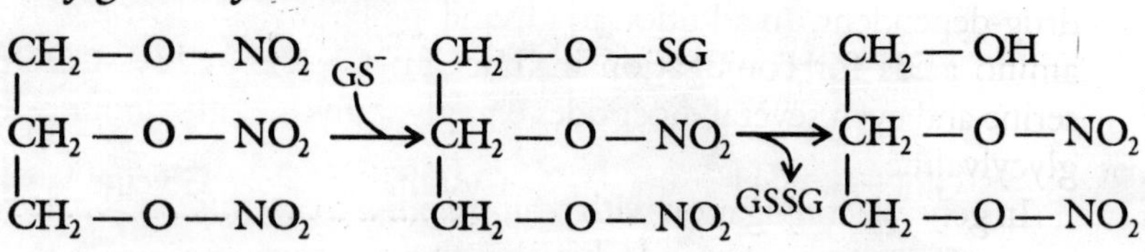

Trinitro glycerine   Glutathione conjugate   Dinitro glycerine

Electrophiles in general are very toxic as they can bind to macromolecules (protein, DNA) and can cause cellular damage and mutations. Hence conjugation of electrophiles with glutathione represents an important detoxification reaction.

Glutathione conjugates can be excreted as such in bile or first they can be converted to mercapturic acid in the kidney and then excreted in urine.

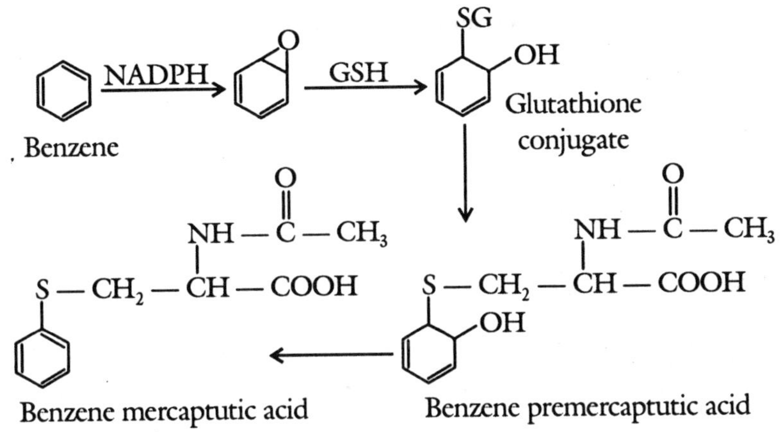

Benzene

Glutathione conjugate

Benzene mercaptutic acid

Benzene premercaptutic acid

3.4.6 Amino Acid Conjugation

Drugs are conjugated with amino acids by two pathways:

1. Conjugation of drugs containing a carboxylic acid group with the amino group of amino acids e.g. glycine, glutamate and taurine. This pathway involves initial activation of drugs with CoA. Acyl-CoA thioether thus formed reacts with amino group of amino acids.

2. Conjugation of drugs containing aromatic hydroxylamine with carboxylic acid groups of amino acids e.g. serine and proline.

The acceptor amino acid used for conjugation is both species and drug-dependent. In addition to glycine, glutamine and taurine, other amino acids for conjugation include ornithine, arginine, histidine, serine and even several dipeptides e.g. glycylglycine, glycyltaurine and glycylvaline.

In general, conjugation with amino acids is a detoxification reaction.

Hippuric acid

3.5 FACTORS AFFECTING METABOLISM OF DRUGS

Numerous factors influence the rate of drug metabolism and are as follows:

♦ Physiochemical properties of the drug
♦ Chemical factors
♦ Biological factors

Physiochemical Properties of the Drug

Physicochemical properties of the drug such as molecular size, pK_a, acid/base characteristics, lipophilicity and steric characteristics influence the drug metabolism. Their exact relationship is not well understood.

Chemical Factors

Enzyme Induction

Enzyme induction is defined as a phenomenon of increased drug metabolizing ability of the enzyme by drugs. Some drugs induce their own metabolism and are called as *auto inducers or self inducers*.

Various mechanisms may be involved in enzyme induction such as:

➢ Increased enzyme synthesis
➢ Decreased rate of enzyme degradation

> Enzyme stabilization
> Enzyme activation

In general enzyme induction results in decreased pharmacological activity, except when metabolites are pharmacologically active.

Some of the examples of enzyme inducers are - alcohol, barbiturates, phenytoin, rifampin etc.

Enzyme Inhibition

Enzyme inhibition is defined as decrease in the drug metabolizing ability of an enzyme. Enzyme inhibition can be of various types, such as:

♦ Competitive inhibition
♦ Noncompetitive inhibition
♦ Repression

Competitive Inhibition

Drugs with structural similarity to natural substrates compete with the natural substrate for active site of an enzyme. This type of inhibition is reversible in nature e.g. succinylcholine inhibits acetylcholine esterase by competing with acetylcholine.

Noncompetitive Inhibition

These type of inhibitors are structurally not related with natural substrates e.g. enzyme inhibition by heavy metals

Repression

Repression may be caused because of the decrease in the rate of synthesis of enzymes e.g. puromycin, actinomycin D or because of the increased degradation of the enzyme e.g. carbon tetrachloride, disulfiram

In general, enzyme inhibition results in prolonged pharmacological action of a drug. Some of the examples of enzyme inhibitors are - monoamine oxidase inhibitors, allopurinol, coumarins etc.

Biological Factors

Species Difference

There are significant differences between species for both Phase I and Phase II reactions. These differences can be quantitative or qualitative.

Because of these differences, extrapolation of animal toxicity data to humans is very difficult. For example, cats are deficient in N-acetyl transferase and UDP-glucuronyl transferase. In rats amphetamine first undergoes aromatic hydroxylation followed by conjugation whereas, in rabbits and guinea pigs oxidative deamination is the main route of elimination for amphetamine. Also, fish generally have a lower metabolic capacity for xenobiotics and birds metabolize xenobiotics less efficiently than mammals.

Genetic Differences

Besides species differences, differences among strains within the same species are also known. *Pharmacogenetics* is the study of intersubject variability in drug response. *Ethnic variation* is the differences observed in the metabolism of a drug among different races and these differences may result because of polymorphism e.g. polymorphism for acetylation of the drug. There are two phenotypes for acetylation reaction: fast acetylators and slow acetylators. Isoniazid demonstrates such polymorphism.

In most European countries, approximately 40% of the population is fast acetylators while 96% of the Eskimos are fast acetylators.

Acetylation phenotype can be a determinant of toxic effects of a drug e.g. in slow acetylators, isoniazid causes neuropathy but in fast acetylators it causes hepatic injury. Hydralazine causes lupus erythematosus in slow acetylators in fast acetylators.

Sex Differences

Sex dependent metabolism is a kind of genetic control but is due to hormonal influences. The sex dependent differences in drug metabolism are because of differences in enzyme concentration, activities and changes in the lipid environment of the enzymes.

Some of the isoenzymes of cytochrome P450 are found to be sex dependent.

In humans it has been shown that women metabolize benzodiazepines slower than men. Overall, sex differences in drug metabolism are of little significance in humans but are of significant importance in laboratory animals such as rats and mice.

Age Differences

Age is an important determinant in the metabolism of the drug. The age dependent differences are mainly because of the differences in the enzyme content, enzyme activity and hemodynamics. For example, in neonates microsomal enzyme system is not fully developed and thus drug metabolism is very slow. Glucuronidation shows an increase in activity upto birth, after which activity decreases to the adult level.

Diet

It is known that total enzyme content and enzyme activity is altered by dietary components. Various nutrients in the diet such as trace elements, minerals, vitamins, proteins, lipids, and carbohydrates and non-nutrients such as tobacco, alcohol and marihuana are known to affect the drug metabolism.

Dietary deficiency of vitamins and minerals will decrease the enzyme activity.

Low protein diet is known to decrease and high protein diet is known to increase the drug metabolism.

Changes in Physiological Factors

Changes in physiological factors because of disease state, hormonal imbalance and pregnancy are known to affect drug metabolizing activity.

Hepatic disease will generally cause a reduction of enzymatic activity. Reduction in blood flow to the liver because of congestive heart failure or myocardial infarction is also known to decrease metabolism of many drugs.

It has been suggested that due to high levels of steroid hormones, drug metabolizing activity is reduced during later stages of pregnancy.

3.6 BIOACTIVATION

In general, biotransformation or metabolism produces more water soluble chemical species and hence increase the excretion. Thus it is expected that duration of toxic effects will be reduced.

Bioactivation reactions are defined as biotransformation reactions which lead to products with higher toxicity/activity than the parent compounds. Reactive compounds generated may belong to two broad categories- electrophiles and free radicals.

Electrophiles are deficient in electron pair and will react with nucleophilic groups in macromolecules such as proteins and DNA. Reactions with DNA produce changes which ultimately lead to cancer.

Examples of xenobiotics which involve formation of an electrophilic reactive intermediate are– aflatoxins which are active as epoxides, vinyl chloride epoxide is formed from vinyl chloride, benzopyrene is converted into a dihydrodiol epoxide.

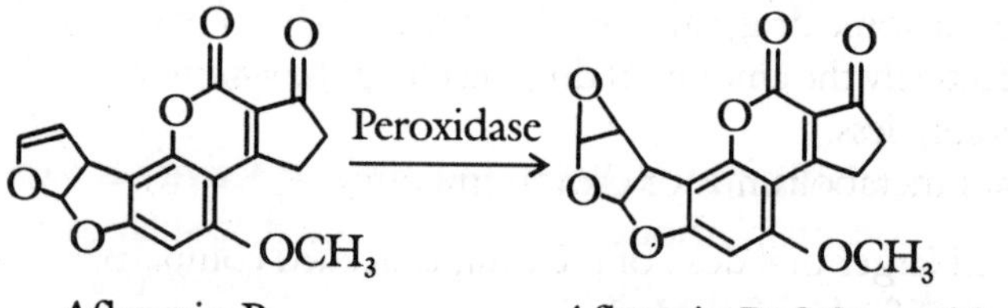

Aflatoxin B_1 Aflatoxin B_1 8,9 epoxide

Inactivation by glutathione conjugation   DNA binding liver tumors

Hepatotoxicity because of paracetamol metabolites is also an example of tissue damage because of electrophiles.

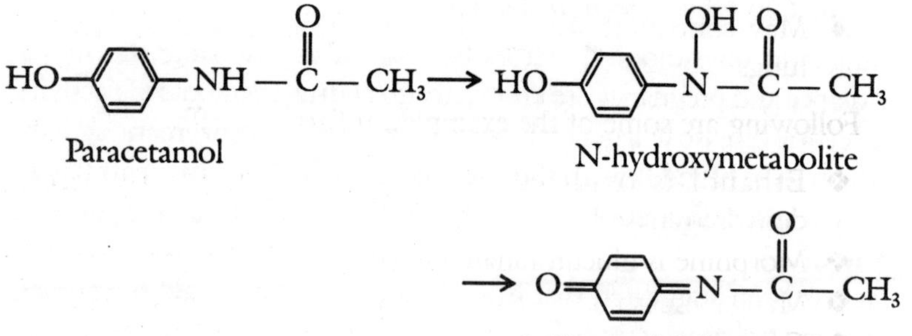

Paracetamol   N-hydroxymetabolite

N-acetyl-P-benzoquinone

covalent binding to macromolecules

Hepatotoxicity

Free radicals contain odd number of electrons and can be anionic, cationic or neutral. Drugs which are known to generate free radicals are quinines, arylamines and nitroaryls. Free radicals produce toxicity by peroxidation.

Protection against free radicals is executed by membrane structure, neutralization by glutathione, antioxidants e.g. vitamins A, E and C and enzymatic inactivation of free radicals.

3.7 FIRST PASS EFFECT

Removal of drugs before entrance into the systemic circulation is referred to as *first pass effect or presystemic elimination*. For example some drugs are removed from the portal circulation very efficiently by the liver or some drugs are metabolized in the wall of the intestine. Hence, effectively the amount of drug reaching the systemic circulation is considerably less.

First pass metabolism is of clinical importance, because:

> Much larger oral dose of the drug is needed compared to other routes of administration

> First pass metabolism shows tremendous individual variations and hence there is great degree of unpredictability when drugs are given orally.

First pass effect has following effects on the toxicity of drugs:

♦ Reduction of toxic effects of drugs that reach the target site by systemic circulation

♦ May contribute to the injury of digestive mucosa, liver and lungs.

Following are some of the examples of first pass effect:

❖ Ethanol is oxidized in the gastric mucosa by alcohol dehydrogenase.

❖ Morphine is glucuronidated in the intestinal mucosa and liver.

❖ Manganese is taken up into the liver and excreted into the bile.

❖ Cyclosporin is returned to intestinal lumen from enterocytes and is also hydroxylated by these cells.

3.8. *IN VITRO* MODELS OF METABOLISM

In modern dug discovery, large numbers of compounds are synthesized in short span of time because of combinatorial chemistry approach. Hence high throughput systems are required to screen these compounds. Identification of metabolic characteristics early in the development process helps in deciding the progress of a particular compound in drug development process. Hence *in vitro* assays are increasingly being used in drug metabolism studies to screen novel chemicals. Also information obtained from these *in vitro* systems can be used as a feedback to design safer and more metabolically stable drugs.

Various aspects of metabolism that can be studied by *in vitro* assay systems are as follows:

* ❖ The rate of metabolism
* ❖ Metabolite profile
* ❖ Identification of metabolites
* ❖ Metabolite stability
* ❖ Identification of enzymes involved in the metabolism
* ❖ Drug-drug interactions
* ❖ Interspecies comparison
* ❖ CYP induction/inhibition

Various *in vitro* methods are available for drug metabolism studies; few of them are discussed below.

Enzyme Preparations

Various enzyme preparations are available viz. simple enzyme preparations, microsomes, liver S9 fractions etc.

Advances in molecular biology have enabled the identification and characterization of a large number of individual CYP genes. Individual CYP enzymes have been expressed transiently or stably in a variety of expression systems, including bacteria, yeast, insect and mammalian cells. Individual CYP isoforms can be used in reaction phenotyping to identify the isoforms responsible for the formation of certain metabolites.

Human liver S9 fractions contain both Phase I enzymes (mainly microsomal) and Phase II enzymes (mainly cytosolic), due to which it is possible to carry out complete drug metabolism studies. It is essential to ensure that sufficient cofactors, reducing equivalents and other requirements for enzymatic reactions are available. These fractions are generally prepared from pools of liver tissue and hence represent average metabolic activities of several donors. S9 fractions have a serious limitation that the overall sensitivity of the system is low. This is because S9 fractions generally contain lower enzyme activities compared to microsomes or supersomes. S9 fractions are commonly used in mutagenicity testing.

Human liver microsomes are the most popular and widely used *in vitro* metabolism system and are commercially available. Because of their low cost they are widely used for screening large number of compounds. While using microsomes it is necessary to ensure that appropriate cofactors are available. Like S9 fractions, microsomes are also prepared from pools of liver tissues. They are formed from smooth endoplasmic reticulum during tissue homogenization and ultracentrifugations. Microsomes are easy to prepare and are stable for extended periods when stored properly (–80°C). Microsomes generally produce primary metabolites from functionalization reactions. Microsomes are useful for the study of metabolic routes and the production of metabolites. Microsomes can be manipulated by induction and inhibition to vary the activity or the levels of isozymes. These are widely used to study various aspects of drug metabolism e.g. metabolic profile, stability, metabolite identification and kinetics. But microsomes have a serious limitation in that they contain only the endoplasmic reticulum-localized enzymes (CYPs, flavin monooxygenases and glucuronosyltransferases) and hence involvement of other enzymes in drug metabolism cannot be studied.

Supersomes are baculovirus-based system. In this system recombinant proteins are expressed in insect cells. Although the system is insect cells based, comparative studies have shown that baculovirus-expressed enzymes are reasonably accurate model and represent *in vivo* situation. Supersomes are generally used to confirm the findings of microsome preparations and to study the involvement of individual enzymes in drug metabolism.

Cell Culture Models

Whole cells will definitely reflect the complete drug metabolism profile and hence extrapolation to *in vivo* situation is much more reliable. Whole cells can be obtained from various sources e.g. primary cells culture, cell lines, differentiated hepatocytes from human stem cells.

Primary Cell Culture

Primary culture of human hepatocytes is the closest system to hepatocytes *in vivo*. It is widely used for drug metabolism studies including mechanistic studies and high-throughput screens. One advantage of hepatocytes is that they are intact cells bearing intact plasma membranes, complete metabolic pathways, physiological cofactor-enzyme levels and active gene expression. Because hepatocytes contain the full range of functionalization and conjugation enzymes, the whole metabolite pattern can be detected. Also, the induction of drug-metabolizing enzymes and possible toxic effects can be studied.

Continuous supply, batch-to-batch variability and quality are the major concerns. Prolonged storage of cryopreserved isolated hepatocytes is possible, but cryopreservation usually results in low cell recovery and alterations in functional activities. However, hepatocytes retain functional drug-metabolizing enzyme activities at least for a short time. Cryopreserved hepatocytes are mainly used for qualitative studies viz. metabolic identification. Their utility in quantitative estimation of drug metabolism has not been well established. Some phenotypic changes e.g. decreased expression of CYPs has also been reported over long time in culture. Many of phenotypic changes can be reduced by modifying culture conditions e.g. use of specialized matrices or co-culture with epithelial cells.

Recently research involving differentiation of human embryonic or adult stem cells into hepatocytes in culture provides many hopes and many constraints placed on primary cultures of hepatocytes may be overcome in the future.

Cell Lines

Cell lines are either obtained from tumour tissue or artificially transformed primary cells. HepG2 (hepatocarcinoma cell line) is one of the oldest and widely used cell lines. Hepatoma cell lines are "stably transformed" and show little or no variation. Over the time these cells alter their phenotype and also show different functionality. It is very important that any cell line used should be validated in-house and growth medium and "age" of the cells should be standardized.

Tissue Slices

Liver tissue slices are most commonly used for drug metabolism experiments. Other tissue slices e.g. brain, heart and kidney have also been tried. This model has certain advantages such as, intact cell-cell junctions, and normal organ architecture. Tissue slices contain complete drug metabolizing enzymes with all the relevant cofactors. Liver slices can be easily and rapidly produced. The tissue slices have certain disadvantages e.g. they cannot be cryopreserved and there is an inadequate penetration of the medium.

Any *in vitro* system described above should be fully validated in-house before actual experiments are carried out. This is because laboratory-to-laboratory variations in terms of techniques and variations within the cell lines are quite common. One of the simplest ways of calibration is to use few compounds (generally ten compounds) whose characteristics *in vivo* are well known.

Besides drug metabolism, *in vitro* systems are very helpful in understanding and predicting likely drug-drug interactions. Liver microsomes have been extensively used for this purpose.

In spite of limitations, use of *in vitro* drug metabolism systems is increasing mainly because of the constraints of time in the drug discovery process. None the less additional work is required to characterize the *in vitro* systems for drug metabolism and its impact on overall drug development. US-FDA has issued a guideline in this respect titled "GUIDANCE FOR INDUSTRY–Drug Metabolism/ Drug Interaction Studies in the Drug Development Process: Studies *In vitro*".

QUESTIONS

1. Write down at least three enzymes involved in drug metabolism involving hydrolysis, reduction and oxidation reactions.
2. Explain following phase I reactions with examples
   (*i*) Hydrolysis
   (*ii*) Oxidation
   (*iii*) Reduction.
3. Explain cytochrome P-450 oxidation reduction cycle.
4. Explain following phase II reactions with examples.
   (*i*) Glucuronidation
   (*ii*) Sulfation
   (*iii*) Acetylation
   (*iv*) Glutathione conjugation reaction
   (*v*) Amino acid conjugation reaction.
5. Write short notes on
   (*i*) Biological factors affecting biotransformation of drugs
   (*ii*) Bioactivation
   (*iii*) First pass effect
   (*iv*) Enzyme induction and inhibition
   (*v*) Isoforms of Cytochrome P450.

4

Excretion

4.1 INTRODUCTION

Elimination includes all the processes in the body that leads to decrease in the amount of foreign substance in the body. Elimination will eventually lead to reduction in the quantity of the drug at site of action and hence will terminate the biological effect of the drug.

Elimination includes excretion and biotransformation. (Biotransformation has already been discussed in the previous chapter).

Drugs are excreted by the body by several routes e.g. renal excretion, fecal excretion, excretion via lungs, excretion via milk, hair, sweat etc.

4.2 RENAL EXCRETION

Renal excretion is one of the most important excretion routes for drugs and their metabolites. More drugs are eliminated from the body by kidney than any other route.

Three main processes are important in renal excretion (Fig. 4.1)

♦ Glomerular filtration
♦ Tubular excretion by passive diffusion
♦ Active tubular secretion

4.2.1 Glomerular Filtration

The kidney receives about 25% of the cardiac output and approximately 20% is filtered at glomeruli. Compounds with molecular weight more than 60,000 are not filtered at glomeruli. The selectivity of the glomerular membrane is related only to the molecular mass of the compound. Protein-drug complexes are too large and do not pass through the pores of glomeruli. Thus, degree of plasma protein binding will affect the rate of filtration.

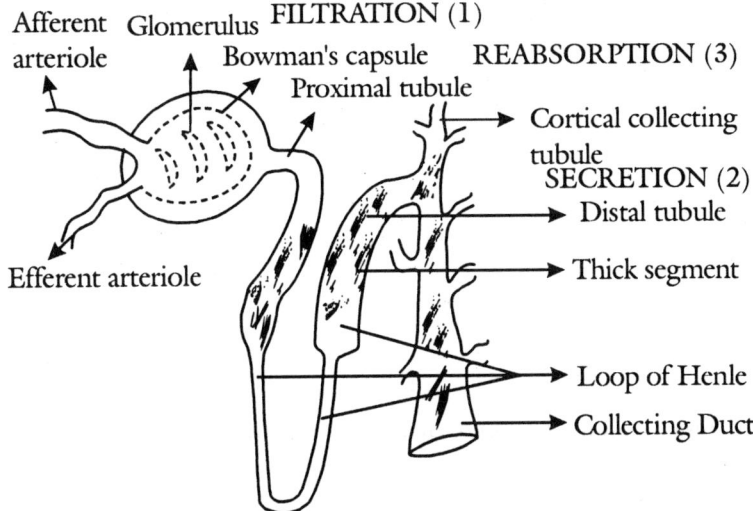

1. Glomerular filtration, 2. Tubular secretion, 3. Reabsorption
   Net excretion = 1 + 2 – 3
   Average rate of urine formation is 1ml/min

Fig. 4.1. Schematic representation of renal excretion

The degree of glomerular filtration depends on three pressures. (1) One of the diriving force for glomerular filtration is the hydrostatic pressure of the blood. Hydrostatic pressure, also called as hematic pressure, in glomerular capillaries is ~55 mm Hg. (2) Pressure of fluid in glomerular capsular space which is ~15 mm Hg and it opposes filtration. (3) Hematic colloid pressure because of plasma proteins e.g. albumin and globumin and is ~30 mm Hg, which also opposes filtration. Thus,

Net filtration pressure = hematic pressure – capsular-space pressure
                          – hematic colloid osmotic pressure

i.e.

Net filtration pressure = 55 – 15 – 30 = 10 mm Hg

Glomerular Filtration Rate (GFR)

A "glomerular substance" is one that is: (1) freely filtered at the glomerulus, (2) neither reabsorbed nor secreted by the tubule. The clearance of such a substance will thus be a measure of the rate at which it is filtered (GFR). GFR can be studied by using compounds such as creatinine, inulin, mannitol and sodium thiosulfate. These compounds are neither secreted nor reabsorbed and are excreted only by filtration.

Inulin is not an endogenous compound and hence has to be infused. It is a nuisance to assay and is of limited practical use. Radio labeled vitamin B_{12}, iothalamate, and EDTA can also be used and are easier to measure but also have to be infused.

The normal range for GFR is 1.25 – 2.10 mL/s 1.73 m^2 and varies with age and sex.

Measurement of GFR

The basic formula for clearance (Cl_x) of a substance X is:

$$Cl_x = \frac{(U_x) \cdot (V)}{P_x} \qquad \qquad ...4.1$$

where,

U_X = Urine concentration of X
V = Urine volume/time
P_X = Plasma concentration of X

For most practical purposes creatinine is an ideal glomerular substance because it is present in the plasma at a constant level as an endogenenous product of muscle metabolism. In severe renal failure and heavy proteinuria, some creatinine may enter the tubular urine by secretion and may overestimate the GFR.

The Serum Creatinine

Creatinine, an end product of muscle metabolism, is excreted solely by the kidneys. Its production rate is proprtional to the patient's muscle mass and is therefore relatively stable over time. The concentration of creatinine in the plasma depends upon two factors.

(1) The rate of creatinine production from muscle depends upon the lean body mass and for practical purposes it is constant from day to day.

(2) The GFR; which determines its rate of elimination.

In adults, the normal range for plasma creatinine is 0.8 to 1.3 mg/dl in men and 0.6 to 1.0 mg/dl in women. Creatinine clearance can also be determined from urine samples. It is usually determined from a 24-hour urine collection because shorter collections give less accurate results. The accuracy of the creatinine clearance may be limited by an incomplete urine collection and increasing creatinine secretion. Calculating the total amount of creatinine in the urine specimen and comparing it to the predicted creatinine excretion can estimate the completeness of a timed collection. Under age 50, men normally excrete 20 to 25 mg/kg lean body weight/day (177 to 221 mmol/kg), whereas women excrete 15 to 20 mg/kg lean body weight/day (133 to 177 mmol/kg).

Deit may have some effect on serum creatinine levels, but is insignificant. For a normal person the serum creatinine concentration reflects the GFR. If the GFR falls by half, the serum creatinine will double. If the serum creatinine is five times the baseline, then GFR is one fifth of normal. For this reason it is simpler merely to follow the serum creatinine levels.

In very small or very muscular individuals or where body weight is changing, then the added accuracy of a measured GFR may be necessary. (*Refer Section 4.3 for more details about creatinine clearance*)

Blood Urea

The blood urea is seldomly used as a measure of renal function because:

1. It varies with the deit, especially protein intake.
2. It is reabsorbed in the tubules and is therefore not a glomerular substance. This results in low estimation of GFR.
3. The reabsorption varies with urine flow and its clearance becomes completely independent of the GFR at low urine flow rates.

However, both serum creatinine and blood urea are approximations with significant potential for error. The limitations of creatinine and urea in assessing GFR are summarized in the Table 4.1.

Table. 4.1: Limitations of Markers of Renal function

	Serum creatinine	Blood urea nitrogen
Production	Constant if muscle mass in constant	Variable, affected by protein intake, liver production, catabolic rate
Filtration	Complete	Complete
Reabsorption	None	40-60% depending on volume status and antidiuretic hormone
Secretion	< 10%	None

Nuclear medicine techniques are also available to measure GFR. ^{99m}Technetium diethylene triamimopentaacetic acid (DTPA) is excreted by glomerular filtration, and GFR can be estimated after a single injection of radioisotope by estimating the amount in plasma samples obtained 60 and 180 minutes after injection. Camera-based clearances are more commonly used because of their convenience. This is done by measuring the increase in counts over the kidney for 3 to 6 minuts and correcting for renal accumulation of radioisotope, tissue depth, and background counts. Recently, iohexol has been evaluated as an exogenous maker of GFR. Iohexol, a nonionic, low osmolar radiocontrast agent, may be measured in minute quantities by high-performance liquid chromatography. Extrarenal elimination is trivial. GFR may be determined by single sample of iohexol clearance 3 to 4 hours after the injection of 3 to 5 mL of iohexol. Importantly renal clearance may be accurately measured in patients with GFR as low as 2 to 3 mL/min.

4.2.2 Tubular Reabsorption and Secretion

There are various active transport systems in the proximal tubule. The drugs can be excreted from plasma into the urine by passive diffusion, but this process is of minor significance. There are two active processes, with low degree of specificity for tubular secretion: *organic anion transporter* and *organic cation transporter*.

The *organic anion transporter* transports organic acids e.g. penicillins, sulfonic acids and acidic metabolites e.g. sulfate conjugates, glucuronides and glycine conjugates. This transporter is localized on the basolateral membrane of proximal tubules. The *organic cation transporter* transports organic bases e.g. morphine and quaternary ammonium compounds. Both systems have low degree of specificity and the finite capacity and hence demonstrate competition between substances that are transported by the same system. For example, penicillin is actively secreted by organic acid system. Thus, by using another acid, which can compete with for renal secretion, half-life and duration of action of penicillin can be increased. In fact, probenecid was successfully introduced for this purpose.

Active reabsorption is mediated via specific transport mechanisms for endogenous compounds such as glucose and amino acids. Thus, drugs show active reabsorption only if they possess close structural relationship with endogenous compounds. Hence, most of the drugs are mainly reabsorbed by passive diffusion. This is particularly true for lipophilic substances and hence are excreted with difficulty. Lipophilic substances are excreted with ease only when first they are biotransformed into polar metabolites. In general, lipophilic drugs are extensively reabsorbed compared to hydrophilic substances. As such very few drugs demonstrate active reabsorption e.g. oxopurinol.

As most of the drugs are either organic acids or bases, the reabsorption mainly depends on ionization constant (pKa) and pH of the urine (Please review Handerson-Hasselbach equation and relationship of pH and pKa from previous chapters).

The effect of pH dependence is some times used for clinical benefits. For example, in case of aspirin poisoning (pKa of aspirin is 3.5), sodium bicarbonate is administered. Sodium bicarbonate makes the urine alkaline and thus promotes the excretion of aspirin. Overdose of sulphonamides produces crystalluria because of precipitation in the renal tubule. This can be avoided by making urine more alkaline and thus increasing the excretion of sulphonamides.

Reabsorption is also affected by urine flow rate. Besides pH dependence, reabsorption of weak acids and weak bases is inversely proportional to the urine flow rate. In fact, in case of intoxication besides modifying pH, forced diuresis by means of increased urine flow by excess fluid intake or diuretics is also used to increase the excretion of drugs.

4.3 CONCEPT OF CLEARANCE

Elimination rate is defined as the amount of substance removed from the circulation per unit time. *Clearance* is the volume of plasma that is cleared of drug per unit time. Clearance has the units of flow, ml/min; thus clearance of 50 ml/min means that 50 ml of blood (or plasma) containing drug is cleared per minute. High values of clearance means efficient and rapid removal of drug.

As elimination rate is the amount of drug removed per unit time, it will go on decreasing as time increases. This is because the amount of drug will go on decreasing with time whereas, clearance will remain constant. This is because, irrespective of amount of drug, volume of blood being cleared of drug per minute will remain constant. The overall effect is decrease in the plasma concentration.

The relationship between clearance, elimination rate and plasma concentration can be expressed as:

$$\text{Clearance (Cl)} = \frac{\text{Elimination Rate } (\mu g / min)}{\text{Plasma concentration } (\mu g / ml)}$$
$$(ml / min)$$

...4.2

Clearance is an additive parameter and *total body clearance* is defined as the sum of clearances by individual organs:

$$Cl = Cl_{renal} + Cl_{hepatic} + cl_{lung} + \ldots \qquad \ldots 4.3$$

or
$$Cl = \frac{\text{Elimination Rate}}{\text{Plasma concentration}}$$

$$= \left(\frac{\text{Elimination rate by renal excretion}}{\text{Plasma concentration}} \right)$$

$$+ \left(\frac{\text{Elimination rate by hepatic metabolism}}{\text{Plasma concentration}} \right)$$

$$+ \left(\frac{\text{Elimination rate by lung excretion}}{\text{Plasma concentration}} \right) + \ldots$$

Renal elimination rate is sum of glomerular filtration and active secretion minus rate of reabsorption. Thus *renal clearance* can be expressed as:

$$Cl_{renal} = \frac{\text{Rate of filtration + Rate of secretion − Rate of reabsorption}}{\text{Plasma concentration}}$$

...4.4

It is important to note that clearance of drug by an organ can not exceed the blood flow to that organ. This is because, rate of overall clearance is limited by the delivery of the drug to that organ via blood.

For a one-compartment model, clearance can also be calculated if volume of distribution and elimination rate constants are known. Thus,

$$Cl = V_d \cdot K_{el} \qquad \ldots 4.5$$

Clearance is generally used as a measure of renal function. Creatinine clearance is widely used for this purpose. Recall that creatinine is a byproduct of muscle catabolism and is amine chemically. Serum creatinine is usually measured in clinical practice for this purpose.

As muscle catabolism and hence creatinine levels differ according to age, weight and sex, different formulas are used to calculate creatinine clearance from serum creatinine concentration.

For children between 1 to 20 years

$$Cl_{cr} = \frac{0.48 \cdot H}{S_{cr}} \cdot \left[\frac{W}{70}\right]^{0.7} \qquad ...4.6$$

For adults above 20 years
Males

$$Cl_{cr} = \frac{(140 - age) \cdot W}{72 \cdot S_{cr}} \qquad ...4.7a$$

Females

$$Cl_{cr} = \frac{(140 - age) \cdot W}{85 \cdot S_{cr}} \qquad ...4.7b$$

where,

Cl_{cr}	= Creatinine clearance (ml/min)
S_{cr}	= Serum creatinine (mg %)
H	= Height (cm)
W	= Weight (Kg)
Age	= in Years

Normal creatinine clearance is 120 to 130 ml/min. Creatinine clearance < 10 ml/min indicates severe renal impairment. Renal function can be expressed as:

$$\text{Renal function (RF)} = \frac{Cl_{cr} \text{ of Patient}}{Cl_{cr} \text{ of normal subject}} \qquad ...4.8$$

Hence

Dose in case of patients with renal impairment = (Normal dose) · (RF)

Some drawbacks and precautions when calculating Cl_{cr} from serum creatinine are as follows:

1. Liver dysfunction is associated with a significant overprediction of Cl_{cr}. These equations should be used with caution in patients with liver disease.

2. Emaciated have low serum creatinine concentrations secondary to decreased muscle mass, resulting in a significant overprediction of Cl_{cr}.

3. Elderly patients may have low serum creatinine concentrations secondary to decreased muscle mass, leading to a possible overprediction of Cl_{cr}.

Relationship Between C_{cr} and K_{el}

The relationship between creatinine clearance and overall drug elimination is shown in Fig. 4.2 (plot of K_{el} versus creatinine clearance). This is often referred to as Dettli plot.

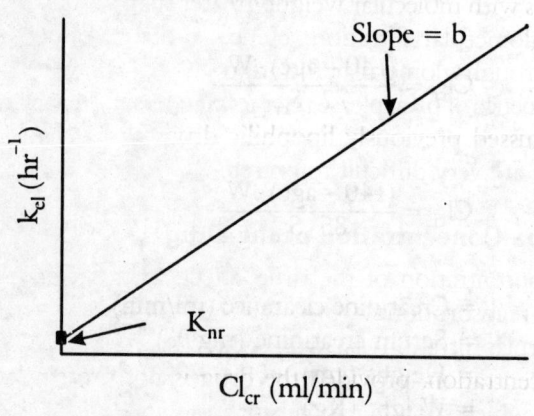

Fig. 4.2. Relationship between Cl_{cr} and K_{el} (Dettli Plot)

The relationship between Cl_{cr} and K_{el} from a number of patients can be determined and then measure the creatinine clearance in a new patient and from the above relationship the elimination rate constant can be estimated and thus an optimum dose and dosing interval for this patient can be calculated.

How to calculate K_{el} for a particular drug and patient?

For this, data previously obtained and published in the literature is used. With this information construct a plot of Cl_{cr} versus K_{el}.

$$K_{el} = K_{nr} + (b \cdot Cl_{cr}) \qquad \ldots 4.9$$

The Y-intercept(K_{nr}) is the nonrenal elimination rate, or which occurs with essentially no renal function. The slope(b) the regression line is the linear relationship between K_{el} and Cl_{cr}.

4.4 FACTORS AFFECTING RENAL EXCRETION

Various factors are known to affect renal excretion and are as follows:

1. Physicochemical Properties of the Drug

Following physicochemical properties of a drug play important role in determining its renal excretion:

- ◆ Molecular size
- ◆ pKa
- ◆ Lipid solubility

Molecular size plays important role in glomerular filtration. Substances with molecular weight greater than 60,000 are not filtered through glomerular filtration. Hence, protein bound drugs are not filtered through glomerular filtration.

For influence of pKa, please refer to Handerson-Hasselbach equation.

As discussed previously lipophilic drugs show renal reabsorption and hence are very difficult to excrete.

2. Plasma Concentration of the Drug

Plasma concentration of the drug affects both glomerular filtration and renal reabsorption.

Glomerular filtration of a drug is directly proportional to the plasma drug concentration, provided the drug is not protein bound.

Drugs, which show renal reabsorption, excretion occur only when concentration in glomerular filtrate is higher than reabsorption capacity.

3. Binding Characteristic of the Drug

As discussed previously only unbound or free drugs are filtered through glomerular filtrate. Thus, as excretion is low, protein bound drugs generally have long half-lives. In other words, drugs with large volume of distribution show poor renal excretion e.g. doxycycline which is 93 % protein bound has clearance of 16 ml/min.

4. Urine pH

For interplay between pH and pKa, please refer to Handerson-Hasselbach equation. For drugs that are weak acids (pKa 3-7) or weak bases (pKa 6-12), the degree of ionisation in tubular fluid is dependent upon pH, for example:

- ◆ **Methamphetamine (weak base, pKa = 10).** Renal excretion is 4 times faster in acidic urine than alkaline urine. It is because at lower pH there is lower ionisation, in turn less reabsorption and greater excretion of methamphetamine.
- ◆ **Phenobarbital (weak acid, pKa = 7.4).** Renal excretion is 7 times faster in alkaline urine. However renal clearance is still only a small fraction of total clearance.

♦ **Salicylic acid (weak acid, pKa = 3.5).** At physiologic pH it is mainly ionised. At pH of 5.0, the amount of non-ionised form is 25 times that present at pH of 7.4. In aspirin overdose, a systemic alkali and tubular acidosis occurs, which enhances tubular reabsorption and therefore prolongs half life of elimination. This can be reversed by giving systemic alkali and fluids and producing an alkaline urine with high flow rate. (Note that haemodialysis is actually used in life-threatening poisoning)

5. Blood Flow to the Kidneys

Renal blood flow plays important role in case of drugs which are excreted by glomerular filtration or renal excretion. Excretion of drugs for which renal flow plays important roles are said to be *perfusion -rate limited*.

6. Biological Factors

Like in metabolism, various biological factors viz. age, sex and species significantly influence drug excretion. In addition, circadian rhythm also plays important role (refer 'Chronopharmacokinetics' in Chapter 11).

In general, females show 10 % lower renal excretion than males, whereas in neonates, renal function is only 60-70 % compared to adults. In old age renal function is reduced and hence renal excretion is also reduced.

7. Pregnancy

Pregnancy leads to significant changes in volume and composition of the body fluids; the plasma volume, the red cell mass and the albumin mass increases. The increase in plasma volume is greatest (up 40%) and there is an increase in the hematocrit and the plasma albumin concentration. Total body volume also increases between 6-8 litres.

Pregnancy has significant effects on renal blood flow and GFR and both increase very early in pregnancy with the GFR increasing up to 50% by the end of the first trimester. Hence, plasma concentration of components handled by filtration falls; for example normal serum creatinine in pregnancy is about 40-50 mmol/L.

8. Drug Interactions

Many drug interactions influence drug excretion and involve following effects:

♦ Forced diuresis
♦ Alteration in urine pH
♦ Alteration in intrinsic clearance
♦ Alteration in renal blood flow
♦ Alteration in binding characteristics
♦ Alteration in active secretion

If the drug is highly protein bound and if other drug displaces it, then excretion of such highly protein bound drug increases. For example, furosemide increases excretion of gentamicin by displacing gentamicin from its protein binding sites. Acidification of urine (e.g. by drugs like ammonium chloride) enhances excretion of basic drugs and alkalinization of urine (e.g. by drugs like bicarbonates) enhances excretion of acidic drugs.

9. Disease States

Renal excretion is one of the most important routes of excretion, and hence renal impairment or renal dysfunction will significantly affect the excretion of drugs. Renal impairment can be caused by various diseases/disorders, such as:

♦ Hypertension
♦ Diabetes
♦ Nephrotoxicity (by aminoglycosides, lead or mercury)
♦ Polynephritis (inflammation of kidney)
♦ Hypovolemia

For example in *uremia* which is associated with decreased glomerular filtration and accumulation of fluids, renal excretion of drugs is reduced. Thus there is an increase in the half-life of the drug and hence accumulation of the drug in the body.

Also refer to 'Dose Adjustments in renal Failure' in Chapter 11.

4.5 NON-RENAL ROUTES OF ELIMINATION

Drugs or xenobiotics and their metabolites are many times excreted by routes other than renal. These other routes of elimination are generally referred to as extrarenal or non-renal routes of elimination and are as follows:

1. Biliary excretion
2. Exhalation
3. Fecal excretion
4. Intestinal excretion
5. Excretion via skin/saliva
6. Excretion via milk
7. Genital excretion

1. Biliary Excretion

Biliary excretion is generally considered as the most important and can be considered as a complementary route to renal excretion. Bile production is carried out by the hepatic cell lining, the bile canaliculi. Blood from GIT first passes through liver. Liver is the main site metabolism, which can remove the drug and their metabolites and excrete them in bile before they can enter general circulation. The transport of drugs and their metabolites from blood to bile is an active process. Generally large molecules with MW > 250-300 are excreted via biliary excretion. Thus, biliary excretion is an important route of elimination for conjugated compounds.

Substances, which are excreted via biliary excretion, are divided into three classes based on their ratio of concentration in bile versus plasma.

> *Class A*: Substances belonging to this class have a ratio of 1 e.g. sodium, potassium, chloride, glucose, thallium, cesium, cobalt and mercury.

> *Class B*: Substances belonging to this class have a ratio greater than 1 (usually between 10-1000) e.g. bile acids, bilirubin, lead, arsenic and manganese.

> *Class C*: Substances belong to this class have a ratio less than 1 e.g. inulin, albumin, zinc, iron, gold and chromium.

Class B compounds constitutes majority of the drugs that are excreted via biliary excretion. These compounds are excreted by active transport mechanism. Mechanism by which compounds belonging to Class A and C are excreted is not known.

In neonates, the hepatic excretory mechanisms are not fully developed due to which some drug may show toxicity, for example, ouabaine shows 40 times more toxicity in neonates than in adult rats.

Biliary excretion shows considerable species variation, and due to which extrapolation of data obtained from animals to humans is very difficult. For example, dogs excrete 3.8 % whereas monkeys excrete 33.6 % of indomethacin in bile. Dogs excrete 52.1 % whereas monkeys excrete 8.1 % of Phase II metabolite of indomethacin.

Enterohepatic Circulation

Drugs and their metabolites enter the duodenum via the common bile duct, and move through the small intestine. The drugs may be reabsorbed into the body from the intestine. Some drugs will be reabsorbed back into the bloodstream and return to the liver by the *enterohepatic circulation* (Fig. 4.3).

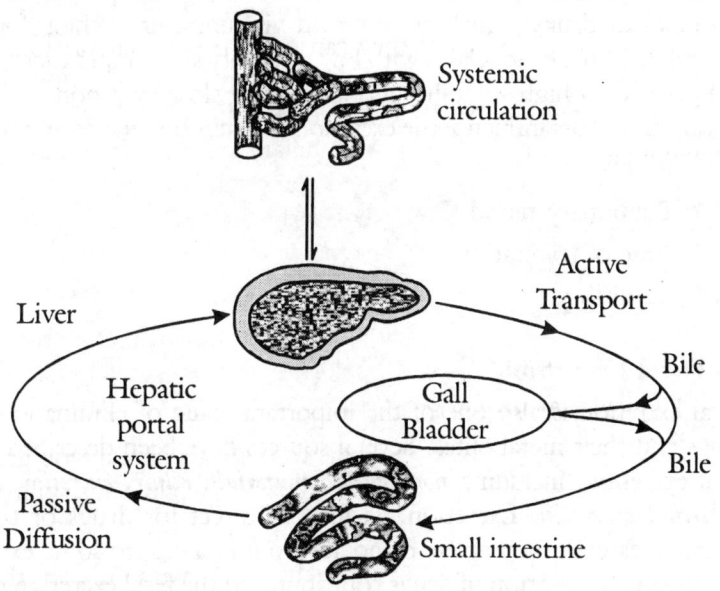

Fig. 4.3. Enterohepatic circulation

The drug then undergoes furher metabolism or is secreted back into bile. This is referred to as enterohepatic cycling and may extend the duration of action of a drug. Enterohepatic circulation has various consequences, such as:

- Active drug secreted into bile may be reabsorbed as "active" drug
- The "active" drug may be re-eliminated in the bile and reabsorbed

Because of this "circulation" drugs that are actively secreted into bile may actually be primarily eliminated from the body via kidneys-e.g. ampicillin.

Drugs like sulfobromophthalein are used to assess biliary function as it is completely eliminated as parent drug in bile.

2. Exhalation

Gases and volatile substances are mainly excreted via lungs by exhalation or pulmonary excretion. Plasma concentration and blood-gas partition coefficient play important role in the excretion of drugs via lungs. Excretion of drugs via lungs is mainly because of simple diffusion. Examples of drugs, which are excreted via lungs, are—chloroform, alcohol, halothane etc. Gases with low solubility show rapid excretion and gases with high solubility in blood show slow excretion.

Various factors influence the excretion of drugs by exhalation route, these includes:

- ❖ Pulmonary blood flow
- ❖ Rate of respiration
- ❖ Solubility

3. Fecal Excretion

Fecal excretion is also one of the important route of elimination of drugs and their metabolites. Several sources have been described for fecal excretion, including *nonabsorbed materials, biliary excretion and intestinal excretion.* Excretion via feces is direct for drugs or their metabolites with incomplete or no absorption. Thus, to some extent nonabsorbable portion of drugs contributes to the fecal excretion e.g. polymers or quaternary ammonium bases, sucrose polyesters, cholestyramine etc. that show limited intestinal absorption. In general fecal excretion is because of biliary excretion.

4. Intestinal Excretion

Intestinal excretion is mainly important for drugs which have low rates of metabolism/low renal clearance/low biliary clearance. Many organic acidic and organic basic drugs show active secretion in the intestine e.g. nicotine and quinine. Many drugs with diverse chemical properties also show intestinal excretion in to feces e.g. digitoxin, hexachlorobenzene, dioxin etc.

5. Excretion via Skin/Saliva

Drug excretion via skin (sweat) and saliva is mainly because of passive diffusion of lipid soluble drugs. Drugs or their metabolites, which are excreted via sweat, are known to cause various dermatological problems such as urticaria, dermatitis or various other allergic disorders. Drugs excreted via sweat are lead, mercury, alcohol and antipyrene.

In general, basic drugs are excreted more in saliva compared to acidic drugs. Although most of the drugs are excreted in saliva by passive diffusion, some of the drugs are known to be actively secreted in saliva e.g. lithium, penicillin and phenytoin. Drugs and their metabolites, which are excreted via saliva, are generally swallowed and thus entire process of absorption of drug starts again.

Overall, excretion of drugs via sweat, saliva, hair or nails is quantitatively of minor importance. Excretion via hair or nails is important for detection of toxicity of arsenic and mercury. "Sweat testing" has been employed for the identification of drug abuse. Saliva testing is also available for drugs like marijuana, cocaine, opiates, amphetamines, methaphetamines and phencyclidine.

6. Excretion via Milk

Excretion of drugs and their metabolites into milk is of great importance because of following reasons:

> ➤ There is danger of drugs to be transferred from mother to infant via breast feeding.
> ➤ Drugs excreted in Cow's milk can be ingested by humans.

Transfer of drugs from plasma to mother's milk is mainly because of passive diffusion and hence depends on following factors:

> ➤ pKa of the drug

> pH partition between plasma (pH 7.4) and milk (pH 6.6)
> Plasma concentration
> Lipid solubility
> Molecular weight.

Because of fat content and presence of calcium in milk, various lipophilic drugs and metals, which can chelate with calcium (e.g. lead), are excreted in milk. Also as milk is slightly acidic compared to plasma, due to which weakly basic drugs concentrate more in milk. Drugs which show high plasma protein binding demonstrate less secretion in milk e.g. diazepam.

The amounts of drug secreted in breast milk is usually very small, but may affect a suckling infant who has less ability to metabolize and excrete drugs.

Breastfeeding Mothers and Medicines—General Guidance

The following principles should be followed when prescribing for breastfeeding mothers:

> Avoid unnecessary use of drugs including the over-the-counter (OTC) products.
> Breastfeeding mothers should seek advice on the suitability of OTC products from physicians.
> Benefit/risk ratio for both mother and infant should be assessed.
> Avoid use of drugs known to cause serious toxicity in adults or children.
> Drugs licensed for use in infants do not generally pose a hazard.
> Neonates (and particularly premature infants) are at greater risk from exposure to drugs via breast milk. This is because of immature excretory functions and the consequent risk of drug accumulation.
> A regimen and route of administration which presents the minimum amount of drug to the infant should be chosen.
> Avoid long-acting preparations, especially those of drugs likely to cause serious side effects (e.g. antipsychotic agents), as it is difficult to time feeds to avoid significant amounts of drug in breast milk.
> Multiple drug regimens may pose an increased risk, e.g. when adverse effects such as drowsiness are additive.

➢ Infants exposed to drugs via breast milk should be monitored carefully for unusual signs or symptoms.

➢ New drugs should be avoided if a therapeutically equivalent alternative that has been more widely used is available.

QUESTIONS

1. Explain renal excretion in details.
2. Explain clearance and its importance.
3. Explain various factors affecting renal excretion.
4. Write note on:
   (a) Biliary excretion
   (b) Excretion of milk
   (c) Exhalation
   (d) Excretion via skin and saliva.

5

Prodrugs

5.1 INTRODUCTION

Prodrug is a pharmacologically inactive chemical derivative that is biotransformed *in-vivo* in to an active drug by an enzymatic or nonenzymatic process(es) to exert therapeutic action. The term "prodrug" or "proagent" was first introduced by Albert in the late 1950s, such compounds have also been called *latentiated drugs, bioreversible derivatives, and congeners.* It is a nonspecific chemical approach to mask undesirable drug properties such as:

♦ Poor solubility.
♦ Poor absorption and distribution.
♦ Lack of site specificity.
♦ Chemical instability.
♦ Toxicity.
♦ Poor patient acceptance (bad taste, odour, pain at injection site, etc.)
♦ Formulation problems.
♦ Prolonged drug release.
♦ Drug targeting, particularly, targeting the prodrugs to a specific enzyme or a specific membrane transport.

5.2 TYPES OF PRODRUGS

1. Carrier-linked Prodrugs

These are compounds that contain an active drug linked to a carrier group. These include covalent linkages such as esters and amides, which can be cleaved by a hydrolytic reaction by enzymatic or non-enzymatic catalysis. Since the carrier is usually lipophilic in nature, the lipophilicity of parent drug is highly modified. The linkage is temporary and the prodrug is mostly inactive or less active than the parent compound. The ideal properties of carrier include:

(i) It should be biologically inactive, nontoxic and nonimmunogenic.

(ii) It should not reduce activity of drug.

(iii) It should minimize the toxicity of host drug.

(iv) It should carry and release the drug to its site of action.

(v) It should protect the drug until it is reached at the site of action.

(vi) It should allow release of drug chemically or enzymatically.

(vii) It should be biodegradable after the release of drug.

($viii$) It should be easy to prepare.

(ix) It should be easy to combine with drug.

Chemical Modification in-vitro

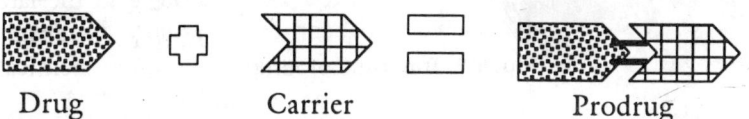

Drug   Carrier   Prodrug

Regeneration of Drug in-vivo

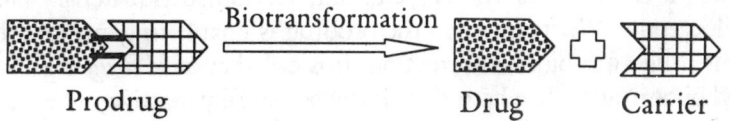

Prodrug   Drug   Carrier

Fig. 5.1. Carrier linked prodrug

Depending on the components involved in prodrug, they can be further classified as:

Bipartate Prodrug: It involves a linkage between a carrier and a drug (Fig. 5.1).

Tripartate Prodrug: It involves linkage of a carrier, linker and drug. Since it involves two attachments it is called as *double prodrug*. Since the release of active drug proceeds through two step trigger mechanisms, it is also called as *cascade latentiation*. When classical carrier-linked prodrugs are ineffective due to stable prodrug linkage, tripartite prodrug can be developed, attaching linker, which assists in the release of active drug (Fig. 5.2).

Chemical Modification in-vitro

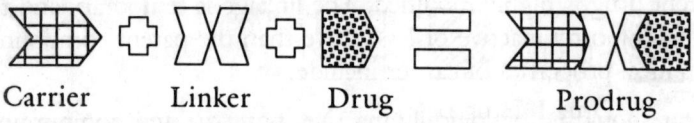

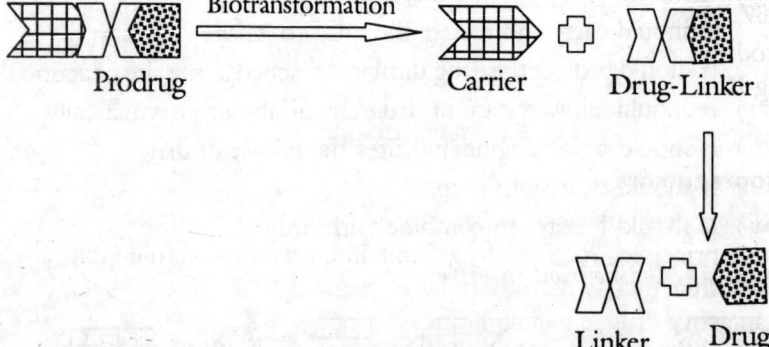

Fig. 5.2. Tripartate prodrug

Hard and Soft Drugs: If the rate of biotransformation of prodrug is faster, it is termed as *soft drug* e.g. tetradecylomethylquatenary salt of pilocarpine. Whereas, when the prodrug is unable to generate the parent drug after biotransformation, it is called as *hard drug* e.g. N-acetyl pilocarpine. The hard drug is therapeutically inactive; where as soft drug can show enhanced absorption and rapid therapeutic as well as toxic effects, if any.

Mutual Prodrug: In this, two synergistic drugs are attached to each other, where one acts as carrier for the other (Fig. 5.3). It may be bipartite or tripartite type. This type of prodrug is useful when simultaneous drug action of two or more drugs is more effective than the single drug. For example sultamacillin, which generates ampicillin, penicillanic acid, sulfone and formaldehyde. The mutual prodrug should release drug components concomitantly, they should have desired or equal rate and extent of bioavailability so as to produce effective plasma-drug concentration, and the distribution and elimination of drug components should be similar.

Chemical Modification in-vitro

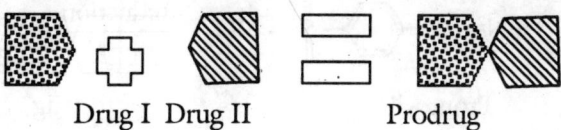

Drug I   Drug II   Prodrug

Regeneration of Drug in-vivo

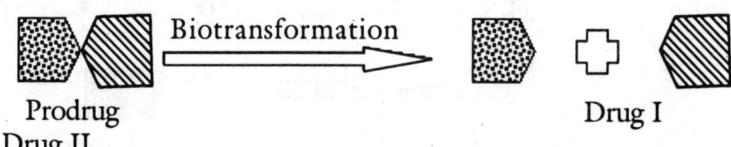

Biotransformation

Prodrug   Drug I
Drug II

Fig. 5.3. Mutual prodrug

2. Bioprecursors

Bioprecursors generate new compound by molecular modification of the active principle. Such prodrugs contain the embryo of the active species within their structure and the biotransformation of which yields an active drug, e.g. fenbufen, losartan. These types of prodrugs do not involve carrier, and the change in the lipophilicity is not significant. Since bioprecursor contains a different structure they can not be biotransformed to active drug by simple cleavage of groups. The drastic structural changes take place to release active drug from bioprecursors and it involves reactions such as oxidation, reduction, phosphorylation, decarboxylation, dehydration etc. Theses reactions are only catalyzed by enzymes. For example, phenacetin produces its analgesic and antipyretic activity because of oxidative activation-O-dealkylation to acetaminophen (Fig. 5.4a); reductive activation of prontosil yields an antibacterial drug suphanilamide (Fig. 5.4b).

Phenacetin   O-dealkylation   Acetaminophen

(a)

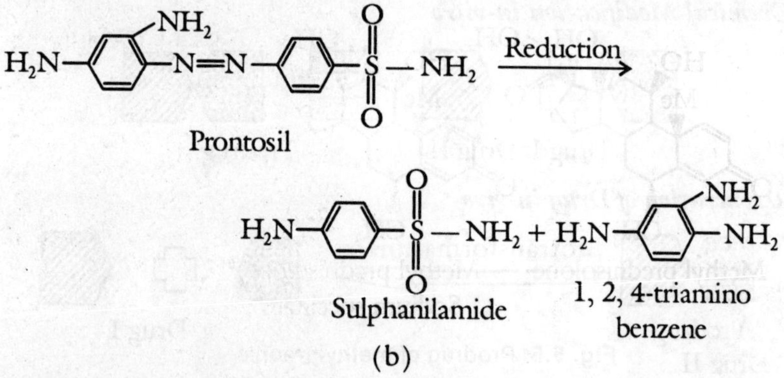

Fig. 5.4. (a) Activation of phenacetin (b) Generation of sulphanilamide

5.3 APPLICATIONS OF PRODRUGS

There are numerous applications of prodrugs as described below.

A. Increase in Solubility

Aqueous solubility of drug is essential to formulate dosage forms. The oral liquid dosage forms and injectables are usually made in aqueous phase. The water solubility increases miscibility of drug in GI fluids after oral administration and thus effectively increases the rate of absorption of the drug. The aqueous injections are easily miscible with blood achieving rapid plasma-drug levels.

The acylation of alcohol and amine groups with carboxylic acids containing amino or additional carboxylate groups increases water solubility, whereas with aliphatic or aromatic carboxylic acids lipophilicity of the drug increases. Esterification of hydroxylic functional groups with succinic acid or phosphoric acid is an excellent way of increasing water solubility of drugs. For example, methylprednisolone has poor water solubility but methylprednisolone sodium succinate is water-soluble. The latter has been used in injections and eye drops. However, it is chemically unstable and it should be used as freeze-dried powder for reconstitution (Fig. 5.5).

Phosphoric acid esters are chemically more stable than succinic acid esters. Riboflavin-5' - phosphoric acid dehydrate has water solubility of 112 g/L at pH 6.9 as compared to 0.06 g/L solubility of riboflavin. Alcohols and phenols can be converted into half-esters such as hemisuccinates, hemiglutarate to increase water solubility.

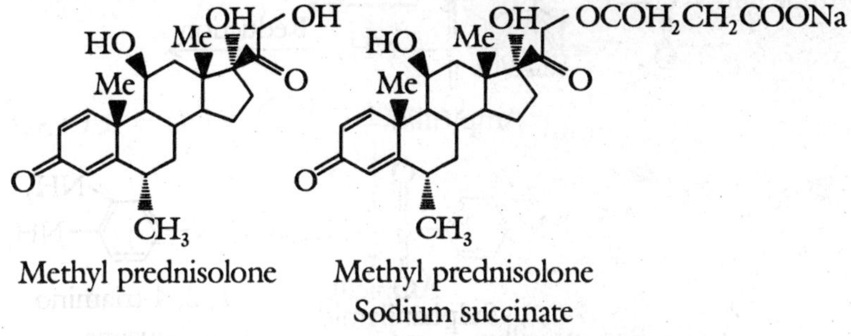

Methyl prednisolone

Methyl prednisolone
Sodium succinate

Fig. 5.5. Prodrug of methylprednisolone

B. Increase in Bioavailability

Increasing lipophilicity of a drug is one of the most important approaches to improve passive transport of the drug. Due to the increased bioavailability it is possible to reduce dose of the drug. Thus the therapy becomes more economical, in addition there is minimization of undesirable effects associated with high dose of the drug.

The amines can be made more lipophilic by conversion to their N-Mannich base or to Schiff base (imines). The N-Mannich base derived from phenylpropanolamine shows 100 times increase in octanol-phosphate buffer partition coefficient as compared to parent amine. N-Mannich base of theophyllin and 5-flurouracil have enhanced transdermal penetration.

Antibiotics such as bacampicillin, pivampicillin are examples of tripartate prodrugs of ampicillin. They contain drug- carrier-linker. The double ester strategy is useful to attach carrier to linker and then to the parent drug. Ampicillin has only 40% drug absorption after oral administration, due to which it requires 2.5 times more dose. Esterification of ampicillin was attempted to increase the lipophilicity. The simple esters of ampicillin were attempted to produce bipartite prodrug. The tripartite prodrug, cyloxymethyl ester of ampicillin viz. bacampicillin and pivampicillin are effective prodrugs. Bacampicillin when administered orally shows 98-99% absorption and in addition, one-half to one-third reduction in dose (Fig. 5.6).

The antiviral drug, acyclovir has poor bioavailability due to its poor solubility, poor GI absorption and biotransformation to inactive metabolite. The 6-deoxyacyclovir, a precursor type of prodrug, is

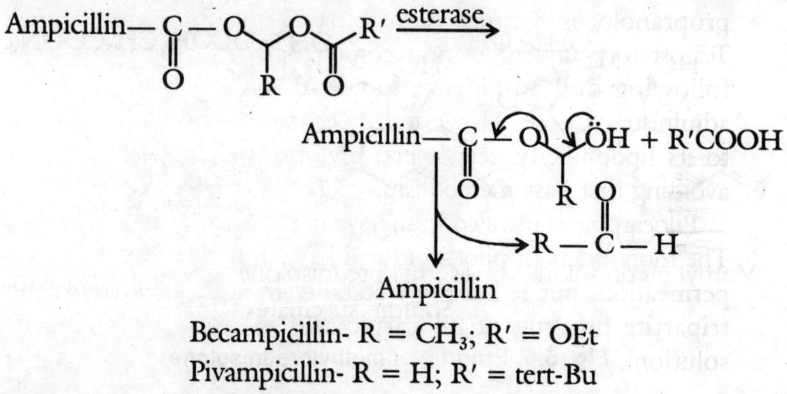

Ampicillin— $\underset{\underset{O}{\|}}{C}$ — O $\underset{R}{\bigvee}$ O — $\underset{\underset{O}{\|}}{C}$ R' $\xrightarrow{\text{esterase}}$

Ampicillin— $\underset{\underset{O}{\|}}{C}$ O $\underset{\underset{O}{\|}}{C}\ddot{O}H$ + R'COOH

$\downarrow$

R — $\underset{\underset{O}{\|}}{C}$ — H

Ampicillin

Becampicillin- R = CH$_3$; R' = OEt

Pivampicillin- R = H; R' = tert-Bu

Fig. 5.6. Prodrugs of ampicillin

oxidized by xanthine oxidase to release acyclovir and is 18 times more water-soluble and 5-6 times more bioavailable after oral administration.

$$6-\text{deoxyacyclovir} \xrightarrow{\text{Xanthine Oxidase}} \text{Acyclovir}$$

The low skin permeability of many steroids containing hydroxyl groups is attributed to its interaction with the skin or binding sites in keratin. Acetonidation or esterification of corticosteroids increases skin permeability. Fluocinolone acetonide is a prodrug of corticosteroid class; it is topically useful in inflammatory and pruritic manifestations. After its percutaneous transport it is activated *in-vivo* by esterase (Fig. 5.7).

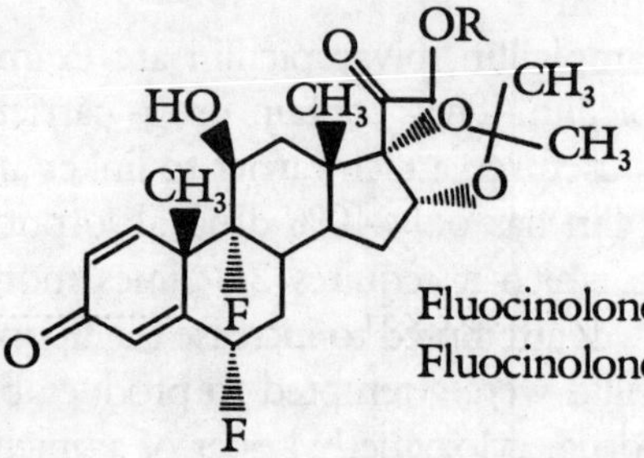

Fluocinolone acetonide- R = H
Fluocinolone - R = COCH$_3$

Fig. 5.7. Prodrug of fluocinolone

C. Chemical Stability

Propranolol, an anti-hypertensive drug, undergoes first pass metabolism after oral administration, but the hemisuccinate ester of propranolol is 8 times more bioavailable than parent molecule. Testosterone undergoes near complete hepatic first pass metabolism following oral administration, with only 3-6 % absorption of administered dose. However, undeconate ester of testosterone, due to its lipophilicity gets selectively absorbed by lymphatic system, avoiding first pass metabolism.

Pilocarpine is instilled in the eye in the form of aqueous eye drops. The monoesters of pilocarpic acid have improved corneal membrane permeation, but it has poor stability in aqueous system. Whereas tripartite prodrug of pilocarpic acid is highly stable in aqueous solution.

D. Reduction in Toxicity

Gastric irritation, ulcer and bleeding are common side effects of the aspirin. These may be attributed to an accumulation of the acid in the gastric mucosal cells. Esterification of aspirin and NSAID agents can suppress these unwanted effects. The conversion of aspirin to salicylic acid is carried out by esterases after absorption from the GI tract. Aspirin-PVP compound is comparatively less toxic. Sulindac is an indene isostere of indomethacin; the former is less irritating and has mild CNS side effects than the indomethacin.

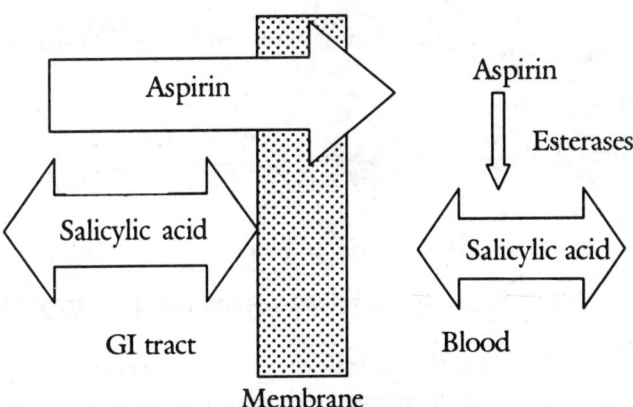

Fig. 5.8. Bioconversion of aspirin

Epinephrine is converted into dipivaloyle epinephrine to minimize ocular and systemic side effects associated with parent drug. Methotrexate, an anti-tumor drug acts equally on healthy cells as well as tumor cells, but its poly (L-lysine) derivative is non-toxic to the healthy cells.

E. Prolonged Action

The drugs having shorter plasma half-life are rapidly cleared from the body and hence frequent dosing is required to maintain therapeutic plasma-drug concentrations. Because of the shorter duration of action, these drugs are good candidates for the development of sustained release dosage form. The sustained release from a particular dosage is possible by (a) fabricating a dosage form to release drug slowly but in a constant fashion, and (b) modifying the drug itself, i.e. prodrug. The first category is the design of sustained release dosage forms using water insoluble or gel forming polymers. The rate of drug release and/ or rate of drug dissolution are mainly rate limiting steps. Conversion of soluble form of drug to insoluble form is the simplest way to produce sustained drug release, e.g. 7,7'-succinylditheophylline, which is a prodrug of theophyllin. Such a technique is mostly used to control drug release over a period of 24 hours. Prodrugs can also be used to prolong drug release for few months or more. The prolonged release over a period of month is achievable if the drug accumulates in fatty tissue and release of drug is slow and constant. Thus, the release of prodrug from site of application and secondly the rate of biotransformation of prodrug to release active drug are two rate determining steps (Fig. 5.9).

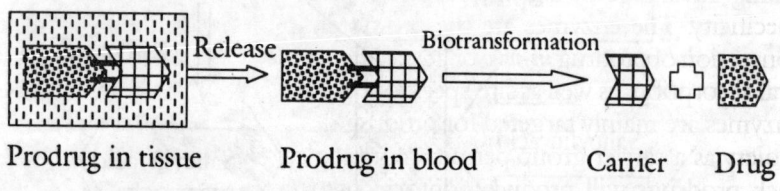

Prodrug in tissue   Prodrug in blood   Carrier   Drug

Fig. 5.9. Prolonged release action using prodrug

Fluphenazine, an anti-psychotic drug has a short duration of action (up to 8 hrs) but its decanoate derivative has duration of action of about a month. A Progestagens contraceptive steroid such as norethysterone enanthate has duration of action up to three months.

The increase in potency and extension of peak plasma concentration of tolmetin sodium, a NSAID is possible by using corresponding glycine conjugate. Poly (oxyethylene) diesters of NSAID agents have prolonged anti-inflammatory action due to higher plasma-half life.

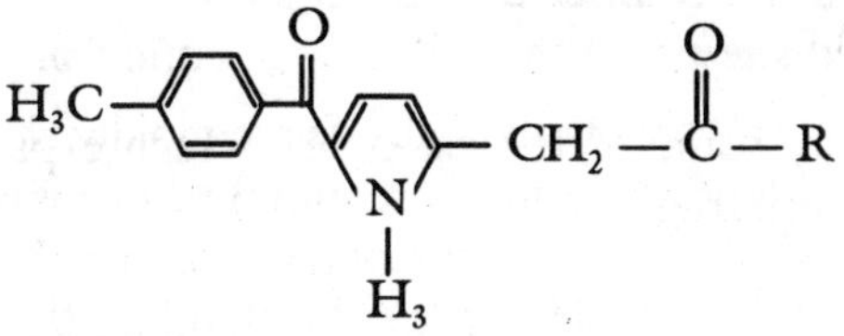

$$H_3C-\bigcirc-\overset{O}{\overset{\|}{C}}-\bigcirc_{\underset{\overset{|}{H_3}}{N}}-CH_2-\overset{O}{\overset{\|}{C}}-R$$

Tolmetin sodium- R = O⁻Na⁺
Tolmetin glycine conjugate-
R = NHCH₂COOH

Fig. 5.10. Prodrug of tolmetin sodium

F. Targeted Drug Delivery

The site-specific drug release enables maximum absorption of administered drug, avoiding toxicity associated with distribution of drug in non-target tissues as well as premature metabolism of drug. The two approaches are widely employed for site specific drug release:

(*i*) Adjustment in hydrophilic-lipophilic properties of drug or coupling the drug with site specific carrier to direct drug to a particular site and

(*ii*) Site specific activation of prodrug to release drug.

Prodrugs can be designed to target specific enzymes or carriers by taking advantage of enzyme-substrate specificity or carrier-substrate specificity. The enzymes are the pre-systemic metabolic sites for the conversion of prodrug *in-vivo* or at specific site. For example, to improve oral absorption, as well as site-specific drug delivery, the gastrointestinal enzymes are mainly targeted for prodrug design. The use of a nutrient moiety as a carrier group permits more logical targeting. In addition, such prodrugs will produce nontoxic nutrient byproducts.

The site-specific drug delivery can be obtained from tissue-specific activation of a prodrug. It is the result of metabolism by an enzyme that is either present at a higher concentration or is unique for the tissue. For example, colon specific drug delivery.

For the site-specific delivery of drugs by using the prodrug approach following factors should be optimized:

1. The prodrug must not be degraded before it reaches to intended site.

2. It must be readily transported to the intended site.
3. It must show selective biotransformation to the active drug at intended site compared to other sites.
4. Intended site/tissue should show retention of the active drug.

Following are some of the examples, which explain site specific application of prodrug.

HLB Concept: The drugs can cross blood -brain -barrier only by passive diffusion (lipoidal drugs) or by an active transport mechanism available for some compounds. Hence, the better approach for brain targeting is to combine hydrophilic drug with lipophilic carrier. The resulting lipoidal prodrug has better penetration in the brain compared to parent drug. After metabolism, the hydrophilic drug released in the brain will remain in the brain for longer time as it can not penetrate blood -brain-barrier and hence can be effluxed easily. β-lactam antibiotics due to their hydrophilicity have slow penetration in brain. The prodrug of penicillin prepared by attaching lipophilic dihydropyridine carrier delivers active antibiotic in brain quite effectively (Fig. 5.11 a and b).

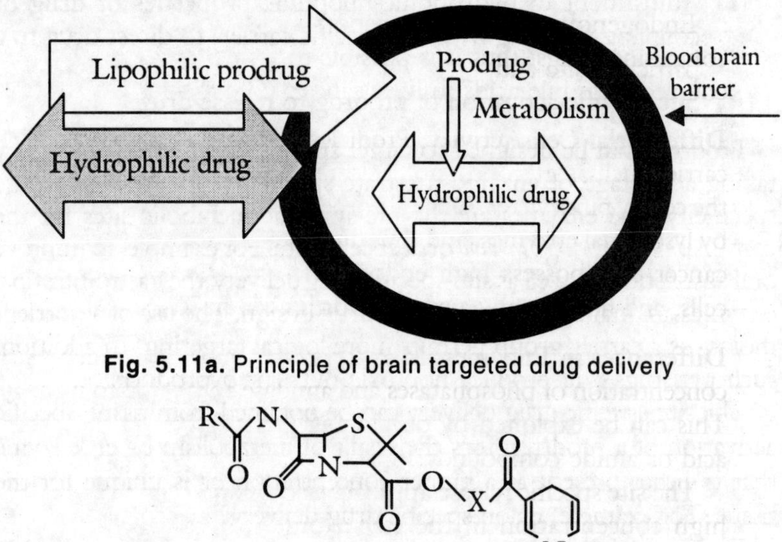

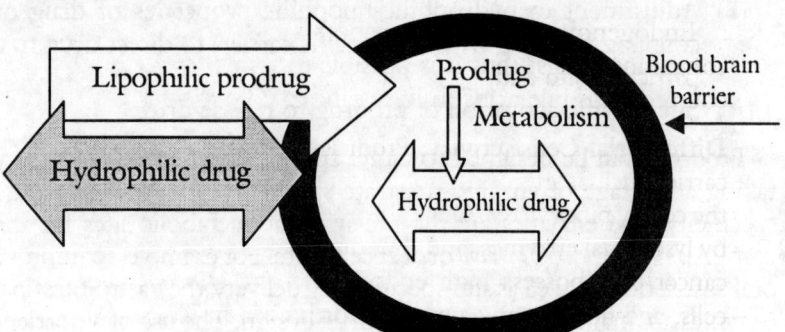

Fig. 5.11a. Principle of brain targeted drug delivery

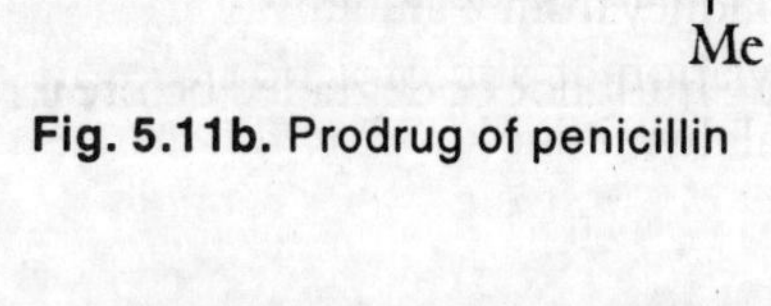

Fig. 5.11b. Prodrug of penicillin

Transport Mechanism: The Parkinson's disease treatment needs high doses of dopamine but dopamine does not crosses the blood-brain barrier. But its prodrug L-dopa can cross blood-brain barrier via L-amino acid active transport. L-dopa is a precursor type of prodrug and undergoes decarboxylation in the brain by dopa decarboxylase to produce dopamine (Fig. 5.12).

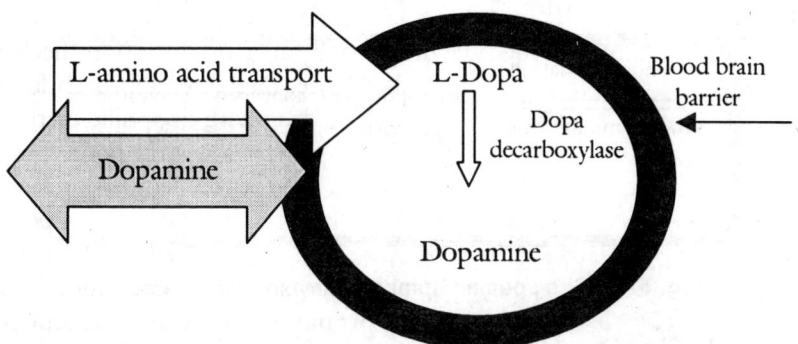

Fig. 5.12. Site specific action release of dopamine in brain

Endogenous bile acid transport system can transport bile salt containing drugs, thus it is possible to target liver, e.g. chlorambucil coupled with bile acids in liver cancer.

Differential Cell Activity: Prodrugs prepared using macromolecular carrier such as glycoprotein, lecithin, albumin, dextran etc. penetrate the cell by pinocytosis. Once absorbed, they are rapidly biotransformed by lysosomal enzymes, and thus drug is delivered inside the cell. Some cancer cells possess high endocytotic activity compared to normal cells, and hence many anticancer drugs can be specifically targeted.

Differences in Enzymes: Many types of tumor cells contain a higher concentration of phosphatases and amidase compared to normal cells. This can be exploited by developing prodrugs based on phosphoric acid or amide compounds.

The site specific release approach is based on presence of enzyme in high concentration in the target organ. For example, γ-glutamyl transpeptidase and L-aromatic aminoacid decarboxylase release dopamine in kidney from γ-glutamyldopa for renal vasodilatation effect.

Phosphorylation at site of action activates acyclovir, an antiviral drug by a viral thymidine kinase to the corresponding monophosphate.

Healthy cells lack this phosphorylation capacity and hence drug is nontoxic to them. Secondly, acyclovir monophosphate undergoes enzymatic conversion in to diphosphate and triphosphate derivatives. The triphosphate acyclovir due to its structural resemblance with that of essential DNA precursor is a selective substrate for viral α-DNA polymerase.

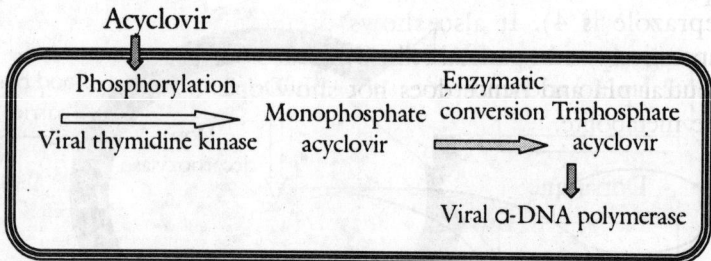

Fig. 5.13. Site specific uptake of acyclovir in infected cell

Colon is unique for azo-reductase and glucosidase activity, which have been exploited for colon targeted drug delivery. These prodrugs remain stable and intact in upper GI tract. Prodrugs of prednisolone, hydrocortisone with β-D-galactosides and β-D-glucosides when taken orally are stable in small intestine (and hence no drug release in small intestine) but are specifically metabolized in colon to release parent drug. Sulphasalzine is a well known drug for the treatment of ulcerative colitis. It is a bioprecursor type of prodrug activated by reduction. Chemically it is 5 -aminosalicylic acid (5-ASA) azo linked at 5 position via a spacer to poly(vinyl amine). This macromolecular synthetic polymer is not absorbed or metabolized in small intestine. In colon, 5-ASA and sulphapyridine are released by azoreduction.

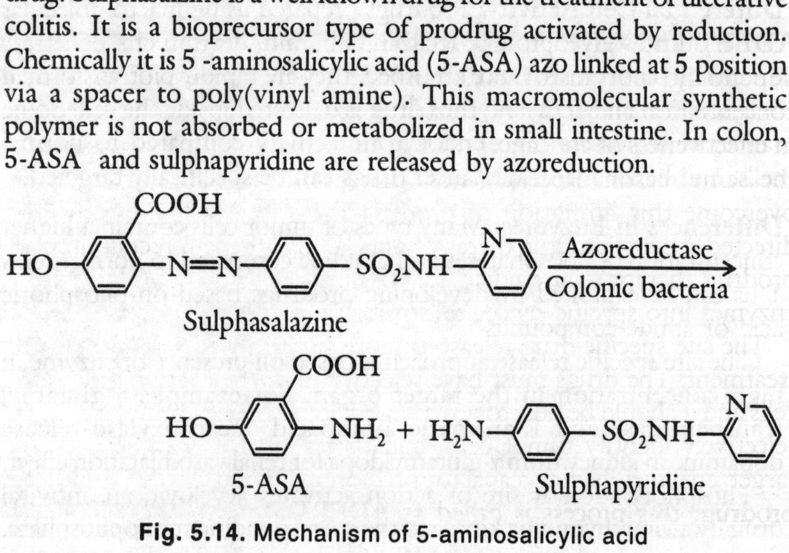

Fig. 5.14. Mechanism of 5-aminosalicylic acid

Stimuli Responsive Activation: The gastric H^+, K^+-ATPase is located on the parietal cell membrane and is responsible for gastric acid secretion. Omeprazole is a precursor type of prodrug, which is converted into a cyclic sulphenamide, an acid secretion inhibitor. This inhibitor inactivates the H^+, K^+-ATPase enzyme by forming disulphide bridges with the its thiol groups. The activation of omiprazole occurs more effectively in acidic environment (pKa of omeprazole is 4). It also shows preferential accumulation in comparatively acidic parietal cells. Omiprazole is relatively more stable at neutral pH and hence does not show significant conversion to active metabolite.

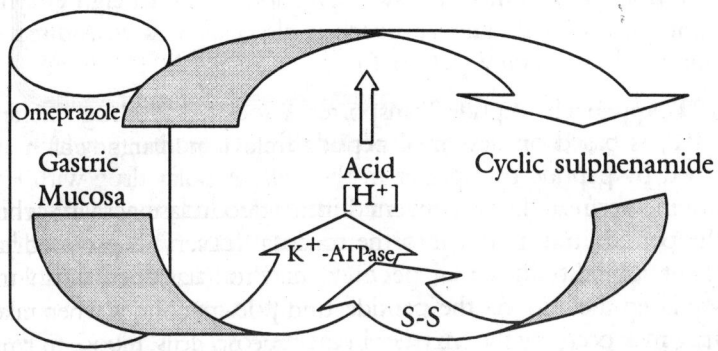

Fig. 5.15. Site specific action of omeprazole

ADEPT and GDEPT Approach: The variability in the enzyme dependant biotransformation is due to the variability in type, concentration and activity of enzymes at particular site. The variation in effectiveness of anticancer drug in animals and human is because of the same reason. Recently, new therapies have been proposed to overcome this limitation of prodrug therapy. ADEPT (antibody-directed enzyme prodrug therapy) and GDEPT (gene-directed enzyme prodrug therapy) are studied for localization of prodrug activation enzymes into specific cancer cells prior to prodrug administration.

The site specific drug release is more significant in anti-neoplastic treatment. The drugs must have selective inhibitory action on cancer cells and it should be non-toxic to healthy cells. Monoclonal antibodies selectively identify tumor cells, and therefore these can be used to target enzymes having capacity of biotransformation of anticancer prodrug; this process is called as ADEPT. Antitumor antibody is conjugated to an enzyme (ATAb-E) not normally present in extracellular fluid or on cell membranes and then these conjugates are localized in the tumor via intravenous infusion. To attain adequate concentration of ATAb-E in the tumor, high plasma and extracellular fluid levels of ATAb-E should be maintained. After that, a prodrug is administered, which is activated by the enzyme delivered to the tumor. For example, phosphoramidase is present in high concentration in cancer cells, which activates cyclophosphamide, an antineoplastic drug.

In GDEPT approach a prodrug-activating enzyme gene is carried by viral vector (e.g. retroviral or adenoviral) into both tumor and normal cells. By linking the foreign gene downstream of tumor-specific transcription units, tumor-specific expression of the foreign enzyme gene can be achieved. This approach is also called as virus-directed enzyme prodrug therapy (VDEPT).

PTAPT Approach: Peptide Transporter Associated Prodrug Therapy (PTAPT) is based on design of peptide linked prodrugs, which are absorbed by peptide transporter in the cells. A polar drug with low membrane permeability is converted into a prodrug that is absorbed via the peptide transporter into the mucosal cells. This prodrug has sufficient solubility in the GI tract and may get absorbed across the intestinal epithelium via the peptide transporters. The activation of prodrug may occur by the enzymes in the mucosal cells, blood, or liver. For example, the effective improvement of the membrane permeability and systemic availability of the polar α-methyldopa through peptidyl prodrugs such as α-methyldopa-Phe, α -methyldopa-Pro.

G. Improvement in Patient Acceptance: Generally patient will not accept a drug with unpleasant odour or taste more readily. The solubility in saliva and in turn the contact with taste buds can be minimized by the esterification of drug with long -chain fatty acids, e.g. clindamycine palmitate is less bitter than the clindamycin.

QUESTIONS

1. Explain various types of prodrugs in detail.
2. Write three applications of prodrugs
3. Write notes on
   (a) Bioprecursors
   (b) Targeted drug delivery in prodrugs
   (c) Carrier molecules used for prodrugs
   (d) Advantages of prodrugs.

6
Pharmacokinetics—
Basic Considerations

6.1 INTRODUCTION

"*Pharmacokinetics* is the discipline dealing with the rates of movement of a drug or its metabolites into the body, out of the body and also which attempts to evaluate the rates of biotransformations of the drug and its metabolites". In addition, pharmacokinetics has applications in drug formulation and treatment regimens.

Therapeutic and toxic effects of drugs depend on the drugs' concentration at the site of action. But in practice, it is not possible to obtain drug concentration in the biological tissues. Therefore, the most widely used procedure is to measure blood or plasma concentration, as it is the most simplest method to get information regarding absorption, distribution, metabolism and excretion (ADME) of the drug.

6.2 DRUG CONCENTRATION-TIME PROFILE

There is a relationship between plasma drug concentration and concentration of drug at the site of action. A typical plasma drug concentration profile is shown in Fig. 6.1.

This profile is obtained by measuring the plasma drug concentration at various time intervals after administration of single dose. Plasma drug concentration is plotted on Y-axis and time on X-axis.

The important pharmacokinetic parameters obtained from Fig. 6.1 are as follows:

1. Peak Plasma Concentration (C_{max})

Maximum concentration obtained in the plasma is called as *peak plasma concentration* (C_{max}). C_{max} depends upon:

- Dose administered (i.e. quantity of drug administered)
- Rate of absorption of drug
- Rate of elimination of drug

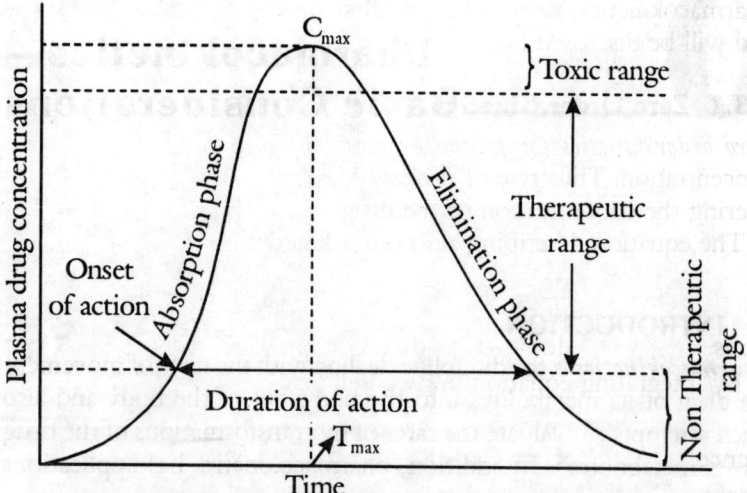

Fig. 6.1. Plasma drug concentration-time profile

The peak of the plasma drug concentration-time profile, which denotes peak plasma concentration, is the point at which rate of absorption and elimination is same. During time period before the peak (left hand side of the peak) absorption dominates whereas time period after the peak (right hand side of the peak) elimination dominates.

2. Time to Reach Peak Concentration (t_{max})

Time to reach peak concentration (t_{max}) is the time required to reach peak plasma concentration (C_{max}), t_{max} is generally expressed in hours. It is an indicator of onset of action.

3. Area Under the Curve (AUC)

Area under the curve (AUC) is generally used to express the bioavailability. AUC is the area under the plasma drug concentration-time profile. AUC represents the amount of drug that enters systemic circulation. AUC is generally expressed as ng/ml·hr or μg/ml·hr AUC is an important parameter in bioequivalence studies.

6.3 ORDERS OF PROCESSES

Processes may be zero order, first order, second order etc. Order depends on the number of variables which determine the rate of reaction. In pharmacokinetics, zero order and first order play an important role and will be discussed here.

6.3.1 Zero Order Kinetics

Zero order kinetics (or process or reaction) is independent of drug concentration. Thus rate of process or reaction can not be altered by altering the concentration of the drug.

The equation describing zero order kinetics is–

$$\frac{dc}{dt} = -K_o \cdot C^o \qquad \qquad ...6.1$$

Thus, $\qquad dc = -K_o \cdot dt \ (A_S \ C^o = 1) \qquad ...6.2$

By integrating equation 6.2 we will get

$$C - C_0 = -K_0 \cdot t$$

Hence $\qquad C = C_0 - K_0 \cdot t \qquad\qquad ...6.3$

where,

K_0 = Zero order rate constant (mg/min)
C_0 = Initial drug concentration
C = Concentration of drug at time t

> *Note: Zero order kinetics is usually seen when reaction system (e.g. enzyme or transport system) is saturated i.e. concentration of drug is in excess of saturating concentration.*

For zero order kinetics, plot of C against t will yield a straight line and a plot of log C against t will yield a curved line.

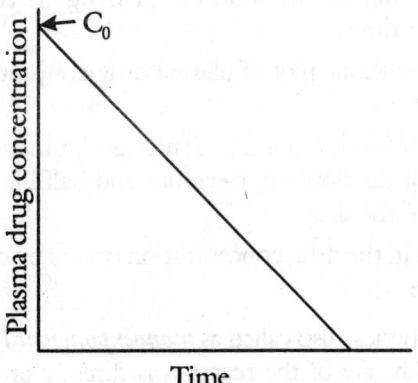

Fig. 6.2. Zero order kinetics (*Slope of the line* = K_0)

As the zero order process continues, concentration will fall. Half-life is the time required for plasma drug concentration to decrease by one half or 50 % i.e.

when $t = t_{1/2}$.

Equation 6.3 can be represented as

$$\frac{C_0}{2} = C_0 - K_0 \cdot t_{1/2}$$

Thus, $t_{1/2} = \dfrac{C_0}{2 \cdot K_0}$ ...6.4

Thus $t_{1/2}$ for zero order kinetics is proportional to C_0.

Following are some of the examples of zero order kinetics.

➤ Conversion of ethanol to acetaldehyde by alcohol dehydro-genase

➤ Metabolism of phenytoin

➤ Elimination of salicylates

➤ Tubular secretion of many drugs

➤ Constant rate IV infusion

➤ Metabolism or enzyme or transport rates under saturated conditions

6.3.2 First Order Kinetics

Following are the characteristics of the first order kinetic processes:

♦ Rate of drug elimination at particular time is directly proportional to the amount of drug in the body at that particular time

♦ Semi logarithmic plot of plasma drug concentration Vs time is a straight line

♦ Pharmacokinetic parameters such as elimination rate constant, volume of distribution, clearance and half life are independent of dose of the drug

♦ Decrease in the drug concentration occurs by constant fraction/ unit time.

First order kinetics, also called as *monoexponential* rate kinetics, is a reaction in which rate of the reaction is directly proportional to the concentration of the drug in the reaction.

For first order kinetics, the change in drug concentration based on time can be expressed as:

$$C = C_0 \cdot e^{-K \cdot t} \qquad \ldots 6.5$$

Where,

C = Concentration at time t
C_0 = Initial concentration
K = Rate constant
t = Time
e = Natural (Naperian) log base

For a diffusion process, K depends on temperature, mobility and permeability.

From equation 6.5 it is apparent that C approaches zero as t approaches infinity. The -ve sign of K in equation 6.5 indicates that concentration decreases as time increases.

The equation 6.5 can be expressed as

$$\log C = \log C_0 - \frac{K \cdot t}{2.303}$$

or

$$\log C = \log C_0 - 0.434 \cdot K \cdot t \qquad \ldots 6.6$$

This is a useful equation as graph plot is in the straight-line form (Fig. 6.3). Thus, extrapolation for the estimation of C_0 is easier and K also can be determined (Slope of the line is $-\dfrac{K}{2.303}$).

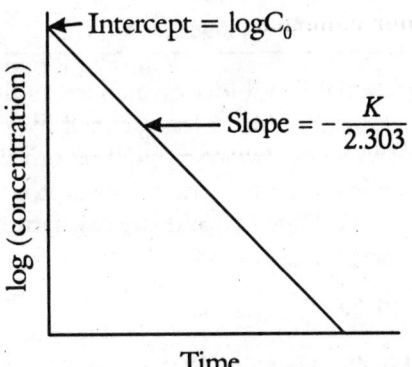

Fig. 6.3. Plot of log concentration versus time for a first order process

It is apparent from Fig. 6.3 that in first order kinetics constant fraction of concentration changes per unit time (unit of K is t^{-1}).

Most commonly used way of expressing rate of change in concentration is half life. Half life is the time required for the concentration to fall to $C_0/2$. It is important to note that *half-life* for a first order process is constant throughout the process and theoretically it never reaches completion. Even at very low concentration change in concentration would be half its value in one half-life.

For all practical purposes, a first order process is considered to be 'complete' if it is more than 95% complete. Hence elimination can be considered to be complete after six half lives have been completed i.e. 98% completion (Table 6.1)

Table 6.1: First order process completeness with increasing half-life

Number of half lives completed	Initial concentration (%)	% completion of process
0	100.00	0.00
1	50.00	50.00
2	25.00	75.00
3	12.50	87.50
4	6.25	93.75
5	3.13	96.87
6	1.56	98.44
7	0.78	99.22
8	0.39	99.61
9	0.195	99.81
10	0.098	99.90

Hence in bioavailability/bioequivalence studies blood sample collection is generally done till at least six half lives are complete.

The half life plays an important role in first order kinetics. Because half-life can be converted to a rate constant or vice versa. The relationship between half life ($t_{1/2}$) and rate constant (K) can be derived as explained below.

Recall equation 6.6

$$\log C = \log C_0 - \frac{K \cdot t}{2.303}$$

or

$$\log \frac{C_0}{C} = \frac{K \cdot t}{2.303}$$

When $t = t_{1/2}$ then $\frac{C_0}{C} = 2$. Hence

$$\log 2 = \frac{K \cdot t_{1/2}}{2.303}$$

$$0.3 = \frac{K \cdot t_{1/2}}{2.303}$$

$$K \cdot t_{1/2} = 0.6909$$

$$t_{1/2} = \frac{0.6909}{K} \qquad \ldots 6.7$$

Generally absorption, distribution and elimination of the drug follow first order kinetics. Radioactive decay is also an example of first order process.

6.3.3 Mixed Order Kinetics

Mixed order kinetics is also termed as *nonlinear kinetics or dose dependent kinetics*. Mixed order kinetics is generally described by *Michaelis Menten Equation*.

Kinetics of most drugs can be satisfactorily explained by first order or zero order kinetics. Some drugs show mixture of first order and zero order kinetics, hence they are considered to follow mixed order kinetics. For example, absorption of ascorbic acid, distribution of naproxen and elimination of riboflavin.

The details of mixed order kinetics will be discussed in Chapter 9.

6.4 PHARMACOKINETIC MODELS

Study of handling of drugs by the body is quite difficult because of the complexities of human anatomy and physiology. Pharmacokinetic models are useful in studying the time course of drug throughout the body.

In pharmacokinetic models, body is considered to be composed of various compartments. It is important to remember that these are not physiologic or anatomic compartments but are virtual or imaginary compartments. One of these compartments is central compartment. This central compartment represents plasma and tissues, which rapidly equilibrate with drugs. The central compartment can be connected to one or more peripheral compartments, which slowly equilibrate with the drugs. It is important to note that the number and size of compartments are determined by the perfusion of the tissues and the organs and by the physicochemical properties of the drug.

In a way, each cell is a small compartment. In pharmacokinetics a compartment means—organs and tissues for which the rates of uptake and subsequent clearance of a drug is similar.

Individual pharmacokinetic models will be discussed in detail in subsequent chapters.

6.5 LAPLACE TRANSFORMATION

The rate equations in previous sections for zero order and first order kinetics are linear equations. The Laplace transformation is generally used for solving linear differential equations. In Laplace transformation Laplace Operator-S replaces time domain of rate expression. Because of Laplace transformation complicated rate expression can be manipulated easily by conventional algebric techniques. By Laplace transformations solutions to differential equations can be found by relatively simple method of algebra by transforming differential equations into algebric equations.

Definition of Laplace transformation is as follows:

$$Lf(t) = \int_0^\infty e^{St} \cdot f(t) \cdot dt$$

where $f(t)$ is time dependent function

Let us see some examples.

i. Transformation of Constant A

The constant is multiplied by e^{-St} and this product is evaluated by integration from time zero to time infinity.

$$L(A) = \int_0^\infty A \cdot e^{-St} \cdot dt$$

$$= A \int_0^\infty e^{-St} \cdot dt$$

$$= A \left[\frac{e^{-St}}{-S} \right]_0^\infty$$

$$= A \left[\frac{e^{-\infty}}{-S} - \frac{e^o}{-S} \right]$$

$$= A \left[0 - \frac{1}{-S} \right]$$

$$= A\left[\frac{1}{S}\right]$$

$$\boxed{L(A) = \frac{A}{S}}$$

ii. Transformation of e^{-at}

Similarly, transformation of exponential function can also be done. Thus, applying Laplace integral for the function e^{-at}:

$$\boxed{L(e^{-at}) = \int_0^\infty e^{-St} \cdot e^{-at} \cdot dt}$$

$$= \int_0^\infty e^{-St-at} \cdot dt$$

$$= \int_0^\infty e^{-(S+a)\cdot t} \cdot dt$$

$$= \left[\frac{e^{-(S+a)\cdot t}}{-(S+a)}\right]_0^\infty$$

$$= \left[0 - \frac{e^0}{-(S+a)}\right]$$

$$\boxed{L(e^{-at}) = \frac{1}{S+a}}$$

iii. Transformation of A.e^{-at}

Suppose the function e^{-at} was multiplied by a constant A, then applying Laplace transformation we will get:

$$\boxed{L(A \cdot e^{-at}) = \int_0^\infty A \cdot e^{-St} \cdot e^{-at} \cdot dt}$$

$$= A\int_0^\infty e^{-St-at} dt$$

$$= A\int_0^\infty e^{-(S+a)\cdot t} \cdot dt$$

$$= A\left[\frac{e^{-(S+a)\cdot t}}{-(S+a)}\right]_0^\infty$$

$$= A\left[0 - \frac{e^0}{-(S + a)}\right]$$

$$\boxed{L(A \cdot e^{-at}) = \frac{A}{S + a}}$$

iv. Transformation of $\dfrac{df(t)}{dt}$

In pharmacokinetics derivative expression $\left(\dfrac{df(t)}{dt}\right)$ is used quite often.

Laplace integral for this expression will be:

$$\boxed{L\left(\frac{df(t)}{dt}\right) = \int_0^\infty e^{-St} \cdot \frac{df(t)}{dt} \cdot dt}$$

By using

$$= \int_a^b h(x) \cdot \frac{dg(x)}{dx} \cdot dx$$

$$= \left[h(x) \cdot g(x)\right]_a^b - \int_a^b \frac{dh(x)}{dx} \cdot g(x) \cdot dx$$

$$\therefore \quad \int_0^\infty e^{-St} \cdot \frac{df(t)}{dt} dt = \left[e^{-St} \cdot f(t)\right]_0^\infty - \int_0^\infty \frac{de^{-St}}{dt} \cdot f(t) \cdot dt$$

$$= \left[0 - e^0 \cdot f(0)\right] - \int_0^\infty \frac{de^{-St}}{dt} \cdot f(t) \cdot dt$$

$$= -f(0) - \int_0^\infty -S \cdot e^{-St} \cdot f(t) \cdot dt$$

$$= -f(0) + \int_0^\infty S \cdot e^{-St} \cdot f(t) \cdot dt$$

$$= -f(0) + \int_0^\infty e^{-St} \cdot Sf(t) \cdot dt$$

$$= -f(0) + L[Sf(t)]$$

(Using definition of Laplace transformation)

$$L\left(\frac{df(t)}{dt}\right) = SLf(t) - f(0)$$

where $f(t)$ is the time dependent function of interest e.g. concentration (C) and $\frac{df(t)}{dt}$ is the derivative of this function. For example, $\frac{dc}{dt}$, and $f(0)$ is the value of $f(t)$ at time zero e.g. initial concentration.

v. Transformation of A.t.e^{-at}

$$L(A \cdot t \cdot e^{-at}) = \int_0^\infty e^{-St} \cdot A \cdot t \cdot e^{-at} \cdot dt$$

$$= A\int_0^\infty e^{-St-at} \cdot t \cdot dt$$

$$= A\int_0^\infty e^{-(S+a)t} \cdot t \cdot dt$$

$$= A\int_0^\infty t \cdot e^{-(S+a)t} \cdot dt$$

$$= A\left[t \cdot \int_0^\infty e^{-(S+a)t} \cdot dt - \int_0^\infty \left\{\int_0^\infty e^{-(S+a)t} \cdot dt \frac{d}{dt}(t)\right\}dt\right]$$

$$= A\left[\left[t \cdot \frac{e^{-(S+a)\cdot t}}{-(S+a)}\right]_0^\infty - \int_0^\infty \frac{e^{-(s+a)\cdot t}}{-(S+a)} \cdot 1 \cdot dt\right]$$

$$= A\left[[0-0] + \int_0^\infty \frac{e^{-(s+a)\cdot t}}{S+a} \cdot dt\right]$$

$$= A\left[0 + \frac{e^{-(s+a)\cdot t}}{-(S+a)(S+a)}\right]_0^\infty$$

$$= A\left[0 + \frac{e^{-(s+a)\cdot t}}{-(S+a)^2}\right]_0^\infty$$

$$= A\left[-\frac{e^{-(s+a)\cdot t}}{(S+a)^2}\right]_0^\infty$$

$$= A\left[-0 + \frac{e^0}{(S+a)^2}\right]$$

$$\boxed{L(A\cdot t\cdot e^{-at}) = A\left[\frac{1}{(S+a)^2}\right] = \frac{A}{(S+a)^2}}$$

vi. Transformation of $\frac{1}{a}(1-e^{-at})$

$$\boxed{L\left(\frac{1}{a}(1-e^{-at})\right) = \int_0^\infty e^{-St}\cdot\frac{1}{a}(1-e^{-at})\cdot dt}$$

$$= \frac{1}{a}\int_0^\infty e^{-St}\cdot(1-e^{-at})\cdot dt$$

$$= \frac{1}{a}\int_0^\infty (e^{-St} - e^{-St}\cdot e^{-at})dt$$

$$= \frac{1}{a}\int_0^\infty (e^{-St} - e^{-(S+a)t})dt$$

$$= \frac{1}{a}\int_0^\infty e^{-St}\cdot dt - \frac{1}{a}\int_0^\infty e^{-(S+a)t}\cdot dt$$

$$= \frac{1}{a}\left[\frac{e^{-St}}{-S}\right]_0^\infty - \frac{1}{a}\left[\frac{e^{-(S+a)t}}{-(S+a)}\right]_0^\infty$$

$$= \frac{1}{a}\left[0 - \frac{e^0}{-S}\right] - \frac{1}{a}\left[0 - \frac{e^0}{-(S+a)}\right]$$

$$= \frac{1}{a}\left[0 + \frac{1}{S}\right] - \frac{1}{a}\left[0 + \frac{1}{(S+a)}\right]$$

$$= \frac{1}{aS} - \frac{1}{a(S+a)}$$

$$= \frac{a(s+a) - as}{as \cdot a(s+a)}$$

$$= \frac{as + a^2 - as}{a^2 s(s+a)}$$

$$= \frac{a^2}{a^2 S(S+a)}$$

$$\boxed{L\left(\frac{1}{a}(1 - e^{-at})\right) = \frac{1}{S(S+a)}}$$

Laplace transforms of some of the important functions are shown in Table 6.2.

Table 6.2: Laplace transforms of some functions

Functions, f(t)	Laplace transforms, (fs)
1	$\dfrac{1}{S}$
A	$\dfrac{A}{S}$
t	$\dfrac{1}{S^2}$
t^m	$\dfrac{m!}{S^{m+1}}$
e^{-at}	$\dfrac{1}{S+a}$
Ae^{-at}	$\dfrac{A}{S+a}$
Ate^{-at}	$\dfrac{A}{(S+a)^2}$
$\dfrac{1}{a}(1 - e^{-at})$	$\dfrac{1}{S(S+a)}$
$\dfrac{A}{a}(1 - e^{-at})$	$\dfrac{A}{S(S+a)}$
$\dfrac{A}{a}e^{-\left(\frac{b}{a}\right) \cdot t}$	$\dfrac{A}{as+b}$
$\dfrac{(B-Aa)e^{-at} - (B-Ab)e^{-bt}}{b-a}(b \neq a)$	$\dfrac{AS+B}{(S+a)(S+b)}$

Functions, f(t)	Laplace transforms, (fs)
$e^{-at}[A + (B - Aa)t]$	$\dfrac{AS + B}{(S + a)^2}$
$\dfrac{1}{b - a}\left(e^{-at} - e^{-bt}\right)$	$\dfrac{1}{(S + a)(S + b)}$
$\dfrac{A}{b - a}\left(e^{-at} - e^{-bt}\right)$	$\dfrac{A}{(S + a)(S + b)}$
$\dfrac{1}{a}t - \dfrac{1}{a^2}\left(1 - e^{-at}\right)$	$\dfrac{1}{S^2(S + a)}$
$\dfrac{A}{a}t - \dfrac{A}{a^2}\left(1 - e^{-at}\right)$	$\dfrac{A}{S^2(S + a)}$
$\dfrac{B}{ab} - \dfrac{Aa - B}{a(a - b)}e^{-at} + \dfrac{Ab - B}{b(a - b)}e^{-bt}$	$\dfrac{(AS + B)}{S(S + a)(S + b)}$
$\dfrac{B}{ab} - \dfrac{a^2 - Aa + B}{a(b - a)}e^{-at} + \dfrac{b^2 - Ab - B}{b(b - a)}e^{-bt}$	$\dfrac{(S^2 + AS + B)}{S(S + a)(S + b)}$
$\dfrac{1}{ab} + \dfrac{1}{a(a - b)}e^{-at} - \dfrac{1}{b(a - b)}e^{-bt}$	$\dfrac{1}{S(S + a)(S + b)}$
$A\left(\dfrac{1}{ab} + \dfrac{1}{a(a - b)}e^{-at} - \dfrac{1}{b(a - b)}e^{-bt}\right)$	$\dfrac{A}{S(S + a)(S + b)}$
$\dfrac{1}{t}(e^{bt} - e^{at})$	$\log\dfrac{S - a}{S - b}$
$\sin bt$	$\dfrac{b}{S^2 + b^2}$
$\cos bt$	$\dfrac{S}{S(S^2 + b^2)}$

QUESTIONS

1. Explain zero order process
2. Explain first order process
3. Explain drug concentration-time profile and define
    (a) C_{max}
    (b) T_{max}
    (c) AUC
4. What is Laplace transformation? Give Laplace transformation of
    (a) Constant A
    (b) e^{-at}
    (c) $A \cdot t \cdot e^{-at}$
5. Write note on:
    (a) Half-life
    (b) Pharmacokinetic models.

7 One Compartment Model

7.1 INTRODUCTION

The one compartment model is the simplest model and considers body as a single homogeneous unit. One compartment model describes the pharmacokinetics of drugs which rapidly equilibrate or distribute evenly between blood and various tissues. This does not mean that drug concentration is same throughout the body. Rather it is assumed that changes in drug concentration in blood (more practically plasma drug concentration) reflect proportional (quantitative) changes in drug concentration throughout the body.

Some times term open (open one compartment model) is used. The term open means that input (intake or administration from any route) and output (elimination by any or all route) are unidirectional (Fig. 7.1).

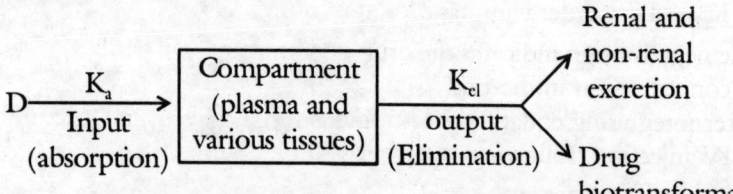

Fig. 7.1. Schematic representation of open one compartment model. (D-Drug, K_a-absorption rate constant, K_{el}-elimination rate constant).

7.2 INTRAVENOUS INJECTION

When drug is administered intravenously (IV), there is no absorption phase and hence peak plasma concentration and distribution occur very rapidly (Fig. 7.2).

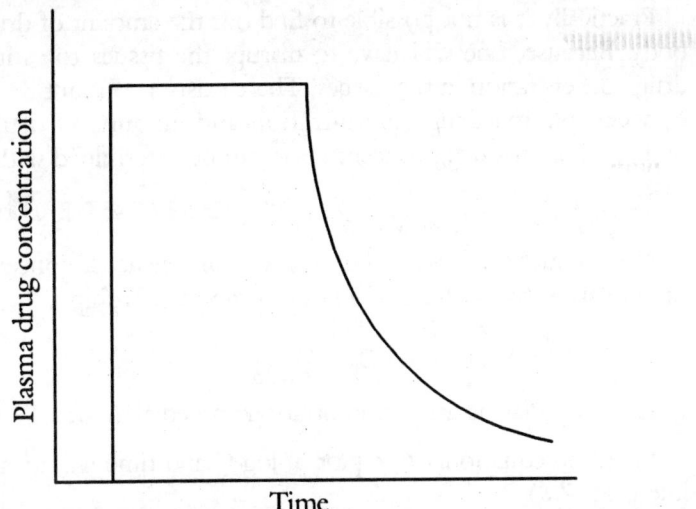

Fig. 7.2. Plasma drug concentration time curve for intravenous injection

As there is no absorption phase, rate of change in drug concentration can be given as:

$$\frac{dx}{dt} = -\text{rate output} \qquad \qquad ...7.1$$

$$\frac{dx}{dt} = -K_{el} \cdot X$$

where,

X = amount of drug in the body at time t after IV injection.

K_{el} = First order elimination rate constant.

The negative sign indicates the drug is being lost from the body i.e. drug concentration in the body is decreasing.

After integrating equation 7.1 to find out the time course of drug after IV injection, following equation will be obtained

$$X = X_0 \cdot e^{-K_{el} \cdot t} \qquad \qquad ...7.2$$

Where, X_0 = Dose of the drug i.e. total amount of drug injected

The logarithmic transformation will give

$$\ln X = \ln X_0 - K_{el} \cdot t \qquad \qquad ...7.3$$

Converting natural logarithm to common logarithm:

$$\log X = \log X_0 - \frac{K_{el} \cdot t}{2.303} \qquad \qquad ...7.4$$

Practically it is not possible to find out the amount of drug in the body. Because, one will have to disrupt the tissues to estimate the drug concentration in the tissues. There exists a constant relationship between plasma drug concentration and amount of drug in the body and plasma drug concentration can be determined with relative ease.

$$X = V_d \cdot C \qquad \qquad ...7.5$$

Now, equation 7.4 can be expressed in terms of concentration-time-relationship instead of amount time relationship

$$\log C = \log C_0 - \frac{K_{el} \cdot t}{2.303} \qquad \qquad ...7.6$$

where, C_0 = Plasma drug concentration immediately after IV injection

Based on equation 7.6, a plot of log C and time will be a straight line (Fig. 7.3)

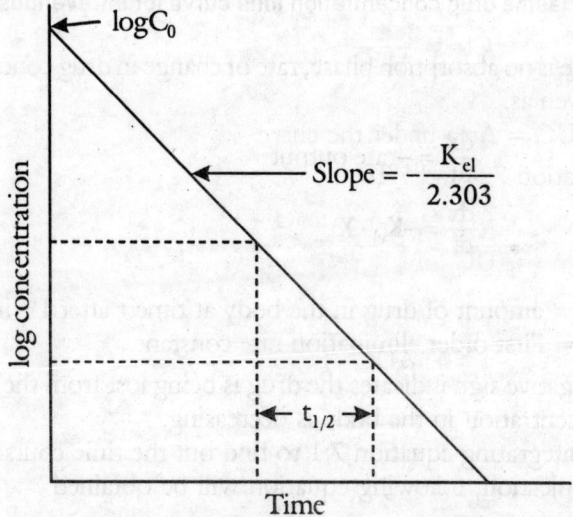

Fig. 7.3. Graphical representation of one compartment kinetics

C_0 can be estimated (log C_0) by extrapolation of the line. As the dose of drug (X) is known, V_d can be calculated by equation 7.5.

K_{el} can be easily determined as slope of the line $= -\dfrac{K_{el}}{2.303}$. K_{el} also can be calculated from the following equation

$$K_{el} = \frac{0.693}{t_{1/2}} \qquad ...7.7$$

(For derivation of equation 7.7 please refer to previous chapter)
where,

$t_{1/2}$ = biological or elimination half life.

Elimination half life of a drug is a function of various factors such as distribution, metabolism and elimination. Hence clearance is a better function than half life for the expression of elimination of drug.

$$Cl_T = K_{el} \cdot V_d \qquad ...7.8$$

where,

$$Cl_T = \text{Total body clearance}$$

or

$$Cl_T = \left(\frac{0.693}{t_{1/2}}\right) \cdot V_d \qquad 7.9$$

Total clearance in one compartment system is

$$Cl_T = \frac{X}{AUC} \qquad ...7.10$$

where,

AUC = Area under the curve

From equation 7.9 and 7.10

$$\frac{X}{AUC} = \left(\frac{0.693}{t_{1/2}}\right) \cdot V_d$$

or

$$V_d = \frac{X \cdot t_{1/2}}{AUC \cdot 0.693}$$

or

$$V_d = \frac{X}{AUC \cdot K_{el}} \qquad ...7.11$$

7.2.1 Urinary Excretion

Urinary excretion data, assuming that at least some fraction of the drug is excreted unchanged in the urine, can be used for studying excretion kinetics.

(*Please review "renal excretion" from the chapter "Excretion"*)

Rate of filtration of drug by glomerular filtration depends upon plasma drug concentration. Glomerular filtration rate (GFR) is more or less constant. Thus,

$$F = C_{pf} \cdot GFR \qquad \qquad ...7.12$$

where,

F = Filtration rate of the drug

C_{pf} = Amount of free drug in plasma

Equation 7.12 can be expressed as

$$F = [C_p (1 - P) \quad GFR] \qquad ...7.13$$

where,

P = Fraction of drug bound to plasma protein.

As discussed previously, creatinine and inulin are used to determine the GFR, because creatinine and inulin are neither secreted nor reabsorbed. As the definition of clearance is "volume of plasma cleared of drug per unit time", the renal clearance can be expressed as

$$Cl_{ren} = \frac{C'_u \cdot V}{C_p \cdot t} \qquad \qquad ...7.14$$

where,

Cl_{ren} = Renal clearance (ml/min).

C'_u = Drug concentration in urine (mg/ml).

t = Time for which urine was collected (min).

V = Urine volume collected during time t (ml).

C_p = Plasma drug concentration (mg/ml).

Clearance will vary according to nature of the drug:

(*i*) For drugs which are filtered but are not reabsorbed or secreted, the excretion ratio will be one and clearance will be 125 ml/min (125 ml/min is GFR)

(*ii*) For drugs which show reabsorption, obviously excretion ratio will be less than one and clearance will be less than 125 ml/min.

(*iii*) For drugs which show tubular secretion, excretion ratio will be more than one and clearance will be much higher than 125 ml/min.

Concept of *hepatic clearance* is more or less similar to renal clearance. Thus hepatic clearance is volume of blood (plasma) cleared of drug per unit time. Hence, hepatic clearance can be expressed as:

$$Cl_H = HBF \cdot \left(\frac{C_{ap} - C_V}{C_{ap}} \right) = HBF \cdot E \qquad ...7.15$$

where,

Cl_H = Hepatic clearance.

HBF = Hepatic blood flow (addition of both portal venous and hepatic arterial blood).

C_{ap} = Mean drug concentration of portal venous and hepatic arterial blood.

C_V = Hepatic venous concentration.

In these circumstances,

$$(E) \text{ Extration ratio} = \frac{C_{ap} - C_V}{C_{ap}}$$

The maximum clearance in the presence of normal hepatic blood flow is called as *total intrinsic clearance* (Cl_{intr}).

The extraction ratio can be expressed as—

$$E = \frac{Cl_{intr}}{HBF + Cl_{intr}}$$

The equation 7.15 can be rewritten as—

$$Cl_H = \left(\frac{Cl_{intr}}{HBF + Cl_{intr}} \right) HBF = HBF \cdot E \qquad ...7.16$$

And intrinsic clearance can be written as—

$$Cl_{intr} = \frac{HBF \cdot E}{1 - E} \qquad ...7.17$$

From above it is clear that hepatic clearance and extraction are function of hepatic blood flow and metabolizing capacity of liver enzymes.

Cl_{intr} can be estimated by following equation

$$Cl_{intr} = \frac{\left(1 - \frac{D_{un}}{f \cdot D}\right) \cdot D}{AUC_0} \qquad ...7.18$$

where,

D_{un} = Total quantity of drug excreted unchanged.

f = Fraction of drug absorbed.

D = Dose of the drug administered.

AUC_0 = Total area under the plasma drug concentration time curve.

Area under the curve (AUC) can be calculated by various methods. To get more accurate determination of AUC it is necessary to collect adequate number of blood samples. Recall that for first order kinetics blood collection till six half lives will provide information about 98% of the process or reaction.

Following are the methods, which can be used to estimate AUC.

(1) **Planimeter:** Planimeter is an instrument for mechanically measuring the area of plane figures that are drawn on rectilinear graph paper.

(2) **Cut and Weigh Method:** Cut the total area under the curve on rectilinear graph paper and accurately weigh it on analytical balance. This total weight is then divided by weight of the unit area of the same paper.

(3) **Trapezoidal Rule:** In brief, the plasma drug concentration time curve is expressed as a series of straight lines, and thus AUC is divided into trapezoids. Area of trapezoid is easy to calculate, and sum of all trapezoidal areas will give true area under the curve (Fig. 7.4).

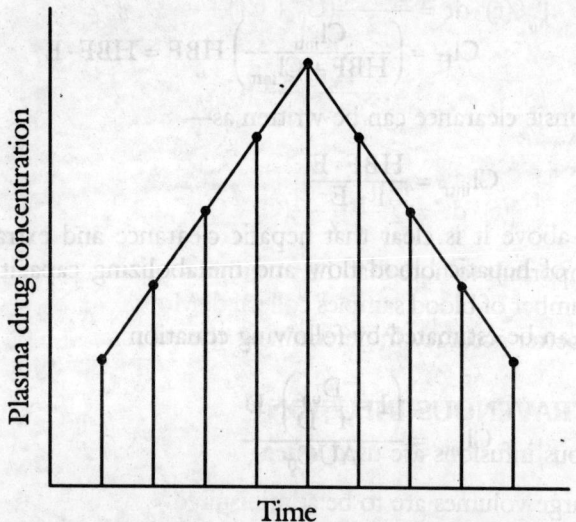

Fig. 7.4. Graphical representation for linear trapezoidal method to estimate AUC

Let us assume that f (t) is a function which describes plasma drug concentration time curve. θ (t) is another function and is linear between two successive plasma drug level time points.

The AUC expressed by $\theta(t)\left(\int_{t_0}^{t_n}\theta(t)\cdot dt\right)$ will be approximately $\int_{t_0}^{t_n}f(t)\cdot dt$

The integral $\int_{t_0}^{t_n}\theta(t)$ is expressed as the sum of total number of trapezoids into which curve is divided (n). Hence,

$$\int_{t_0}^{t_n}\theta(t)\cdot dt = \int_{t_0}^{t_1}\theta(t)\cdot dt + \int_{t_1}^{t_2}\theta(t)\cdot dt...+\int_{t_{n-1}}^{t_n}\theta(t)\cdot dt \quad ...7.19$$

Since it's an area of trapezoid

$$\int_{t_0}^{t_1}\theta(t)\cdot dt = \frac{t_1 - t_0}{2}(C_0 + C_1) \quad ...7.20$$

where,
C_0 and C_1 = Plasma drug concentration at time t_0 and t_1. Similarly,

$$\int_{t_{n-1}}^{t_n}\theta(t)\cdot dt = \frac{t_n - t_{n-1}}{2}(C_{n-1} + C_n) \quad ...7.21$$

Based on equation 7.20 and 7.21; equation 7.19 can be expressed as

$$\int_{t_0}^{t_n}\theta(t)\cdot dt = \frac{t_1 - t_0}{2}(C_0 + C_1) + \frac{t_2 - t_1}{2}(C_1 + C_2)$$

$$...+ \frac{t_n - t_{n-1}}{2}(C_{n-1} + C_n) \quad ...7.22$$

Thus,

$$\int_{t_0}^{t_n}\theta(t)\cdot dt = \sum_{i=0}^{n-1}\frac{t_{i+1} - t_i}{2}(C_i + C_{i+1}) \quad ...7.23$$

It is important to note that the true representation of AUC depends on the number of blood samples collected. More the number of blood samples better accuracy in determining the AUC.

7.3 INTRAVENOUS INFUSION
Intravenous infusions are used when–

➢ Large volumes are to be administered.
➢ Drug has narrow therapeutic range and large fluctuations in plasma concentrations are not desirable.
➢ Drug action is required for longer period.

Note that in case of IV infusion the input of the drug is at a constant rate i.e. zero order kinetics.

Intravenous infusion can be represented by following model:

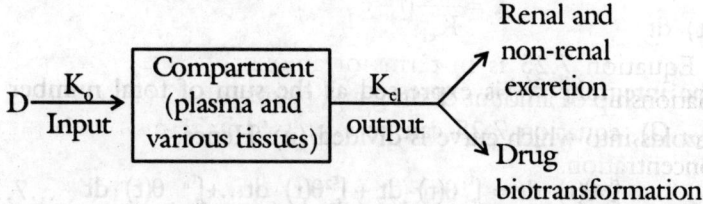

Like in case of IV injection, the concentration of drug is zero in the body at the time of starting infusion. Plasma drug concentration will slowly increase with time and reach a steady state level (plateau). At steady state level (C_{ss}) rate of input of drug i.e. rate of infusion, will be equal to rate of elimination. The plasma drug concentration will start decreasing as soon as infusion is stopped (Fig. 7.5)

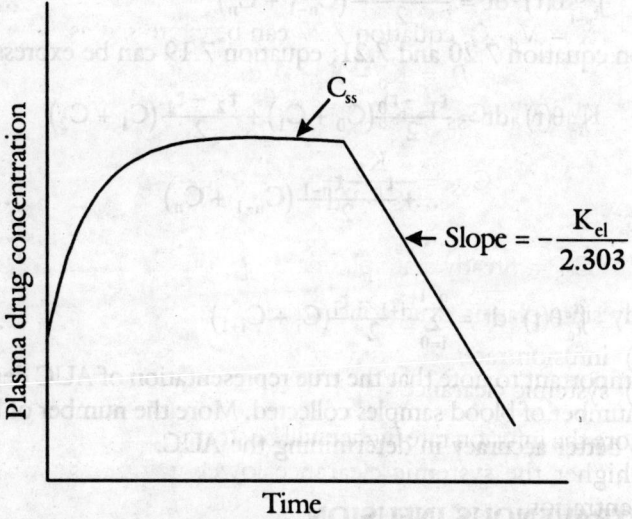

Fig. 7.5. Graphical representation of plasma drug concentration (log scale) versus time for IV infusion (C_{ss} -steady state).

The change in amount of drug with time for IV infusion can be represented as—

$$\frac{dx}{dt} = K_0 - K_{el} \cdot X \qquad \qquad ...7.24$$

where,

K_0 = Rate of drug infusion.

Integrating equation 7.24—

$$X = \frac{K_0}{K_{el}}\left(1 - e^{-K_{el} \cdot t}\right) \qquad ...7.25$$

Equation 7.25 is in terms of amount of drug. Based on the relationship of amount of drug and plasma drug concentration ($X = V_d \cdot C$), equation 7.25 can be expressed in terms of plasma drug concentration.

$$C = \frac{K_0}{V_d \cdot K_{el}}\left(1 \cdot e^{-K_{el} \cdot t}\right) \qquad ...7.26$$

At steady state, there is no change in plasma drug concentration with time i.e. $\frac{dx}{dt} = 0$. Hence equation 7.24 becomes

$$0 = K_0 - K_{el} \cdot X_{SS} \qquad ...7.27$$

where,

$\qquad X_{SS}$ = Steady state amount of drug.

As $\qquad X = V_d \cdot C$, equation 7.27 can be expressed as

$$0 = K_0 - K_{el} \cdot Vd \cdot C_{SS}$$

$$K_{el} \cdot V_d \cdot C_{SS} = K_0$$

$$C_{SS} = \frac{K_0}{K_{el} \cdot Vd} \qquad ...7.28$$

where,

$\qquad C_{SS}$ = Steady state plasma drug concentration.

Steady state plasma drug concentration depends on:

(*i*) infusion rate

(*ii*) systemic clearance

More the infusion rate higher will be steady state drug concentration and higher the systemic clearance lower will be the steady state concentration.

Recall that systemic clearance is $Cl_S = V_d \cdot K_{el}$

Thus equation 7.28 can be expressed as

$$Cl_S = \frac{K_0}{C_{SS}} \qquad ...7.29$$

Elimination rate constant and half life can be calculated for IV infusion. Based on equation 7.26 and 7.28:

$$C = C_{SS}\left(1 - e^{-Kel \cdot t}\right) \qquad ...7.30$$

i.e. $\dfrac{C_{SS} - C}{C} = e^{-K_{el} \cdot t}$ ...7.31

Taking logarithm

$$\log\left(\dfrac{C_{SS} - C}{C_{SS}}\right) = -\dfrac{K_{el} \cdot t}{2.303}$$ ...7.32

Thus semi logarithmic plot of $\left(\dfrac{C_{SS} - C}{C_{SS}}\right)$ versus time will be a straight line (Fig. 7.6)

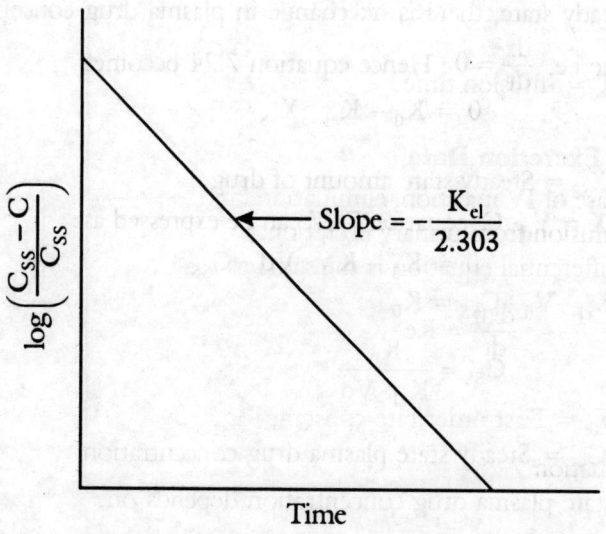

Fig. 7.6. Semi logarithmic plot of $\dfrac{C_{SS} - C}{C_{SS}}$ versus time

Slope of the line is $-\dfrac{K_{el}}{2.303}$ and thus elimination rate constant can be easily estimated. Half life can be determined by following equation:

$$t_{1/2} = \dfrac{0.693}{K_{el}}$$

Volume of distribution can also be calculated by rearranging equation 7.28, thus

$$V_d = \dfrac{K_0}{C_{SS} \cdot K_{el}}$$ ...7.33

Area under the curve is

$$AUC = \frac{K_0 \cdot T}{V_d \cdot K_{el}}$$

...7.34

Recall that $Cl_s = V_d \cdot K_{el}$

Thus,

$$Cl_S = \frac{K_0 \cdot T}{AUC}$$

...7.35

or

$$V_d = \frac{K_0 \cdot T}{K_{el} \cdot AUC}$$

where,

T = Infusion time

Urinary Excretion Data

Like in case of IV injection, elimination kinetics can also be evaluated for IV infusion from urinary excretion.

The differential equation is the same as that for IV injection

$$\frac{dxu}{dt} = Ke \cdot X$$

...7.36

where,

K_e = First order rate constant for renal excretion.

From equation 7.25

$$X = \frac{K_0}{K}\left(1 - e^{-K \cdot t}\right)$$

Substituting above equation for X in equation 7.36 and integrating

$$X_u = \frac{K_e \cdot K_0}{K} \cdot t - \frac{K_e \cdot K_0}{K^2}\left(1 - e^{-K \cdot t}\right)$$

...7.37

At steady state $e^{-Kt} \sim 0$ and hence

$$K_u = \frac{K_e \cdot K_0}{K} \cdot t - \frac{K_e \cdot K_0}{K_2}$$

...7.38

From equation 7.38 the plot of cumulative amount of drug excreted versus time will be as shown in Fig. 7.7.

Slope of the line is $\frac{K_e \cdot K_0}{K}$. Extrapolation of the straight portion of the line on X -axis will be $\frac{1}{K}$.

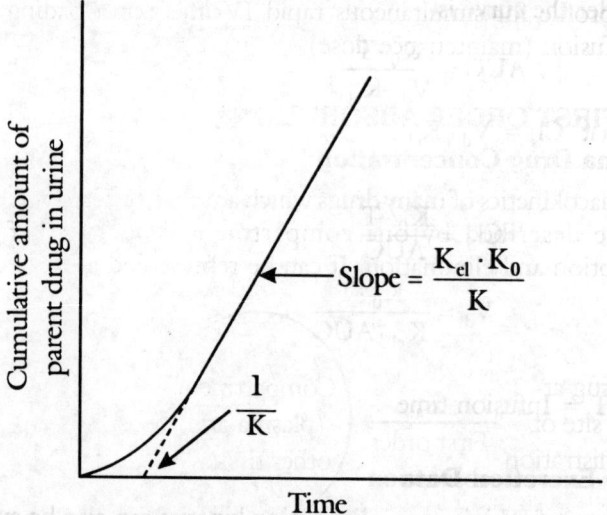

Fig. 7.7. Cumulative amount of parent drug excreted in urine versus time curve for IV infusion

7.4 LOADING AND MAINTENANCE DOSE

In case of drugs with long half lives, time required for reaching steady state is also long. To avoid this and to achieve steady state quicker, an IV *loading dose* is given to achieve desired steady state immediately after injection and is then followed by infusion to maintain the steady state.

It is important to note that, loading dose should be large enough to produce steady state concentration immediately after injection and infusion rate should be adequate to maintain the steady state. Remember that,

$$X = V_d \cdot C$$

Thus loading dose can be calculated as

$$X_{o \cdot L} = C_{SS} \cdot V_d \qquad \ldots 7.39$$

But

$$C_{SS} = \frac{K_0}{K_{el} \cdot V_d}$$

Thus,

$$X_{0 \cdot L} = \frac{K_0}{K_{el}} \qquad \ldots 7.40$$

Thus amount of drug in the body is constant throughout the drug administration. Equation 7.40 expresses plasma drug concentration time profile for simultaneous rapid IV injection (loading dose)and IV infusion (maintenance dose).

7.5 FIRST ORDER ABSORPTION

Plasma Drug Concentration

Pharmacokinetics of many drugs which are administered extravascularly can be described by one compartment model with first order absorption and elimination. It can be represented as

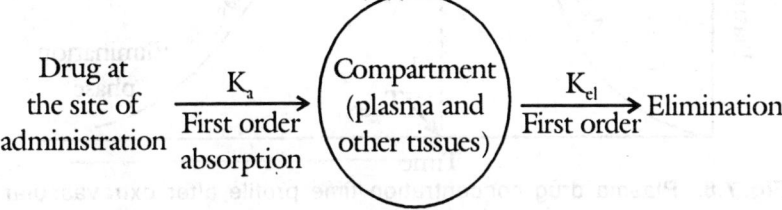

Thus, the drug enters the body by first order process, gets eliminated by first order process and gets distributed as per one compartment model.

$$\frac{dx}{dt} = K_a \cdot X_a - K_{el} \cdot X \qquad \qquad ...7.41$$

where,

K_a = First order absorption rate constant,

X_a = Amount of drug at the absorption site.

After integrating equation 7.41

$$X = \frac{K_a \cdot F \cdot X_0}{K_a - K_{el}} \cdot \left(e^{-K_{el} \cdot t} - e^{-K_a \cdot t}\right) \qquad ...7.42$$

Equation 7.42 is in terms of amount of drug, so converting it into in terms of concentration

$$C = \frac{K_a \cdot F \cdot C_0}{V_d \cdot (K_a - K_{el})} \cdot \left(e^{-K_{el} \cdot t} - e^{-K_a \cdot t}\right) \qquad ...7.43$$

where,

F = Fraction of drug absorbed.

A representative plasma drug profile after the extravascularly administration of drug is shown in Fig. 7.8

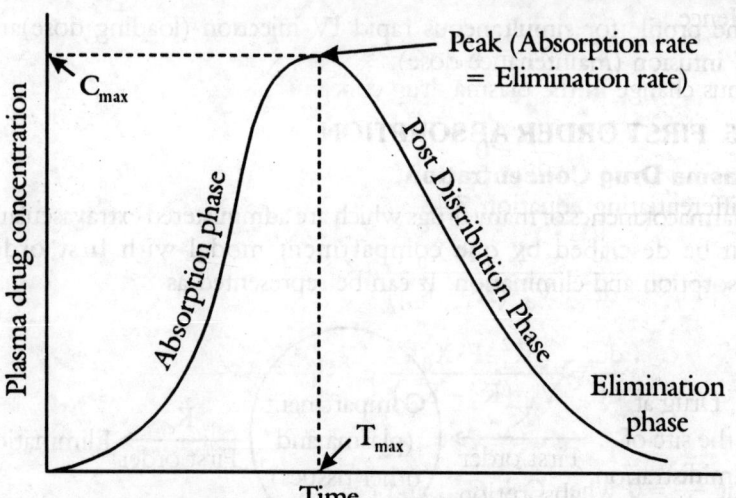

Fig. 7.8. Plasma drug concentration time profile after extravascular administration of drug

But a semi logarithmic plot of plasma drug concentration and time is a biexponential curve (Fig. 7.9)

The terminal portion of biexponential curve is linear and slope of this linear portion is $\dfrac{-K_{el}}{2.303}$.

Determination of C_{max} and T_{max}

At peak plasma concentration, rate of absorption and rate of elimination are same (Fig. 7.8).

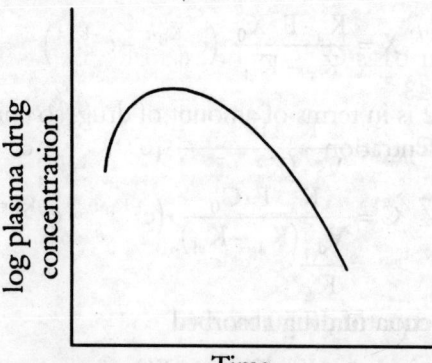

Fig. 7.9. Semi logarithmic plot of plasma drug concentration after extravascular administration of drug

Hence,

$$K_a \cdot X_a = K_{el} \cdot X$$

Thus change in the plasma drug concentration is zero, i.e.

$$\frac{dc}{dt} = 0$$

Differentiating equation 7.43

$$\frac{dc}{dt} = \frac{K_a \cdot F \cdot X_0}{V_d \cdot (K_a - K_{el})} \cdot \left(K_a \cdot e^{-K_a \cdot t} - K_{el} \cdot e^{-K_{el} \cdot t}\right) \quad ...7.44$$

i.e.

$$\frac{dc}{dt} = \frac{K_a^2 \cdot F \cdot X_0}{V_d \cdot (K_a - K_{el})} \cdot e^{-K_a \cdot t} - \frac{K_a \cdot K_{el} \cdot F \cdot X_0}{V_d \cdot (K_a - K_{el})} \cdot e^{-K_{el} \cdot t}$$

$$...7.45$$

But $\frac{dc}{dt} = 0$ when $C = C_{max}$ and $t = t_{max}$, hence

$$\frac{K_a^2 \cdot F \cdot X_0}{V_d \cdot (K_a - K_{el})} \cdot e^{-K_a \cdot t_{max}} = \frac{K_a \cdot K_{el} \cdot F \cdot X_0}{V_d \cdot (K_a - K_{el})} \cdot e^{-K_{el} \cdot t_{max}} \quad ...7.46$$

i.e.

$$\frac{K_a}{K_{el}} = \frac{e^{-K_{el} \cdot t_{max}}}{e^{-K_a \cdot t_{max}}} \quad ...7.47$$

Taking logarithm

$$t_{max} = \frac{2.303}{K_a - K_{el}} \log\left(\frac{K_a}{K_{el}}\right) \quad ...7.48$$

Equation 7.48 implies that as rate of absorption (K_a) increases, t_{max} decreases. It is obvious because $(K_a - K_{el})$ increases much more than $\log (K_a/K_{el})$.

On the similar basis C_{max} can be calculated by substituting t_{max} for t in equation 7.43

$$C_{max} = \frac{K_a \cdot F \cdot X_o}{V_d \cdot (K_a - K_{el})} \cdot \left(e^{-K_{el} \cdot t_{max}} - e^{-K_a \cdot t_{max}}\right) \quad ...7.49$$

From equation 7.47

$$e^{-K_a \cdot t_{max}} = \frac{K_{el}}{K_a} \cdot e^{-K_{el} \cdot t_{max}} \quad ...7.50$$

So substituting equation 7.50 in 7.49

$$C_{max} = \frac{K_a \cdot F \cdot X_0}{V_d \cdot (K_a - K_{el})} \cdot \frac{K_a - K_{el}}{K_a} \cdot e^{-K_{el} \cdot t_{max}} \quad ...7.51$$

But a simpler expression is

$$C_{max} = \frac{F \cdot X_0}{V_d} \cdot e^{-K_{el} \cdot t_{max}}$$ ...7.52

At C_{max} and t_{max}, $K_a = K_{el}$

Hence,

$$X = K_{el} \cdot F \cdot X_0 \cdot t \cdot e^{-K_{el} \cdot t}$$ ...7.53

$$C = \frac{K_{el} \cdot F \cdot X_0 \cdot t \cdot e^{-K_{el} \cdot t}}{V_d}$$ ...7.54

Taking logarithm

$$\log C = \log \frac{(K_{el} \cdot F \cdot X_0 \cdot t)}{V_d} - \frac{K_{el} \cdot t}{2.303}$$ ...7.55

Differentiating equation 7.54

$$\frac{dc}{dt} = \frac{K_{el} \cdot F \cdot X_o}{V_d} \cdot e^{-K_{el} \cdot t} - \frac{K_{el}^2 \cdot F \cdot X_o}{V} \cdot t \cdot e^{-K_{el} \cdot t}$$ ...7.56

At t= t_{max} and C = C_{max}

and $$\frac{dc}{dt} = 0$$

Hence

$$\frac{K_{el} \cdot F \cdot X_0}{V_d} \cdot e^{-K_{el} \cdot t_{max}} = \frac{K_{el}^2 \cdot F \cdot X_0}{V_d} \cdot t_{max} \cdot e^{-K_{el} \cdot t_{max}}$$

i.e. $$1 = K_{el} \cdot t_{max}$$

i.e. $$t_{max} = \frac{1}{K_{el}}$$ ...7.57

Now substituting t_{max} for t in equation 7.54 as per equation 7.57

$$C_{max} = \frac{F \cdot X_0}{V_d} \cdot e^{-1} = \frac{0.37 \cdot F \cdot X_0}{V_d}$$ ...7.58

Urinary Excretion

Evaluation of pharmacokinetic parameters based on urinary excretion after extravascular administration is similar to the one described for IV injection.

Remember that rate of excretion of parent drug in the urine is proportional to the amount of drug in the body. Thus excretion rate of the parent drug can be defined as:

$$\frac{dXu}{dt} = K_{el} \cdot X \qquad \qquad \ldots 7.59$$

where,

X = Amount of drug in the body.

K_{el} = Renal elimination rate constant.

Now recall equation 7.42

$$\frac{dX_u}{dt} = \frac{K_e \cdot K_a \cdot F \cdot X_0}{K_a - K_{el}} \cdot \left(e^{-K_{el} \cdot t} - e^{-K_a \cdot t}\right) \qquad \ldots 7.60$$

i.e. $X_u = \dfrac{K_{el} \cdot K_a \cdot F \cdot X_0}{K_{el}} \left(\dfrac{1}{K_a} + \dfrac{e^{-K_{el} \cdot t}}{K_{el} - K_a} - \dfrac{K_{el} \cdot e^{-K_a \cdot t}}{K_a (K_{el} - K_a)} \right) \qquad \ldots 7.61$

At time = ∞

$$X_u^{\infty} = \frac{K_e \cdot F \cdot X_0}{K_{el}} \qquad \qquad \ldots 7.62$$

Substituting equation 7.62 in equation 7.61

$$X_u^{\infty} - X_u = \frac{X_u^{\infty}}{K_a - K_{el}} \left(K_a \cdot e^{-K_{el} \cdot t} - K_e^{-K_a \cdot t}\right) \qquad \ldots 7.63$$

Note that unless the drug is slowly absorbed it is quite difficult to collect sufficient urine samples during absorption phase.

QUESTIONS

1. Explain various methods used in the determination of AUC.
2. Explain one compartmental pharmacokinetic model for intravenous infusion.
3. Explain one compartmental pharmacokinetic model for intravenous injection.
4. Explain determination of C_{max} and T_{max} after extravascular administration based on one compartment pharmacokinetic model.
5. Explain plasma drug concentration profile after extravascular administration based on one compartment model.
6. Explain urinary excretion based on one compartment model in case of intravenous injection.

8
Multicompartment Model

8.1 INTRODUCTION

Pharmacokinetics of many drugs can be satisfactorily explained by one compartment model. One compartment model is based on the assumption of very rapid distribution and changes in drug concentration are expressed as monoexponential equations. But many drugs show two or more monoexponential components.

In previous section it was assumed that the drug, once administered is mixed instantaneously in the blood and that the drug distributes throughout the body rapidly reaching equilibrium throughout the tissue into which the drug enters. In essence the body was considered to act as a well-mixed container. In most of the situations there is no instantaneous equilibrium between the drug and various tissues of the body. In the next approximation the body is considered to behave as two distinct compartments. These compartments can be called the central compartment and the peripheral compartment. Exact anatomical assignment to these compartments is not always possible. However, generally the rapidly perfused tissues often belong in the central compartment. Thus in open-two compartment model, the entire body is believed to be composed of two compartments and these compartments are in dynamic equilibrium with each other (Fig. 8.1 and 8.2)

Compartment 1 (the central compartment): This can be sampled through blood or plasma or serum. This compartment consists of tissues or organs, which are highly perfused with blood and are in rapid equilibrium distribution with the blood.

Compartment 2 (the peripheral compartment): This cannot normally be sampled. It generally consists of tissues or organs, which are poorly perfused with blood and hence are in slow equilibrium distribution with the blood.

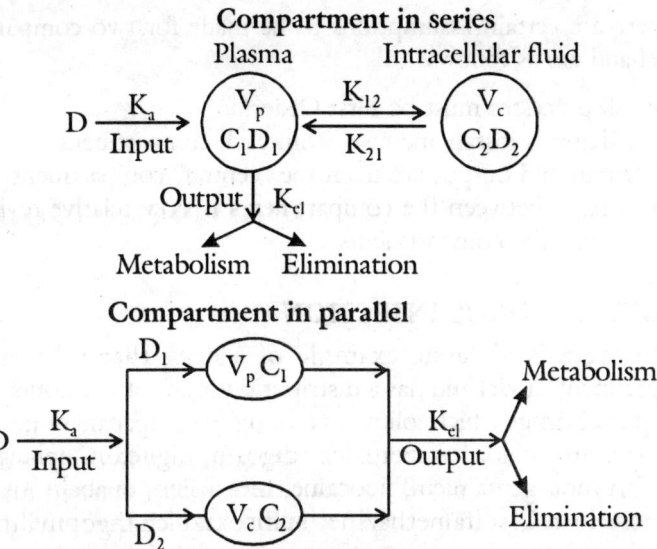

Fig. 8.1. Diagrammatic representation of open two-compartment pharmacokinetic model. (C_1-concentration in compartment 1; D_1 amount of drug in compartment 1; C_2-concentration in compartment 2; D_2-amount of drug in compartment2)

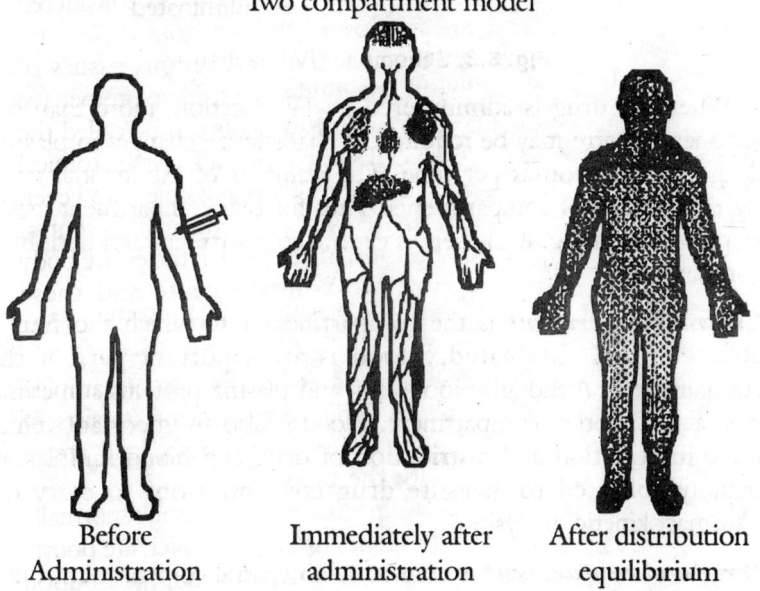

Fig. 8.2. Two compartment model—a whole body view

There are certain assumptions to be made for two compartment model and are as follows:

♦ All processes must be First Order!
♦ Mixing is instantaneous within each compartment.
♦ Input and output are from the "central" compartment.
♦ Mixing between the compartments is slow relative to mixing within the compartments.

8.2 INTRAVENOUS INJECTION

Vancomycin is a classic example of a drug that follows two-compartment model and has a distribution phase of 1-2 hours. Other examples of drugs which follow two or more compartment model are amphetamine, chlordiazeperoxide, digoxin, digitoxin, epinephrine, ethchlorvynol, gentamicin, lidocaine, mehticillin, ouabain, oxacillin, pentaerythritol, sulfamethazine, sulfisoxazole; theophylline and warfarin.

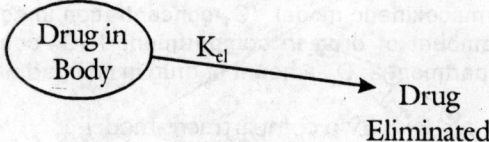

Fig. 8.3. Scheme for IV injection

When the drug is administered by IV injection, more than one exponential term may be required to characterize changes in plasma-drug concentration as per time. The numbers of exponential terms signify number of compartments. Thus for two compartment model (represented in Fig. 8.1) there is central compartment and peripheral compartment.

Central compartment is the compartment into which the drug is absorbed and eliminated. Blood is an important part of this compartment. Although blood cells and plasma proteins sometimes may act as another compartment. Blood is also an important vehicle for transportation and distribution of drug and blood samples are usually collected to measure drug concentrations to carry out pharmacokinetic analysis.

Peripheral compartment is connected to central compartment but is not the part of absorption and elimination of the drug. This compartment generally refers to poorly perfused tissues e.g. muscle, lean tissue and fat.

Thus for IV injection exhibiting two compartment models there will be two phases of change in plasma drug concentration with respect to time. In central compartment, initial decline in the drug concentration will be rapid (distributive phase) but later it will be slow (postdistributive/elimination phase). In peripheral compartment, first there will be increase in the drug concentration followed by a peak (distributive phase) and then followed by a decline in the drug concentration (postdistributive/elimination phase) (Fig. 8.4).

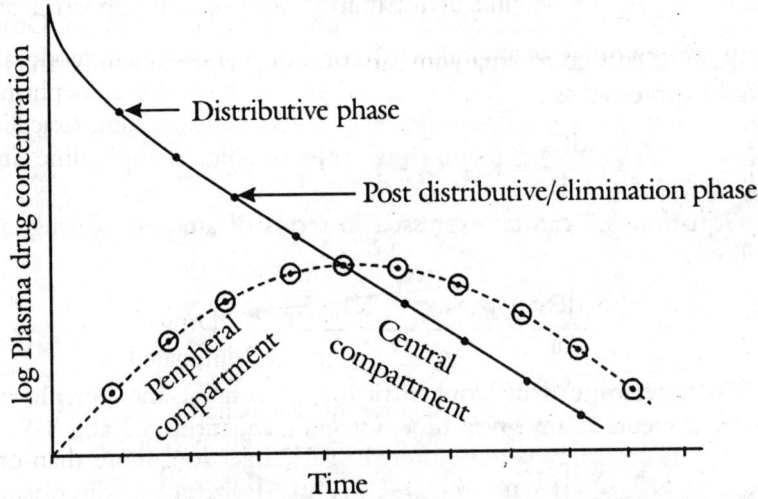

Fig. 8.4. Plasma drug concentration versus time profile after IV injection

Distribution of drug between central and peripheral compartment follows first order kinetics. Thus K_{12} and K_{21} (see Fig. 8.1) are first order rate constants.

The change in drug concentration in central compartment can be expressed as:

$$\frac{dC_c}{dt} = K_{21} \cdot C_p - K_{12} \cdot C_c - K_E \cdot C_c \qquad \ldots 8.1$$

where,

$\frac{dC_c}{dt}$ = Change in drug concentration in central compartment.

C_c = Drug concentration in central compartment.

C_p = Drug concentration in peripheral compartment.

Recall that

$$X = V_d \cdot C$$

Hence, equation 8.1 can be expressed as:

$$\frac{dC_c}{dt} = \frac{K_{21} \cdot X_p}{V_p} - \frac{K_{12} \cdot X_c}{V_c} - \frac{K_E \cdot X_c}{V_c} \qquad \ldots 8.2$$

where,

X_c = Amount of drug in central compartment.
X_p = Amount of drug in peripheral compartment.
V_c = Volume of distribution of central compartment.
V_p = Volume of distribution of peripheral compartment.

Rate of change of drug concentration in peripheral compartment can be expressed as:

$$\frac{dC_p}{dt} = K_{12} \cdot C_c - K_{21} \cdot C_p \qquad \ldots 8.3$$

Equation 8.3 can be expressed in terms of amount of drug, as follows:

$$\frac{dC_p}{dt} = \frac{K_{12} \cdot X_c}{V_c} - \frac{K_{21} \cdot X_p}{V_p} \qquad \ldots 8.4$$

To determine drug concentration in central and peripheral compartments at any given time, integrate equations 8.2 and 8.4.

$$C_c = \frac{X_0}{V_c}\left[\left(\frac{K_{21} - \alpha}{\beta - \alpha}\right) \cdot e^{-\alpha \cdot t} + \left(\frac{K_{21} - \beta}{\alpha - \beta}\right) \cdot e^{-\beta \cdot t}\right] \qquad \ldots 8.5$$

$$C_p = \frac{X_0}{V_p}\left[\left(\frac{K_{12}}{\beta - \alpha}\right) \cdot e^{-\alpha \cdot t} + \left(\frac{K_{12}}{\alpha - \beta}\right) \cdot e^{-\beta \cdot t}\right] \qquad \ldots 8.6$$

where,

X_0 = Dose of IV injection.
α = First order constant for rapid distributive phase.
β = First order constant for slow elimination phase.
α and β depends on K_{12}, K_{21} and K_E.

Figure 8.3 shows a plasma drug concentration versus time curve of a drug, which follows two-compartment system when administered by IV injection. It can be expressed by biexponential equation.

$$C = A \cdot e^{-\alpha \cdot t} + B \cdot e^{-\beta \cdot t} \qquad ...8.7$$

where,

A; B = Corresponding zero time intercepts

Equation 8.7 can be resolved into its components by *method of residuals*.

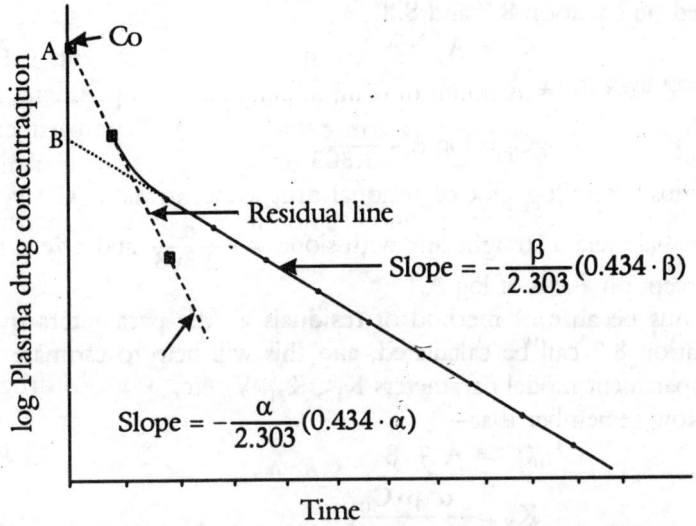

Fig. 8.5. Plasma drug concentration profile versus time after IV injection.
(□ ·························□ Indicates residual values)

Initial decline because of distribution is much more rapid compared to the later postdistributive/elimination phase. In other words, α is much larger than β. Thus $A \cdot e^{-\alpha \cdot t}$ will approach zero more rapidly than $B \cdot e^{-\beta \cdot t}$. Hence, equation 8.7 will become:

$$C' = B \cdot e^{-\beta \cdot t} \qquad ...8.8$$

Taking logarithm,

$$\log C' = \log B - \frac{\beta \cdot t}{2.303} \qquad ...8.9$$

As shown in Fig. 8.3 semilog plot of plasma drug concentration versus time will have a linear terminal phase with the slope $= -\dfrac{\beta}{2.303}$ (or $0.434 \cdot \beta$) which when extrapolated to zero yields an intercept of $\log B$.

The half-life for elimination phase will be:

$$t_{1/2} = \frac{0.693}{\beta} \qquad ...8.10$$

Substraction of the concentration-time values based on extrapolated line from the actual plasma-concentration-time values will give series of residual-concentration time values (C_r). This can be expressed as:

$$C_r = C - C' \qquad \qquad ...8.11$$

Based on equation 8.7 and 8.8

$$C_r = A \cdot e^{-\alpha \cdot t} \qquad \qquad ...8.12$$

Taking logarithm

$$\text{Log}\,C_r = \log A - \frac{\alpha \cdot t}{2.303} \qquad \qquad ...8.13$$

Thus a semilog plot of residual drug concentration (C_r) versus time will yield a straight line with slope $= -\dfrac{\alpha}{2.303}$ and a zero time intercept on Y-axis of log A.

Thus because of method of residuals all the parameters in the equation 8.7 can be calculated, and this will help to estimate two compartment model parameters K_{12}, K_{21}, V_d etc.

Now remember that—

$$C_0 = A + B \qquad \qquad ...8.14$$

$$K_E = \frac{\alpha \cdot \beta \cdot C_0}{A \cdot \beta + B \cdot \alpha} \qquad \qquad ...8.15$$

$$K_{12} = \frac{A \cdot B + (\beta - \alpha)^2}{C_0(A \cdot \beta + B \cdot \alpha)} \qquad \qquad ...8.16$$

$$K_{21} = \frac{A \cdot \beta + B \cdot \alpha}{C_0} \qquad \qquad ...8.17$$

β is elimination rate constant for entire body. And K_E is the elimination rate constant for central compartment.

Based on Fig. 8.5 AUC can be calculated as:

$$AUC = \frac{A}{\alpha} + \frac{B}{\beta} \qquad \qquad ...8.18$$

Apparent volume of distribution for central compartment is

$$V_C = \frac{X_0}{C_0} \qquad \qquad ...8.19$$

Which can be represented as:

$$V_C = \frac{X_0}{K_E \cdot AUC} \qquad \qquad ...8.20$$

Apparent volume of distribution for peripheral compartment is:

$$V_p = \frac{V_c \cdot K_{12}}{K_{21}}$$ ...8.21

At steady state

$$V_{d\text{-ss}} = V_c + V_p$$ ...8.22

or $$V_{d\text{-ss}} = \frac{X_0}{\beta \cdot AUC}$$ ...8.23

And hence systemic clearance will be:

$$Cl_T = \beta \cdot V_d$$ ...8.24

8.2.1 Urinary Excretion Data

It is possible to determine pharmacokinetic parameters from urinary excretion data. Thus based on renal clearance and renal excretion rate constant, it is possible to characterize kinetics of renal excretion. Renal clearance (Cl_r) is the volume of blood flowing through the kidney per unit time which is cleared off drug. Cl_r is the urinary excretion rate divided by plasma drug concentration at the midpoint of the urine collection.

$$Cl_r = \frac{\frac{dX_u}{dt}}{C}$$ ...8.25

But

$$\frac{dX_u}{dt} = K_e \cdot X_c$$ ...8.26

Based on equation 8.26, equation 8.25 can be written as

$$Cl_r = \frac{K_e \cdot X_c}{C}$$ ...8.27

Recall that

$$V_c = \frac{X_c}{C}$$

Hence,

$$Cl_r = K_e \cdot V_c$$ ...8.28

Thus, renal clearance is a product of renal excretion rate constant and apparent volume of distribution of central compartment.

Total body clearance or systemic clearance (Cl_T) is nothing but the summation of all clearances e.g. renal clearance + hepatic clearance + lung clearance ...

$$Cl_r = \frac{\frac{dX_E}{dt}}{C} \qquad \qquad ...8.29$$

where,

$$\frac{dX_E}{dt} = \text{Rate of drug elimination by all routes of elimination,}$$

and

$$\frac{dX_E}{dt} = Cl_T \cdot C$$

Integrating for $\frac{dX_E}{dt}$

$$[X_E]_0^\infty = Cl_T \cdot \int_0^\infty C \cdot dt = Cl_T \cdot AUC \qquad ...8.30$$

where,

$[X_E]_0^\infty$ = Total amount of drug eliminated between time zero and infinity

Infact, $[X_E]_0^\infty$ must be equal to X_0 (total amount of drug administered or dose of IV injection).

8.3 INTRAVENOUS INFUSION

Open two-compartment model for IV infusion can be shown as in Fig. 8.6.

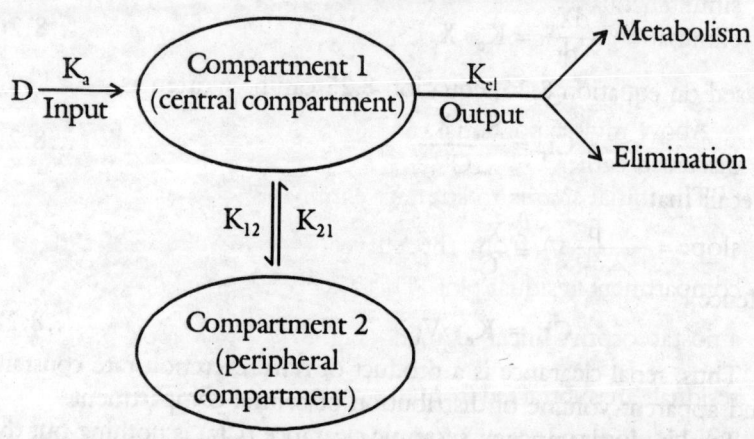

Fig. 8.6. Diagrammatic representation of open two-compartment pharmacokinetic model for IV infusion

Remember that drug administration by IV infusion is at constant rate i.e. zero order kinetics and can be represented as:

$$C = \frac{K_0}{V_c \cdot K_E}\left[1 + \left(\frac{K_E - \beta}{\beta - \alpha}\right) \cdot e^{-\alpha \cdot t} + \left(\frac{K_E - \alpha}{\alpha - \beta}\right) \cdot e^{-\beta \cdot t}\right] \quad ...8.31$$

Steady state will be reached at time = infinity; hence equation 8.31 can be written as

$$C_{ss} = \frac{K_0}{V_c \cdot K_E} \quad ...8.32$$

But $\quad V_C \cdot K_E = V_d \cdot \beta$

Hence,

$$C_{ss} = \frac{K_0}{V_d \cdot \beta} = \frac{K_0}{Cl_T} \quad ...8.33$$

The loading dose in order to obtain C_{ss} before the start of the infusion can be calculated as:

$$X_{0,L} = C_{ss} \cdot V_c = \frac{K_0}{K_E} \quad ...8.34$$

8.4 FIRST ORDER ABSORPTION (EXTRAVASCULAR ADMINISTRATION)

After extravascular administration in a two compartment model, three simultaneous processes are encountered– absorption, distribution and elimination. It can be represented as:

$$C = A \cdot e^{-\alpha \cdot t} + B \cdot e^{-\beta \cdot t} - C_p^{o^{-K_a \cdot t}} \quad ...8.35$$

Above multiexponential can be resolved by method of residuals as discussed earlier.

The initial step is to subtract elimination line (Fig. 8.7 solid line, slope $= -\frac{\beta}{2.303}$) from the curve. This will leave behind a two compartment residual plot. This two compartment residual plot has a postabsorptive linear segment (Fig. 8.7, ✕—✕ slope $= -\frac{\alpha}{2.303}$). If residuals are subtracted from this plot, a line with the slope of $-\frac{K_a}{2.303}$ will be produced (Fig. 8.7, ...)

Intercept A and B are same as described before. C_p^o is the Y-axis intercept of absorption residual line and theoretically equals to A + B.

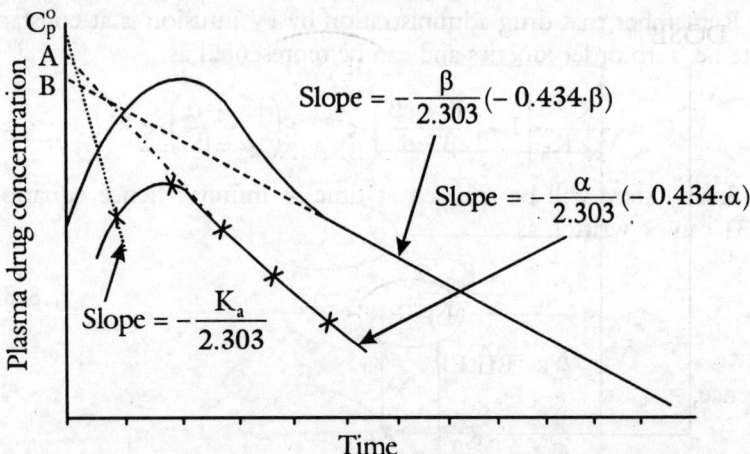

Fig. 8.7. Semilog plot of plasma drug concentration versus time for two compartment model after extravascular administration

8.5 MULTICOMPARTMENT MODEL

One and two compartment models are helpful in understanding the processes of pharmacokinetics, but they are crude approximation of complex body processes. For more accuracy, the body can be subdivided into a larger number of compartments. Figure 8.8 is an example of a nine compartment research model for mercury. Note that separate compartments are now included for major organ systems. Input to the model is oral (into the gut) and elimination is through excretion in the hair, urine, and faces. The model studied actually had 18 compartments– nine for each of two chemical forms of mercury.

If nine compartment are better than two, why not use more sophisticated version skipping the simpler ones?

Using computers, the mathematical equations for nine and 18 compartment models can be solved readily. However, the behaviour of these larger models is vastly more complex than that of a one or two compartment model.

DOSE

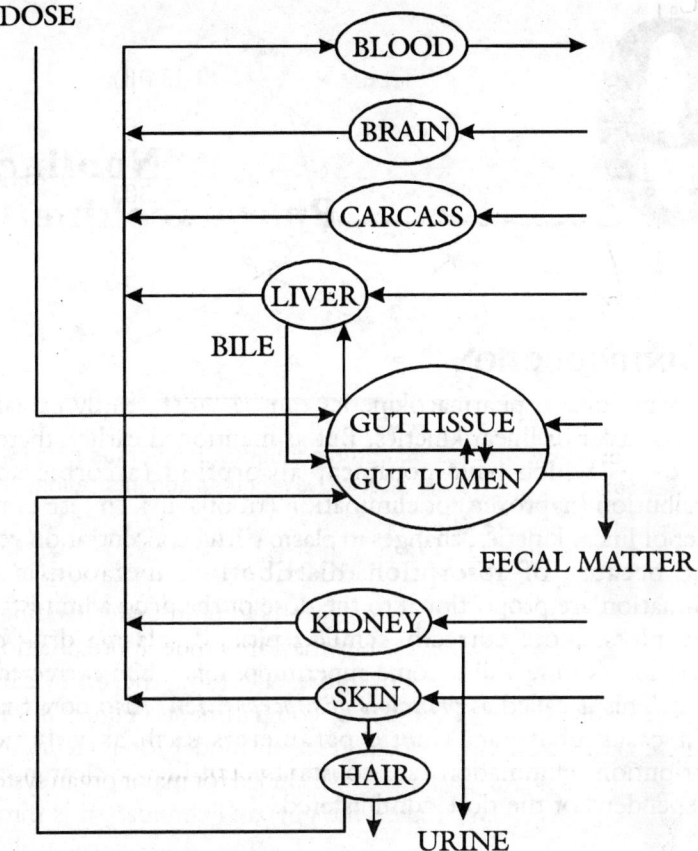

Fig. 8.8. Nine compartment model of mercury

QUESTIONS

1. Explain pharmacokinetics of IV injection based on two-compartment model.
2. What is method of residuals?
3. Explain urinary excretion data for IV injection in relation to two-compartment model.

9

Nonlinear Pharmacokinetics

9.1 INTRODUCTION

For many drugs, pharmacokinetics can be satisfactorily explained by first-order or linear kinetics. But as mentioned earlier, there are few drugs which have nonlinear absorption (ascorbic acid), distribution (naproxen) or elimination (riboflavin). In case of first-order or linear kinetics, changes in plasma drug concentration versus time because of absorption, distribution, metabolism and elimination are proportional to the dose of the drug administered. Such plots, more correctly semilog plots of plasma drug concentration vs time will become superimposable when corrected for doses. This is called as *principle of superposition*. Also note that in such cases pharmacokinetic parameters such as volume of distribution, elimination rate constants, half-life or clearance are independent of the dose administered.

9.2 MICHAELIS MENTEN EQUATION

Many biological processes are mediated by enzymes or transport carrier systems. These systems have limited capacities and hence are saturable. Kinetics of such processes are described by *Michaelis-Menten equation;* also called as *dose dependent kinetics*:

$$\frac{-dc}{dt} = \frac{V_{max} \cdot C}{K_m + C} \qquad \qquad ...9.1$$

where

$\dfrac{-dc}{dt}$ = Rate of decline of drug concentration with respect to time.

V_{max} = Theoretical maximum rate of the process.

K_m = Michaelis-Menten constant.

9.2.1 Explanation of Derivation of Michaelis–Menten Equation

Michaelis-Menten equation was initially used in enzyme kinetics:

$$\text{Enzyme + Substrate} \underset{K_2}{\overset{K_1}{\rightleftharpoons}} \text{Enzyme-Substrate Complex}$$

$$\xrightarrow{K_3} \text{Enzyme + Product}$$

$$E + S \underset{K_2}{\overset{K_1}{\rightleftharpoons}} [ES] \xrightarrow{K_3} E + P \qquad ...9.2$$

There are certain assumptions, such as

♦ ES is a steady state complex
♦ When enzyme is saturated i.e. substrate concentration higher than enzyme concentration, all enzyme is in the form of ES complex
♦ Under saturating conditions, rate of formation of product will be maximum i.e. $V_{max} = K_3 \cdot [ES]$

At equilibrium (steady state):

$$V_{\text{formation of ES complex}} = V_{\text{breakdown of ES complex}}$$

where,

$$V_{\text{formation of ES complex}} = K_1 \cdot [E] \cdot [S]$$
$$V_{\text{breakdown of ES complex}} = K_2 \cdot [ES] + K_3 \cdot [ES]$$
$$= [ES]\,(K_2 + K_3)$$

Hence,

$$K_1 \cdot [E] \cdot [S] = [ES]\,(K_2 + K_3) \qquad ...9.3$$

Divide equation 9.3 by K_1

$$[E] \cdot [S] = [ES] \cdot \left(\frac{K_2 + K_3}{K_1}\right) \qquad ...9.4$$

But,

$$K_m = \frac{K_2 + K_3}{K_1}$$

where,

K_m = Michaelis-Menten constant.

Hence equation 9.4 can be written as:

$$[E] \cdot [S] = [ES] \cdot K_m$$

or

$$[E] = K_m \cdot \frac{[ES]}{[S]} \qquad ...9.5$$

Remember that [E] is the concentration of free enzyme i.e. amount of enzyme available for the reaction and can be expressed as:

$$[E] = [E_t] - [E_c]$$

where, $[E_t]$ = concentration of total enzyme.

$[E_c]$ = concentration of enzyme in [ES] complex.

Thus equation 9.5 can be expressed as:

$$[E_t] - [E_c] = K_m \cdot \frac{[ES]}{[S]} \qquad \ldots 9.6$$

Dividing above equation by [ES]

$$\frac{[E_t] - [E_c]}{[E_s]} = \frac{K_m}{[S]}$$

i.e.

$$\frac{[E_t]}{[E_c]} - 1 = \frac{K_m}{[S]}$$

i.e.

$$\frac{[E_t]}{[E_c]} = 1 + \frac{K_m}{[S]}$$

i.e.

$$\frac{[E_t]}{[E_c]} = \frac{[S] + K_m}{[S]} \qquad \ldots 9.7$$

When substrate concentration is higher than enzyme concentration i.e. enzyme is saturated, thus,

$$[E_t] = [ES]$$

and rate of the reaction is maximum (V_{max})

Remember that,

$$V_{max} = K_3 \cdot [ES]$$

Hence,

$$V_{max} = K_3 \cdot [E_t] \text{ or } [E_t] = \frac{V_{max}}{K_3} \qquad \ldots 9.8$$

When substrate concentration is lower than enzyme concentration i.e. enzyme is not saturated, thus,

$$[E_t] \neq [E_c]$$

thus,

$$V = K_3 \cdot [ES]$$

or

$$[ES] = \frac{V}{K_3} \qquad \ldots 9.9$$

Hence,

$$\frac{[E_t]}{[E_c]} = \left(\frac{\dfrac{V_{max}}{K_3}}{[ES]} \right)$$

or $$\frac{[E_t]}{[E_c]} = \left(\frac{\dfrac{V_{max}}{K_3}}{\dfrac{V}{K_3}} \right)$$

i.e. $$\frac{[E_t]}{[E_c]} = \frac{V_{max}}{V}$$

Based on above, equation 9.7 can be written as:

$$\frac{V_{max}}{V} = \frac{K_m + [S]}{[S]}$$

or $$\frac{V}{V_{max}} = \frac{[S]}{K_m + [S]} \qquad \ldots 9.10$$

or $$V = \frac{V_{max} \cdot [S]}{K_m + [S]} \qquad \ldots 9.10a$$

Equation (9.10 a) is Michaelis Menten equation (Fig. 9.1).

In nonlinear pharmacokinetics, V is rate of change of drug concentration $\left(-\dfrac{dc}{dt} \right)$ and [S] is drug concentration (C).

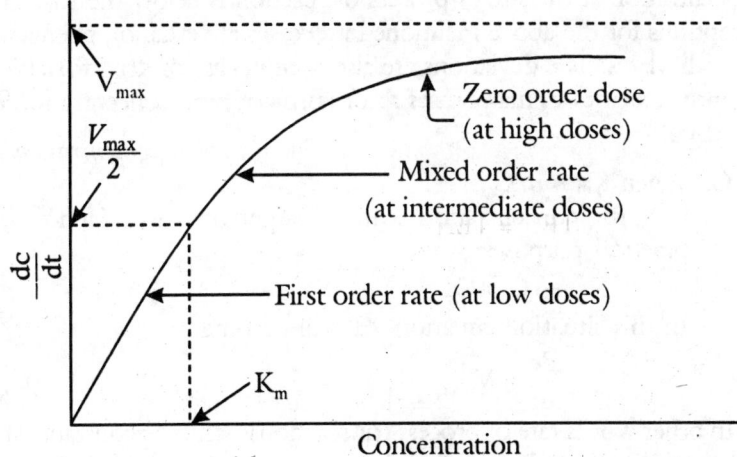

Fig. 9.1. Graphical representation of Michaelis Menten equation

Consider following situations

A. When $K_m = C$

In this situation equation 9.1 will become

$$-\frac{dc}{dt} = \frac{V_{max} \cdot C}{2 \cdot C}$$

i.e. $\qquad -\frac{dc}{dt} = \frac{V_{max}}{2}$ $\qquad\qquad$ ...9.11

In other words K_m is equal to the drug concentration at which the rate of process or rate of reaction is equal to one-half of the theoretical maximum rate of the process (or reaction)

B. When $K_m >> C$

i.e. K_m is much larger than C. Hence, for practical purposes:

$$K_m + C \approx K_m$$

In this situation equation 9.1 will become—

$$-\frac{dc}{dt} = \frac{V_{max} \cdot C}{K_m}$$ $\qquad\qquad$ ...9.12

Equation 9.12 is similar to the equation which describes first-order elimination of the drug, where first-order rate constant $K_E = \frac{V_{max}}{K_m}$. The fact that elimination of most drugs follow first order kinetics suggests that the plasma drug concentration more specifically, drug concentration at the site of process or reaction is below the K_m. The exceptions for the above mentioned processes are ethanol, phenytoin and salicylates. The deviations are also seen in case of drug toxicities, as drug toxicities in many cases are because of high concentration of the drug.

C. When $K_m << C$

i.e. drug concentration is much larger than K_m. Hence, for practical purposes:

$$K_m + C \approx C$$

In this situation equation 9.1 will become

$$-\frac{dc}{dt} = V_{max}$$ $\qquad\qquad$ ...9.13

In other words rate of process (or reaction) occurs at constant rate, V_{max} and is independent of drug concentration. Thus it is identical to zero order kinetics. For example, metabolism of ethanol.

From Fig. 9.1 it can be seen that initially at low concentration, change in drug concentration $\left(-\dfrac{dc}{dt}\right)$ is linear with change in total concentration i.e. first order kinetics. As concentration increases $-\dfrac{dc}{dt}$ is neither linear nor independent with change in total concentration i.e. mixed order kinetics. Finally, when total concentration is very high, $-\dfrac{dc}{dt}$ is independent of total concentration i.e. zero order kinetics

Consider IV injection of drug, which is eliminated by capacity-limited process.

Rearrangement of equation 9.1 will give

$$V_{max} \cdot dt = -\frac{dc}{C}(C + K_m) \qquad \qquad ...9.14$$

After integration we will get

$$V_{max} \cdot t + i = -C - K_m \cdot \ln C \qquad \qquad ...9.15$$

i is integration constant. At t = 0, C = C_0, thus

$$i = -C_0 - K_m \cdot \ln C \qquad \qquad ...9.16$$

Substituting equation 9.16 in equation 9.15

$$t = \frac{(C_o - C)}{V_{max}} + \frac{K_m}{V_{max}}\left(\ln \frac{C_o}{C}\right) \qquad \qquad ...9.17$$

Changing to common logarithm

$$\log C = \log C_o + \frac{(C_o - C)}{2.303 \cdot K_m} - \frac{V_{max}}{2.303 \cdot K_m} \qquad \qquad 9.18$$

From equation 9.18 it is apparent that plot of log plasma drug concentration versus time will be a curve with terminal linear segment having slope $= \dfrac{V_{max}}{2.303 \cdot K_m}$ (Fig. 9.2).

Kinetic parameters V_{max} and K_m can be calculated by various methods. It is necessary to determine the rate of change of plasma drug concentration with time. For this, blood samples are generally collected at various time intervals and the data is plotted. One of the most widely used plot is *Lineweaver-Burk plot*, also called as *double reciprocal plot*– plot of $\dfrac{1}{dc/dt}$ versus $\dfrac{1}{C_m}$.

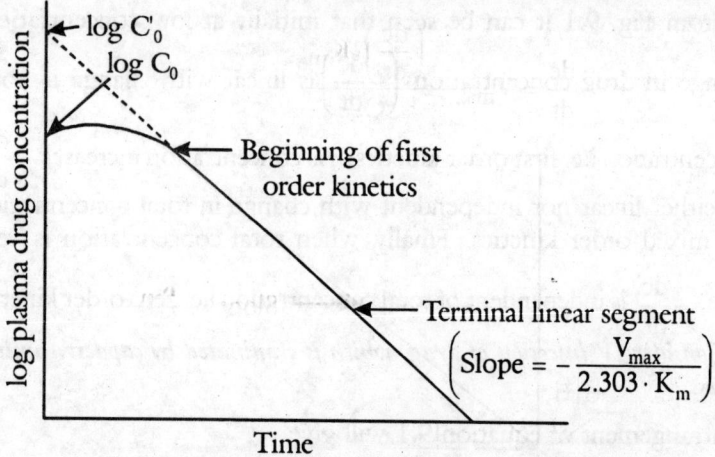

Fig. 9.2. Plot of log plasma drug concentration versus time when drug is administered as IV injection with capacity limited process

Lineweaver-Burk expression is

$$\frac{1}{\left(\dfrac{dc}{dt}\right)} = \frac{K_m}{V_m \cdot C_m} + \frac{1}{V_m} \qquad \text{...9.19}$$

(Basically the reciprocal of equation 9.1)

where,

C_m = plasma drug concentration at the midpoint of sampling interval

Plot of the reciprocal of $\dfrac{dc}{dt}$ versus the reciprocal of C_m yields a straight line with Y-intercept = $\dfrac{1}{V_{max}}$ and slope = $\dfrac{K_m}{V_{max}}$ (Fig. 9.3)

Sometimes in double reciprocal plot the points are too crowded. To over come this problem, two more plots are used which are more reliable: *Hanes-Woolf plot* (equation 9.20) and the *Woolf-Augustinsson-Hofstee plot* (equation 9.21)

$$\frac{C_m}{\left(\dfrac{dc}{dt}\right)} = \frac{K_m}{V_{max}} + \frac{C_m}{V_{max}} \qquad \text{...9.20}$$

$$\frac{dc}{dt} = V_{max} - \frac{\left(\dfrac{dc}{dt}\right) \cdot K_m}{C_m} \qquad \qquad ...9.21$$

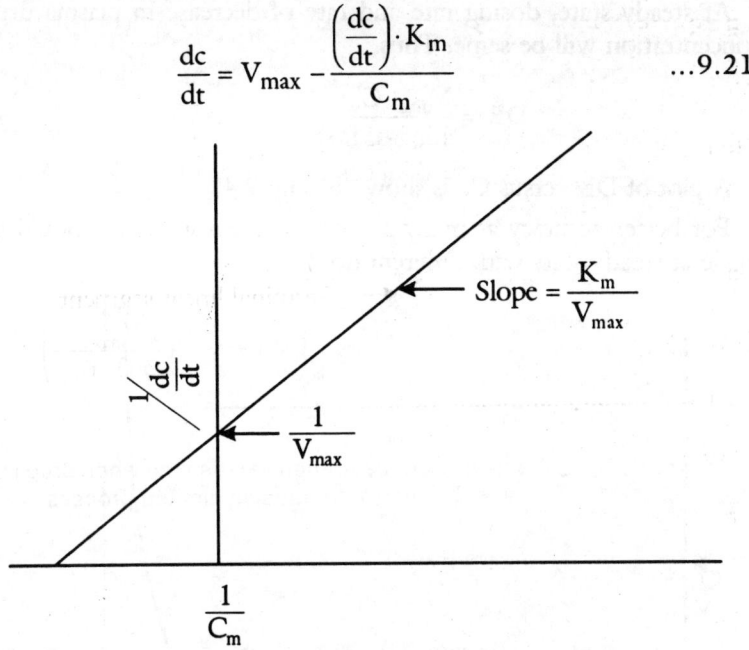

Slope $= \dfrac{K_m}{V_{max}}$

$\dfrac{1}{V_{max}}$

$\dfrac{1}{\frac{dc}{dt}}$

$\dfrac{1}{C_m}$

Fig. 9.3. Lineweaver-Burk plot (double reciprocal plot)

Equation 9.20 and 9.21 are formed by rearrangement of equation 9.19. Thus, based on equation 9.20, plot of $\dfrac{C_m}{dc/dt}$ versus C_m will be a straight line with slope $= \dfrac{1}{V_{max}}$ and an intercept of $\dfrac{K_m}{V_{max}}$.

Based on equation 9.21, plot of $\dfrac{dc}{dt}$ versus $\dfrac{dc/dt}{C_m}$ will be a straight line with slope $= -K_m$ and an intercept of V_{max}.

In case of IV infusion or multiple dosing, the administration of the drug is at the constant rate (zero order process).

$$DR = C_{ss} \cdot Cl_T \qquad \qquad ...9.22$$

where,

$\quad$ DR = dosing rate, K_0 for IV infusion (zero order rate constant)

or $\quad$ DR = $(F \cdot X_0)/\tau$ for multiple dosing regimen

$\quad$ where, F = available fraction.

$\qquad$ X_0 = oral dose.

$\qquad$ τ = dosing time intervals.

At steady state, dosing rate and rate of decrease in plasma drug concentration will be same. Thus,

$$DR = \frac{V_{max} \cdot C_{ss}}{K_m + C_{ss}} \qquad \ldots 9.23$$

A plot of DR versus C_{ss} is shown in Fig. 9.4

For better accuracy as many as possible measurements should be made at steady state with different doses.

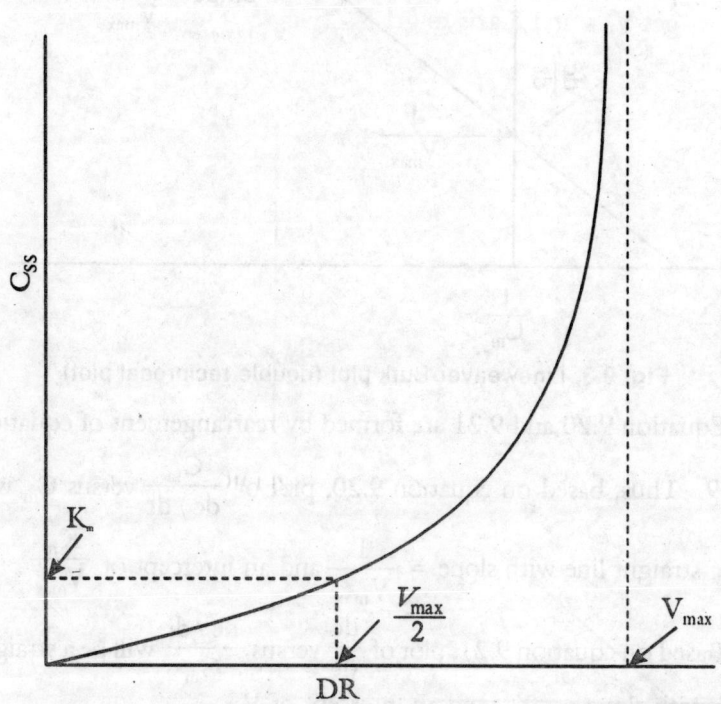

Fig. 9.4. Plot of DR versus C_{ss} for a drug with nonlinear kinetics

K_m and V_{max} can be graphically computed by:

A. Lineweaver-Burk plot

Take the reciprocal of equation 9.23

$$\frac{1}{DR} = \frac{K_m}{V_{max} \cdot C_{ss}} + \frac{1}{V_{max}} \qquad \ldots 9.24$$

Thus plot of $1/DR$ versus $1/C_{ss}$ will be a straight line with

$$\text{slope} = \frac{K_m}{V_{max}} \text{ and Y-intercept} = \frac{1}{V_{max}}$$

B. Direct Linear Plot

With two different dosing rates DR1 and DR2, two steady states will be obtained, C_{ss1} and C_{ss2}. On graph, C_{ss1}–DR1 and C_{ss2}-DR2 points are joined with straight lines. The intersection point of these two lines is extrapolated on Y-axis (DR-axis) to get V_{max} and X-axis to get K_m (Fig. 9.5).

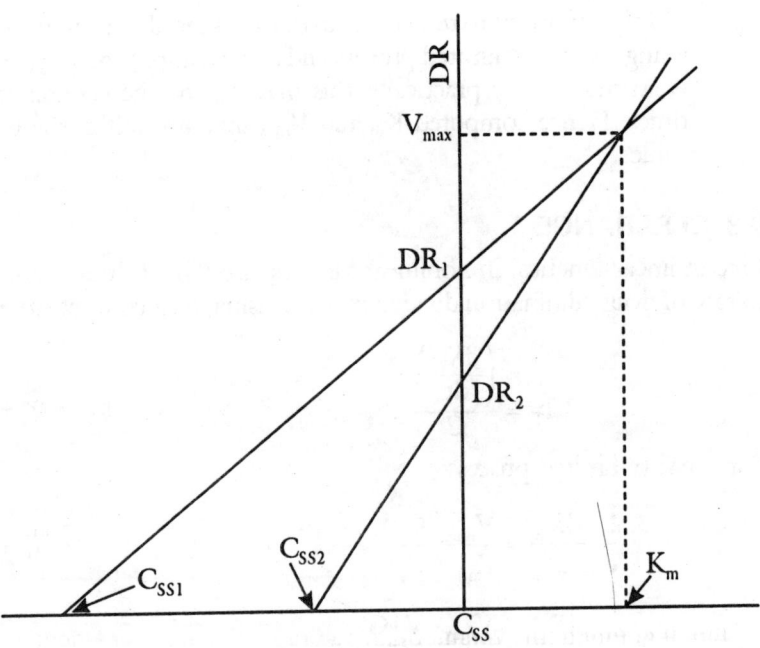

Fig. 9.5. Direct linear plot of steady state concentrations when drug is given at two different rates

C. Recall equation 9.23

$$DR = \frac{V_{max} \cdot C_{ss}}{K_m + C_{ss}}$$

Rearrange the equation

$$DR \, (K_m + C_{ss}) = V_{max} \cdot C_{ss}$$

i.e. $$DR \cdot K_m + DR \cdot C_{ss} = V_{max} \cdot C_{ss}$$

i.e. $$DR \cdot C_{ss} = V_{max} \cdot C_{ss} - DR \cdot K_m$$

Divide both sides of the above equation by C_{ss}

$$DR = V_{max} - \frac{DR \cdot K_m}{C_{ss}} \qquad \qquad ...9.25$$

Thus, plot of DR versus DR/C_{ss} will be a straight line with slope = $-K_m$ and Y-intercept = V_{max}.

It is important to remember that, for all the above discussion a single capacity limited process and a one compartment system is assumed. But practically, this may not be the case all the time. Hence computed K_m and V_{max} may not reflect the real values.

9.3 CLEARANCE

Like in linear kinetics, in nonlinear kinetics also Cl_T of drug is equal to rate of drug elimination divided by the plasma drug concentration.

$$Cl_T = \frac{\left(\dfrac{dX_E}{dt}\right)}{C} \qquad \qquad ...9.26$$

For capacity limited process

$$\frac{1}{V} \cdot \frac{dX_E}{dt} = \frac{V_{max} \cdot C}{K_m + C} \qquad \qquad ...9.27$$

i.e. $$\frac{dX_E}{dt} = \frac{V_{max} \cdot V \cdot C}{K_m + C} \qquad \qquad ...9.28$$

Divide both sides of the above equation by C

$$\frac{\left(\dfrac{dX_E}{dt}\right)}{C} = \frac{V_{max} \cdot V}{K_m + C} \qquad \qquad ...9.29$$

Substituting equation 9.29 in equation 9.26

$$Cl_T = \frac{V_{max} \cdot V}{K_m + C} \qquad ...9.30$$

When $K_m >> C$; *plasma drug concentration is less than* K_m
Then,

$$K_m + C \approx K_m$$

Hence,

$$Cl_T = \frac{V_{max} \cdot V}{K_m} \qquad ...9.31$$

When $C >> K_m$; *plasma drug concentration is more than* K_m
Then,

$$K_m + C \approx C$$

Hence,

$$Cl_T = \frac{V_{max} \cdot V}{C} \qquad ...9.32$$

From equation 9.31 it is apparent that at very low plasma drug concentration, clearance is independent of drug concentration. From equation 9.32 it is apparent that at higher plasma drug concentration, clearance is inversely proportional to concentration. In other words as plasma drug concentration increases, clearance of the drug from plasma decreases.

Half life of the drug by nonlinear clearance is:

$$t_{1/2} = \frac{0.693 \cdot V}{Cl_T} \qquad ...9.33$$

i.e.

$$Cl_T = \frac{0.693 \cdot V}{t_{1/2}}$$

Substitute above equation in equation 9.30

$$\frac{0.693 \cdot V}{t_{1/2}} = \frac{V_{max} \cdot V}{K_m + C}$$

i.e.

$$t_{1/2} = \frac{0.693 \cdot V \cdot (K_m + C)}{V_{max} \cdot V}$$

i.e.

$$t_{1/2} = \frac{0.693 \cdot (K_m + C)}{V_{max}} \qquad ...9.34$$

From equation 9.34 it is apparent that at very low concentration, half-life of the drug is independent of plasma drug concentration (as $K_m + C \approx K_m$). But at very high concentration, half life will be proportional to concentration i.e. as plasma drug concentration increases half life of the drug will also increase (as $K_m + C \approx C$).

9.4 AREA UNDER THE CURVE

For a first order kinetics, area under the plasma drug concentration versus time curve is proportional to the amount of drug administered i.e. dose of the drug. For drugs which follow capacity limited process, area under the curve is not proportional to the amount of drug administered but as dose increases area also increases proportionally.

Recall equation 9.1

$$-\frac{dc}{dt} = \frac{V_{max} \cdot C}{K_m + C}$$

Rearrange above equation

$$-dc \cdot (K_m + C) = V_{max} \cdot C \cdot dt$$

i.e.

$$C \cdot dt = -dc \cdot \frac{(K_m + C)}{V_{max}}$$

i.e.

$$C \cdot dt = \frac{K_m}{V_{max}} \cdot dc - \frac{C}{V_{max}} \cdot dc \qquad \qquad ...9.35$$

Integrating above equation

$$\int_0^\infty C \cdot dt = -\int_{C_0}^0 \frac{K_m}{V_{max}} \cdot dc - \int_{C_0}^0 \frac{C}{V_{max}} \cdot dc \qquad ...9.36$$

$$\int_0^\infty C \cdot dt = -\frac{K_m}{V_{max}}\Big|_{C_0}^0 - \frac{C^2}{2 \cdot V_{max}}\Big|_{C_0}^0 \qquad ...9.37$$

($C = C_0$ at t = 0) and $\int_0^\infty C \cdot dt$ is area under the curve

$$\int_0^\infty C \cdot dt = \frac{K_m}{V_{max}} \cdot C_0 + \frac{C_0^2}{2 \cdot V_{max}}$$

$$\int_0^\infty C \cdot dt = \frac{C_o}{V_{max}}\left(K_m + \frac{C_o}{2}\right) \qquad \ldots 9.38$$

At very low doses $K_m \gg \dfrac{C_o}{2}$. Thus equation 9.38 will be

$$\int_0^\infty C \cdot dt = \frac{K_m}{V_{max}} \cdot C_o$$

as $\qquad K_m + \dfrac{C_o}{2} \simeq K_m$

But $C_o = \dfrac{X_o}{V_d}$; V_d is apparent volume of distribution

Thus,

$$\int_0^\infty C \cdot dt = \frac{K_m \cdot X_0}{V_{max} \cdot V_d} \qquad \ldots 9.39$$

Thus $\int_0^\infty C \cdot dt$ (area under the curve) is proportional to the amount of drug administration. It also suggests that in nonlinear situation, area shows a more dependence on dose.

At very high doses $\dfrac{C_o}{2} \gg K_m$

Thus equation 9.38 will be

$$\int_0^\infty C \cdot dt = \frac{C_o^2}{2 \cdot V_{max}}$$

And as $\qquad C_o = \dfrac{X_o}{V_d}$

$$\int_0^\infty C \cdot dt = \frac{X_0^2}{2 \cdot V_d^2 \cdot V_{max}} \qquad \ldots 9.40$$

Thus area is proportional to the square of the amount of drug administered. Hence even a small increase in the dose will significantly increase the area under the curve.

9.5 ENZYME INDUCTION

Auto induction, where drug induces its own metabolism is also an example of nonlinear kinetics. Many drugs are known to induce their own metabolism e.g. barbiturates. Usually this enzyme induction is because of new protein synthesis (new enzyme synthesis) and not because of change in substrate affinity towards enzyme. In normal situation, rate of synthesis and rate of degradation of the enzyme are mainly responsible for rate of change of enzyme levels. Hence

$$\frac{dE}{dt} = S - K \cdot E \qquad \qquad ...9.41$$

where,

S = Rate of enzyme synthesis. Under normal circumstances it is assumed to be zero order.

K = First order rate constant for enzyme degradation.

At steady state $\frac{dE}{dt} = 0$. Hence,

$$E = \frac{S}{K} \qquad \qquad ...9.42$$

When there is enzyme induction, a new steady state will exist – E'

$$E' = \frac{S'}{K'} \qquad \qquad ...9.43$$

The rate of change of enzyme levels as E approaches E' will be represented as

$$\frac{dE}{dt} = S' - K' \cdot E \qquad \qquad ...9.44$$

i.e. $$\frac{dE}{S' - K' \cdot E} = dt \qquad \qquad ...9.45$$

After integration

$$t + i = -\frac{1}{K'} \ln(S' - K' \cdot E_t) \qquad \qquad ...9.46$$

where, E_t = Concentration of enzyme at time t

When t = 0, E_t = E_0 i.e. enzyme levels prior to administration of drug, meaning prior to enzyme induction. Thus,

$$i = -\frac{1}{K'} \ln(S' - K' \cdot E_o) \qquad \qquad ...9.47$$

Substituting equation 9.47 in equation 9.46

$$-K' \cdot t = \ln \frac{S' - K' \cdot E_t}{S' - K' \cdot E_o} \qquad \ldots 9.48$$

Converting above equation in exponential form

$$e^{-K' \cdot t} = \frac{S' - K' \cdot E_t}{S' - K' \cdot E_o} \qquad \ldots 9.49$$

i.e.
$$E_t = \frac{S'}{K'} - \frac{S' - K' \cdot E_o}{K'} e^{-K' \cdot t} \qquad \ldots 9.50$$

According to equation 9.42, $E_o = \dfrac{S}{K}$. Thus,

$$E_t = \frac{S'}{K'} - \left(\frac{S'}{K'} - \frac{S}{K} \right) e^{-K' \cdot t} \qquad \ldots 9.51$$

From equation 9.51 it is apparent that enzyme levels during induction depends on:

♦ Preinduction levels;
♦ Induced steady state enzyme levels;
♦ Rate constant for enzyme degradation.

Enzyme induction is an example of time-dependent and not dose dependent or concentration dependent pharmacokinetics. It involves physiological and biochemical changes in the organs associated with the metabolism/elimination of the drug.

QUESTIONS

1. Explain Michaelis-Menten equation in detail.
2. Explain following situations in relation to Michaelis-Menten equation
   (a) $K_m = C$
   (b) $K_m >> C$
   (c) $K_m << C$
3. What is enzyme induction?
4. Explain clearance in relation to nonlinear pharmacokinetics.
5. Explain various graphical methods used for the computation of K_m and C_{max}.
6. Give details of AUC in relation to nonlinear pharmacokinetics.

10

Non-Compartmental
_____Analysis

10.1 INTRODUCTION

Non-compartmental methods can be used to determine pharma-cokinetic parameters without fitting the pharmacokinetic data to any specific compartment model. Thus, non-compartmental analysis does not assume any compartmental model for drug or its metabolites. As long as linear kinetics is assumed, non-compartmental analysis can be applied to any compartment models. As a matter of fact, we have already used non-compartmental analysis without specifying it for the estimation of various parameters viz. clearance and (apparent) volume of distribution.

The non-compartmental model and its parameters are also called as "model independent." Both the non-compartmental and compartmental models do have assumptions; most assumptions for the compartmental model also apply to non-compartmental models such as linear constant co-efficient. Non-compartmental models are now increasingly used to predict bioavailability, excretion and the apparent volume of distribution. Non-compartmental model can be schematically shown as in Fig. 10.1

There is a direct entry of drug into central compartment and also from non-central or peripheral compartments and any number of recirculations of the drug can occur. Also the elimination of drug and its metabolites can be from central or non-central compartments. The various model parameters are calculated according to _statistical moment theory_ (see below).

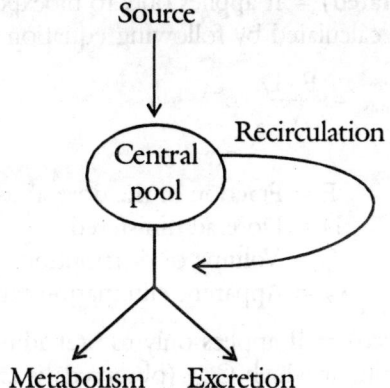

Fig. 10.1. Non-compartmental model

10.2 PLASMA CONCENTRATION—TIME CURVE PARAMETERS

The typical plasma concentration vs time curve after single dose administration can be shown as in Fig. 10.2

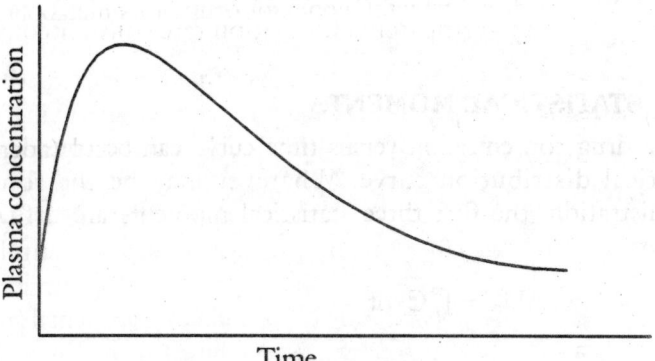

Fig. 10.2. Plasma concentration vs time curve

The various parameters of this curve are as follows:

♦ $C_{initial}$ = It is the initial concentration extrapolated to time zero after IV administration

$$C_0 = \Sigma C_n \qquad \qquad \dots 10.1$$

♦ $C_{max}(observed)$ = It applies only to oral administration and is the maximum concentration observed.

◆ C_{max}(**calculated**) = It applies only to bioexponential oral data and can be calculated by following equation

$$C_{max} = \frac{F \cdot D}{V_d} \cdot e^{-\lambda_Z \cdot t_{max}} \qquad \qquad ...10.2$$

where,

F = Fraction of the dose absorbed.
D = Dose administered.
V_d = Volume of distribution.
λ_Z = Apparent elimination rate constant.

◆ t_{max}(**observed**) = It applies only to oral administration and is the time point at which C_{max} (observed) is reached.

◆ t_{max}(**calculated**) = It applies only to biexponential oral data and can be calculated by following equation

$$t_{max} = \frac{2.303}{\lambda_a - \lambda_Z} \cdot \left(\log \frac{\lambda_a}{\lambda_Z} \right) \qquad \qquad ...10.3$$

where,

λ_a = Apparent absorption rate constant.
λ_Z = Apparent elimination rate constantconstant.

10.3 STATISTICAL MOMENTS

Plasma drug concentration versus time curve can be considered as statistical distribution curve. Whatever may be the route of administration, the first three statistical moments are defined as follows:

$$AUC = \int_0^\infty C \cdot dt \qquad \qquad ...10.4$$

$$MRT = \frac{\int_0^\infty t \cdot C \cdot dt}{\int_0^\infty C \cdot dt} = \frac{AUMC}{AUC} \qquad \qquad ...10.5$$

$$VRT = \frac{\int_0^\infty t^2 \cdot C \cdot dt}{\int_0^\infty C \cdot dt} = \frac{\int_0^\infty (t - MRT)^2 \cdot C \cdot dt}{AUC} \qquad ...10.6$$

where,

MRT = Mean residence time of a drug in the body.
VRT = Variance of mean residence time of a drug in the body.

AUC, MRT and *VRT* are called as *zero, first* and *second* moment of plasma drug concentration versus time curve. AUMC (area under the (first) moment curve) is area under the curve of a plot of the product of concentration and time versus time from zero to infinity. The equation for $AUMC_{0-t}$ can be written as follows:

$$AUMC_{0-t} = \sum_{1-0}^{n-1} \frac{t_{i+1} - t}{2}(C_i t_i + C_{i+1} \cdot t_{i+1})$$

$$+ \frac{C_{last} \cdot t_{last}}{\lambda_z} + \frac{C_{last}}{\lambda_z^2} \qquad ...10.7$$

where,

λ_z = Apparent elimination rate constant.

These moments can be calculated by *trapezoidal rule* (Refer to Chapter "One Compartment Model") from plasma drug concentration versus time curve.

The question is—how to estimate area under the curve from time zero to infinity?

In general, in a pharmacokinetic study blood samples will be collected till time t', when the plasma drug concentration will be C'. So first calculate the area under the curve from time zero to t' by trapezoidal rule. To this AUC add the area under the curve from time t' to infinity. This will be estimated as:

$$\int_{t'}^{\infty} C \cdot dt = \frac{C'}{\lambda_n} \qquad ...10.8$$

where,

λ_n = (2.303.Slope) 2.303 time the slope of terminal portion of log plasma drug concentration versus time plot.

The total AUC will be the sum of two partial areas described above i.e. from time zero to t' and from time t' to infinity.

10.4 BIOAVAILABILITY

Bioavailability is described as fraction (F) of an oral dose, which reaches the systemic circulation.

Remember that for an intravenous dose bioavailability is unity. Thus,

$$F = \frac{D_{IV} \cdot AUC_{oral}}{D_{oral} \cdot AUC_{IV}} \qquad ...10.9$$

If dose of intravenous and oral administration is same, then F is the ratio of zero moments after oral and intravenous administration. Meaning ratio of AUC after oral and intravenous administration.

10.5 CLEARANCE

By this time reader must be aware that clearance is one of the most important pharmacokinetic parameter.

Clearance is generally calculated after intravenous administration, except in circumstances when complete oral dose is known to reach systemic circulation (100 % bioavailability).

Clearance can be expressed as:

$$Cl = \frac{D_{IV}}{AUC} \qquad \qquad ...10.10$$

For single dose oral administration (having less than 100% bioavailability), systemic clearance based on AUC_{0-t} trapezoid calculation is

$$Cl = \frac{F \cdot D}{AUC_{0-t}} \qquad \qquad ...10.11$$

where,

F = Fraction of the dose absorbed.

D = Dose administered.

Systemic clearance normalized by body weight can be calculated as:

$$Cl_{normalized} = \frac{Cl}{Body\,weight\,(Kg)} \qquad \qquad ...10.12$$

10.6 HALF LIFE

Statistical moment analogous to half-life is the first moment i.e. mean residence time (MRT). MRT represents the time for 63.2% of the dose to be eliminated and can be expressed as:

$$MRT_{IV} = \frac{1}{K_{el}} \qquad \qquad ...10.13$$

where,

K_{el} = First-order elimination constant after intravenous administration.

Thus,
$$t_{1/2} = 0.693 \cdot MRT_{IV} \qquad \ldots 10.14$$

MRT depends on the route of administration of the drug. MRT after intravenous administration will always be shorter than that after the extravascular administration.

10.7 ABSORPTION

For calculating statistical moment for rate of absorption, differences in the mean residence time after intravenous and extravascular administration are used.

$$MAT = MRT_{EV} - MRT_{IV} \qquad \ldots 10.15$$

where,

MAT = Mean absorption time.

MRT_{EV} = Mean residence time after extravascular administration.

MRT_{IV} = Mean residence time after intravenous administration.

For a first order process

$$MAT = \frac{1}{K_a} \qquad \ldots 10.16$$

where,

K_a = First order absorption rate constant.

Hence,

$$t_{1/2\ (ab)} = 0.693 \cdot MAT \qquad \ldots 10.17$$

where,

$t_{1/2\ (ab)}$ = Absorption half life.

For a zero order process

$$MAT = \frac{T}{2} \qquad \ldots 10.18$$

where,

T = Time required for complete absorption.

For biexponential oral data after single dose administration, t_{max} can be calculated by following equation

$$t_{max} = \frac{2.303}{\lambda_a - \lambda_z} \cdot \log \frac{\lambda_a}{\lambda_z} \qquad \ldots 10.19$$

where,

λ_a = Apparent absorption rate constant.

λ_z = Apparent elimination rate constant.

AUC_{0-t} (i.e. not extrapolated to infinity) can be calculated by trapezoid rule using following equation

$$AUC_{0-t} = \sum_{i=0}^{n-1} \frac{t_{i+1} - t_i}{2} (C_i + C_{i+1}) \qquad \ldots 10.20$$

where,

n = Number of data points.

Whereas, AUC_∞ (i.e. total AUC) can be calculated by combining AUC_{0-t} with an extrapolated value by following equation:

$$AUC_\infty = AUC_{0-t} + \frac{C_n}{\lambda_z} \qquad \ldots 10.21$$

where,

C_n = Last concentration.

λ_z = Apparent elimination rate constant.

10.8 VOLUME OF DISTRIBUTION

Apparent volume of distribution is the valuable pharmacokinetic parameter to describe the distribution of the drug in the body.

As per statistical moment theory, for intravenous injection, volume of distribution is the product of clearance and mean residence time. Thus,

$$V_d = Cl \cdot MRT \qquad \ldots 10.22$$

i.e.

$$V_d = \frac{D_{IV} \cdot AUMC}{(AUC)^2} \qquad \ldots 10.23$$

Apparent volume of distribution based on AUC_{0-t} trapezoid calculation and elimination rate for single oral dose administration is:

$$V_d = \frac{F \cdot D}{AUC_{0-t} \cdot \lambda_z} \qquad \ldots 10.24$$

where,

F = Fraction of dose absorbed (bioavailability).

D = Dose administered.

λ_z = Apparent elimination rate constant.

Apparent volume of distribution normalized by body weight can be calculated as:

$$V_{d-normalized} = \frac{V_d}{Body\ weight\ (kg)} \qquad ...10.25$$

From above discussion it is apparent that statistical moment theory is helpful in adequately characterizing the pharmacokinetics of the drug.

Non-compartmental analysis of the data thus allows the estimation of most of the basic pharmacokinetic parameters for characterizing the disposition of the drug. One of the main advantages of non-compartmental model is that there is no assumption of any number of compartment(s) for drug or metabolite. Also, the drug is free to recirculate and there is no need to identify body compartment associated with this. Hence, all the moments are completely independent and can be easily calculated.

Some of the non-compartmental models are as follows:

♦ **Logan plot:** It is the graphical analysis of reversible system in order to calculate the total distribution volume

♦ **Patlak plot:** It is the graphical analysis of irreversible system.

♦ **Bolus/infusion optimization:** In this, the bolus/infusion ratio for an equilibrium study can be calculated based on a bolus study.

♦ **Tissue/plasma ratio:** In this the ratio of tissue binding to plasma concentration is calculated so as to estimate the total distribution volume.

Many commercial computer softwares are available for non-compartmental analysis of the pharmacokinetic data. *WinNonlin®* allows the calculation of model independent parameters based on plasma or urine data from single dose or steady state design. Another one, *PK Solutions®* uses two techniques, one based on the concentration-time profile (AUC is calculated by applying trapezoidal rule), and second technique based on the method of residuals.

However, non-compartmental analyses do not adequately treat non-linear cases. They also do not describe the time course of the drug in the blood. In addition, non-compartmental models are mathematically complex and can lead to extrapolation errors, because AUC, MRT and VRT are dependent on time. Hence longer the sampling time better is the prediction. Todate, non-compartmental analysis has been used only for toxicokinetics. Nonetheless it is an exciting and emerging field and in future will definitely play an important role in pharmacokinetics.

QUESTIONS

1. What are zero, first and second statistical moments? And how they are calculated?
2. In brief, explain the statistical moments for following parameters
   (a) Bioavailability
   (b) Clearance
   (c) Absorption
   (d) Volume of distribution
   (e) Half-life.

11

Applications of Pharmacokinetics

In addition to their academic and theoretical importance, pharmacokinetic principles are also effectively applied in clinical practice. Some of the important applications of pharmacokinetic principles are discussed below.

11.1 DOSE ADJUSTMENT IN RENAL FAILURE

Elimination of the drug shows considerable inter-individual variations. These variations can be physiological or pathological e.g. renal insufficiency.

Creatinine clearance and serum creatinine levels are generally used to determine renal function. These are helpful for predicting clearance or half life of the drug. The reason creatinine is a good marker of renal function is that, it is produced in the body as an end product of muscle metabolism and its elimination is almost equal to glomerular filtration rate. In addition, elimination of number of drugs shows good correlation with elimination of creatinine clearance.

The total first order elimination rate can be expressed as:

$$K_{el} = K_r + K_{nr} \qquad \qquad ...11.1$$

where,

K_{el} = Elimination rate constant.

K_r = Rate constant for renal excretion.

K_{nr} = Rate constant for non-renal excretion.

Thus,

$$K_{el} = aCl_r + K_{nr} \qquad \qquad ...11.2$$

where,

a = proportionality constant, assuming drug elimination is directly related to creatinine clearance.

Hence plot of Cl_r versus K_{el} will be linear (Fig. 11.1)

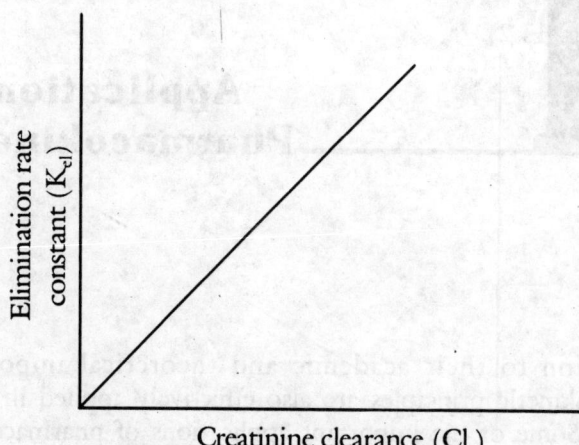

Fig. 11.1. Plot of Cl_r versus K_{el}

Practically it is not always possible to determine creatinine clearance as it requires urine collection for 24 hours. Thus *serum creatinine levels* are widely used instead of creatinine clearance to estimate renal function.

$$C_c = \frac{PR}{Cl_{cr}} \qquad \qquad ...11.3$$

where,

C_c = Serum creatinine concentration.

PR = Production rate of creatinine.

i.e.

$$Cl_r = \frac{PR}{C_c} \qquad \qquad ...11.4$$

Substituting equation 11.4 in equation 11.2

$$K_{el} = \frac{a \cdot PR}{C_c} + K_{nr} \qquad \qquad ...11.5$$

Recall that

$$K_{el} = \frac{0.693}{t_{1/2}}$$

Hence,

$$\frac{1}{t_{1/2}} = \frac{a \cdot PR}{0.693 \cdot C_c} + \frac{K_{nr}}{0.693} \qquad \qquad ...11.6$$

Thus plot of $\dfrac{1}{C_c}$ versus $\dfrac{1}{t_{1/2}}$ (or $\dfrac{1}{C_c}$ versus K_{el}) will be a straight line (Fig. 11.2).

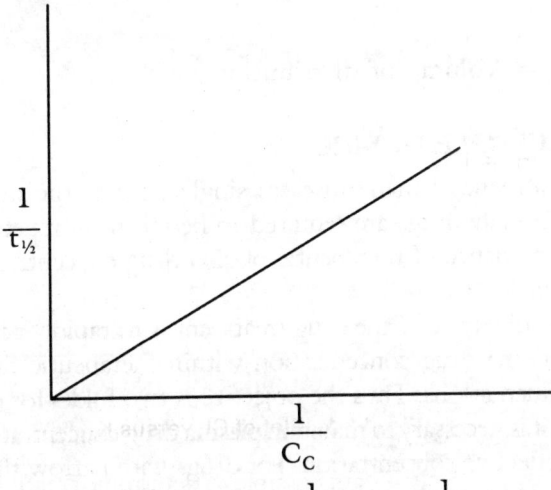

Fig. 11.2. Plot of $\dfrac{1}{C_c}$ versus $\dfrac{1}{t_{1/2}}$

Assume here that production rate of creatinine is constant. As creatinine is an end product of muscle metabolism, its production rate will depend on muscle mass. Hence sex, age and body weight will play an important role. Thus,

$$Cl_{cr} = \frac{Wt \cdot (144 - age)}{71 \cdot C_c} \qquad ...11.7$$

where,

C_c = Is in mg/dl.
Cl_{cr} = Is in ml/min.
Wt = Body weight in Kg.

Maintenance dose can be calculated as follows:

$$X_o = \frac{C' \cdot Cl_{cr} \cdot \tau}{F} \qquad ...11.8$$

where, X_o = Maintenance dose
C' = Average steady state plasma drug concentration.
Cl_{cr} = Creatinine clearance (estimated from equation 11.7).
τ = Dosing interval.
F = Fraction of the dose absorbed.

Equation 11.8 can also be represented as

$$X_o = \frac{C' \cdot V_d \cdot \tau}{1.44 \cdot F \cdot t_{1/2}} \qquad \text{...11.9}$$

where,

V_d = Volume of distribution.

11.2 MULTIPLE DOSING

For the treatment of many diseases single dose of the drug is not sufficient. Usually drugs are required to be taken on repetitive basis for the maintenance of therapeutic plasma drug concentrations over the treatment period.

The basic objective of the drug treatment is to rapidly achieve and maintain plasma drug concentration within therapeutic range with minimum fluctuations. Thus the objective is two fold—for drugs like antibiotics, it is necessary to maintain plasma drug concentration above minimum effective concentration. For drugs with narrow therapeutic range, it is necessary to ensure that plasma drug concentrations do not reach toxic levels.

Consider an oral multiple dosing regimens. When the first dose is administered, there is an increase in plasma drug concentration followed by a peak and then a decline in plasma drug concentration. When the second dose is administered, plasma drug concentration will again increase and reach a higher level than the one with first dose. This increase will continue till a steady state plasma drug concentration is achieved (Fig. 11.3).

Obviously at steady state, input and output of the drug will be equal.

How much drug accumulates in the body relative to the first dose can be calculated as follows:

$$R = \frac{1}{1 - e^{(-0.693\tau)/t_{1/2}}} \qquad \text{...11.10}$$

where,

R = Accumulation factor (depends on dosing interval and half life).

τ = Dosing interval.

Thus smaller the $\tau/t_{1/2}$ ratio, greater will be the accumulation.

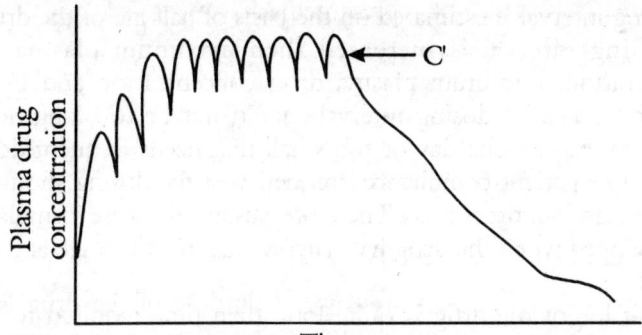

Fig. 11.3. Plasma drug concentration-time profile after multiple dosing regimen (C'– average steady state plasma drug concentration)

From first order kinetics ~90% of steady state will be reached within four half lives. But actual time required to reach steady state will depend on half life of the drug. Average steady state plasma drug concentration (C') will depend on:

♦ Maintenance dose, X_0
♦ Fraction of the dose absorbed, F
♦ Dosing interval, τ
♦ Clearance

$$C' = \frac{F \cdot X_o}{Cl \cdot \tau} \qquad \qquad ...11.11$$

i.e.
$$C' = \frac{1.44 \cdot F \cdot X_o \cdot t_{1/2}}{V_d \cdot \tau} = \frac{AUC}{\tau} \qquad ...11.12$$

where,

V_d = Volume of distribution,

AUC = Area under the plasma drug concentration versus time curve after single maintenance dose.

From equation 11.11 and 11.12 maintenance dose can be calculated as follows

$$X_o = \frac{C' \cdot Cl \cdot \tau}{F}$$

$$= \frac{C' \cdot V \cdot \tau}{1.44 \cdot F \cdot t_{1/2}} \qquad \qquad ...11.13$$

Dosing interval is estimated on the basis of half life of the drug. If the dosing interval is increased then maximum plasma drug concentration, minimum plasma drug concentration and C` will decrease. However, dosing interval should not be too long, ideally should not exceed one day or too small that needs frequent dosing. For a better patient compliance, frequency of the dosing should not be more than four times a day. Therefore, sustained release formulations are developed when the drug has narrow therapeutic range and short half life.

If half life of the drug is quite long then time required to reach steady state concentration will be very long. To shorten this time period *loading dose* can be administered, which will be followed by maintenance dose.

$$X'_0 = X_0 \cdot R \qquad \qquad ...11.14$$

where,

X'_0 = Loading dose.

R = Accumulation factor

Substituting equation 11.10 in equation 11.14

$$X'_0 = X_0 \cdot \frac{1}{1 - e^{-(0.693\tau/t_{1/2})}} \qquad ...11.15$$

During multiple dosing, maximum plasma drug concentration (C_{max}) and minimum plasma drug concentration (C_{min}) can be calculated after n^{th} dose as follows:

$$C_{n,max} = C_0 \left[\frac{1 - e^{-n \cdot K_{el} \cdot \tau}}{1 - e^{-K_{el} \cdot \tau}} \right] \qquad ...11.16$$

$$C_{n,min} = C_0 \left[\frac{1 - e^{-n \cdot K_{el} \cdot \tau}}{1 - e^{-K_{el} \cdot \tau}} \right] e^{-K_{el} \cdot \tau} \qquad ...11.17$$

Fluctuation is defined as the ratio of C_{max}/C_{min}; larger the ratio more is the fluctuation.

11.3 INDIVIDUALIZATION

Generally drug dosing and/or dosing adjustments are based on population data. But *intersubject variability* is known to exist for many drug responses. Meaning of intersubject variability is when different doses are required to produce same pharmacological response in different individuals. *Clinical Pharmacokinetics* uses pharmacokinetic principles in designing dosage regimens for individual patients.

Intersubject variability can be of two types:

1. *Pharmacokinetic variability*: It is due to differences in the drug concentration at the site of action and are because of the differences in absorption, distribution, biotransformation and excretion.

2. *Pharmacodynamic variability*: In this case, pharmacological response varies from individual to individual at a given dose.

Let us Design a Dosing Regimen

Consider a drug which follows first order kinetics and one compartment model. Elimination rate constant or half life and volume of distribution can be calculated in a patient.

$$C_{max} = \frac{K_0}{V_d \cdot K_{el}}(1 - e^{-K_{el}t}) + C_0 e^{-K_{el}t} \qquad ...11.18$$

where,

C_{max} = Maximum plasma drug concentration,
K_0 = Zero order infusion rate,
K_{el} = Elimination rate constant,
V_d = Volume of distribution,
C_0 = Initial drug concentration,
t = Time for which infusion is given.

i.e. $$V_d = \frac{K_o(1 - e^{-K_{el}t})}{K_{el}(C_{max} - C_o e^{-K_{el}t})} \qquad ...11.19$$

By collecting blood samples, C_0, C_{max} and K_{el} can be determined. C_o will be zero as this is the first time infusion has been administered, and now V_d can be calculated.

C_{max} and C_{min} can be calculated at steady state as follows:

$$C_{ss,max} = \frac{K_o(1 - e^{-K_{el}t})}{V_d \cdot K_{el} \cdot (1 - e^{-K_{el}\tau})} \qquad ...11.20$$

where,

τ = Dosing interval.

Based on equation 11.20, infusion rate can be estimated to achieve maximum steady state concentration.

$$K_o = V_d \cdot K_{el} \cdot C_{ss, max} \cdot (1 - e^{-K_{el} \cdot \tau})/(1 - e^{-K_{el} \cdot t}) \quad ...11.21$$

Minimum steady state concentration can be calculated as:

$$C_{ss, min} = C_{ss, max} \cdot e^{-K_{el}(\tau - t)} \quad\quad ...11.22$$

Let us consider some specific cases of individualization.

A. Obese Patients

It is obvious that volume of distribution of the drug will depend on body weight, as body weight is directly related to the volume of body fluids.

Ideal body weight (IBW) is calculated as follows:

$$IBW_{Men} = 50 \text{ Kg} \pm 1 \text{Kg}/2.5 \text{ cm}$$
$$\text{above or below 150 cm in height} \quad ...11.23$$
$$IBW_{Women} = 45 \text{ Kg} \pm 1 \text{Kg}/2.5 \text{ cm}$$
$$\text{above or below 150 cm in heigh} \quad ...11.24$$

Any person is considered as obese if the body weight is more than 25% above the IBW.

If the drug is not getting distributed in excess body volume i.e. no significant change in V_d, then dose calculation should be based on IBW e.g. digoxin.

If the drug is polar in nature, then it will show less distribution in obese, as extracellular fluid of adipose tissue is less compared to lean tissue. Then dose will be more than IBW but less on the basis of per kg total body weight e.g. gentamicin

For drugs which show similar extent of distribution both in lean and adipose tissue, dose should be administered based on the total body weight. Thus dose will be higher but because of larger V_d it will be same on per kg total body weight basis e.g. caffeine.

For drugs which are lipid soluble, distribution will be more in adipose tissue. Thus V_d will be larger for obese. Hence will require larger dose on total body weight basis e.g. phenytoin, diazepam.

B. Dosage Calculations In Neonates, Infants and Children

For adults the dosing regimens are usually calculated on the population basis. To determine doses for neonates, infants and children, body surface area is preferred over body weight. In children body surface area has a good correlation with dosage requirement, cardiac output, renal blood flow and glomerular filtration.

Various ways to calculate doses for neonates, infants and children are as follows:

1. Young's Rule (For children 2 years and above)

$$\left(\frac{Age(yr)}{Age(yr)+12}\right) \cdot \frac{Adult}{dose} = (Approx.) \; Child's \; dose \quad ...11.25$$

2. Clark's Rule

$$\left(\frac{Weight(lb)}{150}\right) \cdot \frac{Adult}{dose} = (Approx.) \; Child's \; dose \quad ...11.26$$

3. Fried's Rule (For infants upto 2 years old)

$$\left(\frac{Age(months)}{150}\right) \cdot \frac{Adult}{dose} = (Approx.) \; Infant's \; dose \quad ...11.27$$

4. Square Meter Surface Area
   Surface area (SA) in square meters can be calculated by Mosteller's equation

$$SA\left(in\,m^2\right) = \frac{(height \cdot weight)^{\frac{1}{2}}}{60} \quad ...11.28$$

$$\left(\frac{SA\,of\,child}{SA\,of\,adult}\right) \cdot Adult\,dose = (Approx.) \; Child's \; dose \quad ...11.29$$

But average body SA for adult is $1.73m^2$, hence equation 11.29 can be written as:

$$\left(\frac{SA\,of\,child}{1.73}\right) \cdot Adult\,dose = (Approx.) \; Child's \; dose \quad ...11.30$$

If the dose of the drug is prescribed as amount of drug/body SA (m^2) then individual dose can be calculated as:

$$Dose = (Amount\,of\,drug/m^2) \times Body\,SA\,(m^2) \quad ...11.31$$

A relationship also exists between body SA and body weight and is as follows:

$$SA\,(m^2) = Body\,weight\,(kg)^{0.7}$$

Hence,

$$(Approx.)\,Child's\,dose = \left(\frac{Body\,wieght\,of\,child\,(kg)}{70}\right)^{0.7} \cdot Adult\,dose \quad ...11.32$$

C. Hemodialysis

Hemodialysis is used in severe renal failure i.e. in uremic patients, to remove urea, creatinine, uric acid, phosphate and other endogenous waste materials. Hemodialysis may also result in drug loss from the body and hence may require additional dose adjustments.

Following factors affect the hemodialyzability of a drug:

1. **Molecular size:** Larger the molecular size poor is the dialyzability of a drug
2. **Blood flow:** Less the blood flow less is the dialyzability of a drug
3. **Dialyzate flow:** Less the dialyzate flow less is the dialyzability of a drug
4. **Aqueous solubility:** Less the aqueous solubility less is the dialyzability of a drug
5. **Volume of distribution/protein binding:** Larger the volume of distribution or more the drug is protein bound less is the dialyzability of a drug.

The fraction of the drug removed by dialysis can be calculated as follows:

$$f = \left(\frac{t_{1/2} - (t_{1/2})d}{t_{1/2}} \right) \cdot \left(1 - e^{-0.693 \cdot T / (t_{1/2})d} \right) \qquad ...11.33$$

where,

f = Fraction of the drug removed by dialysis.

$t_{1/2}$ = Half life of the drug in absence of dialysis.

$(t_{1/2})d$ = Half life of the drug during dialysis.

T = Duration of dialysis.

Amount of drug removed from the body by dialysis, this will also be the amount of drug to be administered at the end of the dialysis to maintain the therapeutic concentration, can be calculated as follows:

$$X_d = f \cdot C \cdot V_d \qquad ...11.34$$

where,

X_d = Amount of drug removed from the body by dialysis.

f = Fraction of the drug removed by the dialysis.

C = Predialysis plasma drug concentration.

V_d = Predialysis volume of distribution of the drug.

Peritoneal dialysis is similar to hemodialysis. In peritoneal dialysis peritoneal membrane is used, whereas in hemodialysis synthetic membrane is used. Although peritoneal membrane is more permeable, peritoneal dialysis appears to be less effective than hemodialysis. This is because certain lipophilicity is required to be dialyzed by peritoneal membrane.

A similar technique, hemoperfusion technique, is used in removing the drug in case of drug overdose.

D. Monitoring Drug Therapy

Ideally rationale drug therapy requires individualization of the dosage regimen on an individual basis. *Monitoring of drug therapy* involves evaluation of drug response in a particular individual at the recommended dosage regimen. This management involves a well defined clinical response called as *therapeutic endpoint*. Monitoring therapeutic end point is quite easy for many drugs e.g. antihypertensives, oral hypoglycemics, antianginal agents, analgesics, anticoagulants, and antihyperlipidemics or for drugs used for reducing serum uric acid levels.

For many other drugs therapeutic end point is not quite clear and toxic concentrations are also just slightly more than therapeutic concentrations. For such drugs *toxic end point* is considered for therapeutic regimens e.g. dryness of mouth in response to atropine.

Monitoring of drug therapy can also be done by monitoring plasma drug concentrations (pharmacokinetic monitoring). This approach is particularly useful when—

♦ There is no definite therapeutic point or is absent.
♦ Chances of clinical failures are high because of unpredictable absorption or pharmacokinetic variable.

Monitoring drug therapy is quite useful in deciding the dosage regimen in presence of hepatic or renal insufficiency. It is important to note that this is just an aid and not a substitute for careful clinical observations in the management of drug therapy.

E. Sustained Drug Delivery

For the treatment of many diseases it is necessary to achieve the therapeutic concentrations immediately and then to maintain those concentrations for the duration of the treatment. Conventionally this can be achieved by appropriately selecting dose size and frequency of administration. This conventional approach has certain limitations, such as:

> Even at steady state, fluctuations in plasma drug concentrations are present. So at the most average steady state concentrations remain constant.
> Because of fluctuations, plasma drug concentrations may reach toxic levels or below effective concentration level.
> For drugs with shorter half lives, frequent doses are required to achieve steady state. Thus too many doses may lead to poor patient compliance.

Because of these limitations, *extended release* preparations are formulated. These formulations are designed to eliminate/reduce the cyclical plasma concentrations seen after conventional treatment. Various terms are used to describe these systems e.g. delayed release, repeat action, prolonged release, sustained release, extended release, controlled release and modified release.

In this discussion *controlled release* term will be used to describe a dosage form which continuously releases drug at desired rates so as to prolong therapeutic action. Consider that drug used in modified release dosage form follows open one compartment model. Then drug disposition can be represented as shown in Fig. 11.4.

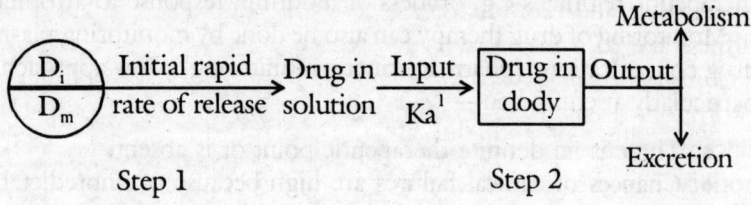

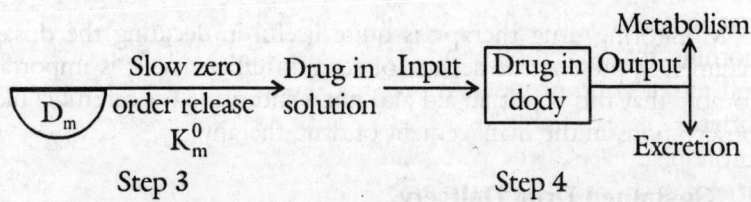

Fig. 11.4. Drug disposition for controlled release dosage form. D_i = initial dose of the drug in formulation; D_m = maintenance dose in formulation; K_a^1 = first order absorption rate constant; K_m^0= Zero order rate constant for drug release.

The initial loading dose (Di) is immediately released from the controlled dosage form. This helps in immediately achieving the therapeutic drug concentration. After this, maintenance dose of the drug (D_m) is release at a much slower but at a constant rate. This helps to maintain the constant plasma drug level.

F. Chronopharmacokinetics

Conventional strategies of drug delivery systems have been based on the assumption that biological functions display constancy over time (Homeostatic theory). But *chronobiological* studies have proved circadian rhythm for almost all body functions viz. heart rate, blood pressure, body temperature, hormonal concentration, gastric secretions and renal functions. Besides physiological functions and pathological states of the disease also have circadian rhythm. For example, asthma attacks are more pronounced at night. It is well known that patients with asthma experience asthmatic attacks at night e.g. dyspnoea and peak expiratory flow values have been found to become worse during night. Symptoms of allergy e.g. runny nose, stuffy nose, wheezing and sneezing are most frequent in the morning before breakfast. Ischaemic heart diseases manifest more frequently between 9 to 11 at night, rise in blood pressure is significantly more before awakening in both hypertensive and normotensive individuals. In rheumatoid arthritis, stiffness and pain are more on awakening and early morning hours.

Chronopharmacokinetics is the study of temporal changes in drug absorption, distribution, metabolism and elimination. Plasma drug concentrations are significantly affected by acid secretion, intestinal motility, intestinal blood flow, protein binding, enzyme activity and urinary pH. By chronopharmacokinetics, it has been demonstrated that in general drugs show higher bioavailability when taken in morning than when taken in evening. For example, for nifedipine, oral nitrates and propranolol C_{max} is almost twice and T_{max} is also shorter after morning doses than evening doses. This chronopharmacokinetic pattern is may be because of comparatively faster gastric emptying and better intestinal perfusion in the morning. Indomethacin and ketoprofen also show similar pattern. These observations are clinically relevant as high plasma concentrations correlate with high occurrence of adverse effects.

In *chronopharmacotherapy* drug administration (dosing regimen) is synchronized with biological rhythms so as to maximize therapeutic effect and minimize incidences of adverse effects.

Thus with the help of chronopharmacokinetics, drug delivery is based on circadian rhythm of disease and hence drug effect can be optimized and side effects can be reduced.

QUESTIONS

1. Explain application of pharmacokinetic principles in:
   (a) Renal failure
   (b) Multiple dosing
   (c) Individualization of dosing in obese patients
   (d) Individualization of dosing in infants/children.

2. Write short notes on:
   (a) Hemodialysis
   (b) Monitoring drug therapy
   (c) Sustained drug delivery
   (d) Chronopharmacokinetics.

12

Bioequivalence

12.1 INTRODUCTION

In order to elicit desired therapeutic effect the drug, an active substance, should be:

♦ Delivered at the site of action
♦ Delivered in an effective concentration
♦ Delivered during the desired period

It is absolutely essential that the performance of the dosage form containing the drug is reproducible in the body so as to predict the uniform therapeutic effect. It is necessary that the bioavailability of the drug from a dosage form is known and importantly, is reproducible. This is especially important when a product is substituted for another. Of course one of the best way to compare two products is by clinical studies. But performing clinical studies is extremely cumbersome and expensive. Hence bioequivalence studies are generally used to compare two products so as to confirm their biological equivalence. Bioequivalence is a comparison of bioavailability of two or more drug products i.e. formulations containing the same active ingredient are said to be bioequivalent if their rates and extent of absorption are same.

Bioavailability and bioequivalence are receiving increasing attention because of the increased availability and importance of generic drugs in today's pharmaceutical market. As a matter of fact, bioequivalence study is an important part of ANDA (Abbreviated New Drug Application). ANDA is required to be submitted to Food and Drug Administration by a pharmaceutical manufacturer who intends to introduce a generic drug in the market.

Bioequivalence is not a straightforward thing for all the drugs. Many drugs are known to be notorious for demonstrating *bioinequivalence*. Initial observations of bioinequivalence were seen with drug products containing vitamins, aspirin, tetracycline and tolbutamide from different manufacturers. But digoxin is a classic example and debate involving bioequivalence of digoxin still continues. Bioequivalence problems of digoxin are of importance because of its narrow therapeutic index. Many other drugs possessing narrow therapeutic index also suffer from bioinequivalence. In 1973 Ad Hoc Committee on Drug Product Selection of the American Pharmaceutical Association published a list of drugs that show bioinequivalence. Based on this list, drugs have been divided into three categories: "high", "moderate" and "low" risk. Some of the drugs belonging to these categories are listed in Table 12.1.

Table 12.1: Drugs with bioinequivalence potential

High Risk Potential	Moderate Risk Potential	Low Risk Potential
Aminophylline	Amphetamine	Acetaminophen
High doses of aspirin	Ampicillin	Codeine
Bishydroxycoumarine	Chloramphenicol	Hydrochlorthiazide
Digoxin	Chlorpromazine	Ephedrine
Phenytoin	Digitoxin	Isoniazid
Para-amino salicylic acid	Erythromycin	Meprobamate
Prednisolone	Griseofulvin	PenicillinVK
Prednisone	Oxytetracyclin	Sulfisoxazole
Quinidine	Penicillin G	
Warfarin	Pentobarbital	

12.2 IMPORTANT DEFINITIONS

Before proceeding into details of bioequivalence study, it is important to get familiarized with various terminologies.

Drug Product

Drug product means a finished dosage form formulation e.g. capsules, tablets, oral solution etc. containing the active substance (drug) with or without inactive ingredients (excipients).

Pharmaceutical Equivalents

Two products are called as pharmaceutical equivalents if they contain same amount of the active substance (drug) in the same dosage form, which have the comparable standards. It is important to note that pharmaceutical equivalence does not necessarily means bioequivalence.

Pharmaceutical equivalents may contain different inactive ingredients such as color, flavour, excepients and even may have different shape. Because of differences in these and/or manufacturing process, products from different manufacturers can show variable absorption pattern.

Pharmaceutical Alternatives

Two products are pharmaceutical alternatives if they contain the same drug molecule but in different chemical form e.g. different salt or different dosage form or strength.

Bioavailability

Bioavailability means the rate and extent to which the drug is absorbed from a dosage form and thus becomes available at the site of action. The term "absolute bioavailability" is used when a dosage form is compared with an intravenous administration. Intravenous administration is taken as 100% bioavailable. In "comparative bioavailability" two different formulations other than intravenous are compared e.g. tablets vs. oral solution.

Bioequivalence

Bioequivalence means the absence of a significant difference in the rate and extent of drug being available at the site of action. It is assumed that drug is administered at the same molar dose under the similar conditions in an appropriately designed study.

Bioequivalents

Two products are considered to be bioequivalent, if they are pharmaceutical equivalents or alternatives and if their bioavailability is similar after administration of same molar dose. Hence their effects in terms of efficacy and safety will be essentially same.

Essentially Similar Products

A product is considered to be "essentially same" to original (Innovator product) if it is same in qualitative and quantitative composition in terms of drug, formulation type and in addition it is bioequivalent.

Therapeutic Equivalents

Two products are considered to be therapeutic equivalent if they contain same active substance and have same efficacy and safety.

Generally bioequivalence is the widely accepted proof to confirm the therapeutic equivalence of two products.

12.3 BIOEQUIVALENCE STUDY PARAMETERS

Two products are said to be bioequivalent when they demonstrate similar rate and extent of drug release. This means that amount of drug molecules released and rate (speed) at which they are released should be similar. To study these characteristics of two drug products inside the body (*in vivo* situation), following parameters are usually used for the comparison.

AUC: Area under the plasma drug concentration-time curve. AUC provides the information regarding amount of drug in plasma i.e. extent of release.

C_{max}: Maximum plasma drug concentration. C_{max} partly depends on the rate of drug release from the formulation

T_{max}: Time required to reach maximum plasma drug concentration. T_{max} is also dependent on the rate of drug release from the formulation.

$T_{1/2}$: Elimination half-life. $T_{1/2}$ provides the information regarding elimination of the drug from the body.

Recall that these parameters and their calculations have been discussed in detail in earlier chapters.

Besides above-mentioned parameters, which are usually studied in a bioequivalence study, many times following additional parameters are also studied.

Normalized C_{max}

C_{max} and t_{max} are known to show significant intra-subject variability and hence normalized C_{max} is used in some cases. Normalized C_{max} is calculated by following equation:

$$\text{Normalized } C_{max} = \frac{C_{max}}{AUC}$$

...12.1

Studies have demonstrated that normalized C_{max} shows less intra-subject variability compared to C_{max}.

Mean Residence Time (MRT)

Mean residence time (MRT) provides an idea about the time a drug molecule spends in the body before it gets excerted. To calculate MRT, first area under the moment curve (AUMC) is calculated by following equation:

$$AUMC_{0-t} = \sum_{i=1}^{t}\left(\frac{t_i C_i + t_{i-1} \cdot C_{i-1}}{2}\right)\left[t_i - t_{i-1}\right] \quad ...12.2$$

From equation 12.2 it can be seen that calculation of AUMC is very much similar to AUC. The only difference is that in AUMC there is a multiplication of drug plasma concentration by time. $AUMC_{0-\infty}$ can be calculated from $AUMC_{0-t}$. Now MRT can be calculated by following equation.

$$MRT = \frac{AUMC_{0-\infty}}{AUC_{0-\infty}} \quad ...(12.3)$$

Plasma Trough Fluctuation (%)

This parameter is generally used in the bioequivalence study of sustained release formulations. Sustained release formulations are designed in such a way so as to maintain steady state plasma drug concentration for extended periods of time. Hence bioequivalence study of sustained release formulations mainly involves the comparison of steady state plasma drug concentrations obtained form two drug products.

Therefore, in this case, two additional parameters are taken in to consideration:

C_{min}– Lowest plasma drug concentration just before the next dose, and %PTF– Percent change in the plasma drug concentration between two dose administrations is calculated by following equation:

$$\%PTF = \frac{C_{max} - C_{min}}{C_{average}} \quad ...12.4$$

where, $C_{average}$ = Average plasma drug concentration during the dosing period.

12.4 BIOEQUIVALENCE STUDY PROTOCOL

Any bioequivalence study is always driven by a study protocol. Bioequivalence study protocol should include following components-

- ➤ Title
  - ◆ Principal investigator or study director
  - ◆ Project or protocol number and date
- ➤ Study objective
- ➤ Study design
  - ◆ Design
  - ◆ Drug Products
    - ❖ Test product
    - ❖ Reference product
  - ◆ Dosage regimen
  - ◆ Sample collection schedule
  - ◆ Housing of subjects
  - ◆ Fasting and meal schedule
  - ◆ Analytical method
- ➤ Study population
  - ◆ Subjects
  - ◆ Subject selection
    - ❖ Medical history
    - ❖ Physical Examination
    - ❖ Laboratory tests
  - ◆ Inclusion and exclusion criteria
  - ◆ Restrictions during study
- ➤ Clinical procedures
  - ◆ Dosage and drug administration
  - ◆ Biological sampling
  - ◆ Handling of biological samples
- ➤ Ethical considerations
  - ◆ Institutional Review Board
  - ◆ Informed consent
  - ◆ Indications for withdrawal of subjects
  - ◆ Adverse reactions
  - ◆ Emergency procedures
- ➤ Facilities
- ➤ Data analysis
  - ◆ Validation of analytical procedure
  - ◆ Statistical methods used
- ➤ Appendix

12.5 STUDY DESIGN

A bioequivalence study should be designed in such a way so as to identify treatment effects that are produced after administration of drug products i.e. formulation effects. Basically there are two types of study designs—crossover and parallel. Generally a crossover design is used in practice. In this design both test and reference products are compared in each subject i.e. each subject acts as his/her own control. Hence inter-subject variables such as, age, weight, metabolism etc are minimal. Because of the minimal inter-subject variability, crossover design is widely used for routine bioequivalence studies. In this design first subjects are randomly divided into two groups and sequence of drug is randomly assigned. If there are two formulations - Test formulation (T) and reference formulation (R), in Period I Group I will receive T followed by R (it is just an example, it can be other way round i.e. Group I may receive R followed by T). The time period between the administrations of two formulations will be sufficiently long considering adequate washout period. *Washout period* is essential to ensure complete elimination of drug before the next administration. Ten (10) half-lives ensures more than 99% of elimination and hence washout period should be at least 10 half lives. Period II will start after the completion of washout period. Now in Period II, Group I will receive R following by T.

If a drug requires washout period of 7 days (half-life ~16 hours), then sequence of administration of two formulations can be shown as in Table 12.2

Table 12.2: Sequence of administration in a bioequivalence study (Period I and II)

Group	Period I (Day 1)	Period II (Day 8)
I	T	R
II	R	T

Thus *sequence* of administration (treatment) for Group I is T-R and for Group II is R-T. In other words, any two-formulation trial is a two-sequence trial. As can be noticed from Table 12.2, two-formulation trial is also always a two period trial. Thus in Period I, 50% subjects (Group I) receive T and 50% subjects (Group II) receive R. In Period II order is reversed.

The number of subjects in a study is based on the statistical parameters. Although 24 subjects are usually preferred, a study should never have less than 12 subjects.

The blood sampling should be scheduled in such way so as to cover at least 80% of the area under the plasma concentration curve. The blood sampling schedule should also be planned in such a way so as to provide adequate estimation of C_{max} and t_{max}.

12.6 SUBJECTS

Bioequivalence studies are usually performed with healthy volunteers (subjects). As far as possible an attempt should be made to include subjects of both the sexes. Usually subjects should be between 18-55 years old. Subjects should weigh within the normal range according to accepted normal values for the Body Mass Index.

It is important to reduce the intra and inter-subject variability. The products are usually administered after the over night fasting. Also, meals taken during the course of the study should be standardized. It is important to note that even the fluid intake including water should be standardized, as fluid intake significantly influences gastric emptying time. It is essential that during the course of study, subject should not be taking any medications including over the counter products. During the course of study, subject should not be allowed to have alcoholic or xanthine containing beverages e.g. coffee, tea, cola flavored soft drinks etc., as they are known to affect circulatory, GI, liver or renal functions. Subjects enrolled in a study preferably should be non-smokers. If they are smokers then this should be noted in their medical history.

12.7 BIOANALYSIS OF SAMPLES

The details of bioanalytical techniques can be found in next chapter (Chapter 13).

It is important that bioanalytical method used should have required specificity, accuracy, sensitivity and precision. It is absolutely essential to validate the method and validation results should be included in the study report. Generally the bioanalytical method should have following characteristics:

> ➤ Adequate stability of stock solutions and analyte(s) in biological fluid under processing and storage conditions.
> ➤ Specificity
> ➤ Accuracy
> ➤ Precision
> ➤ Low limit of quantification

Generally measurement of metabolites (biotransformation products) is not essential. But if the drug is a prodrug then measurement of concentration of metabolite is essential.

12.8 REFERENCE AND TEST PRODUCT

Generic product or test product, which is a pharmaceutical equivalent, is usually compared with reference product. Reference product is generally the "Innovator product" (product of a company who first invented this product). In some cases instead of innovator product another well established product available in the market could be used. But choice of reference product other than innovator product should be justified by the principal investigator.

Before proceeding to bioequivalence studies both test products and reference products are tested for *in vitro* dissolution profile. It is essential that both the product should have comparable dissolution profile. The products from the same batch should be used for dissolution study and bioequivalence study.

12.9 STATISTICAL METHODS

Generally statistical method for testing bioequivalnce is based upon the 90% confidence interval for the ratio of the means (Test/Reference), for a particular parameter under consideration. Pharmacokinetic parameters e.g., AUC, C_{max} etc. derived from the data should be analyzed using ANOVA. The data needs to be transformed prior to analysis using a logarithmic transformation. Also, summary statistics such as, median, minimum and maximum should be given.

It is important to note that 90% confidence interval for a particular parameter under consideration should be within an acceptable range of 0.8 - 1.25 i.e. 80-125%. It means that a product is considered to be bioequivalent if the difference between two formulations is less than ±20% i.e. average rate and extent of a bioavailability of the test formulation is within 20% that of reference formulation.

12.10 REPORTING

Bioequivalence study report should provide complete documentational evidence regarding study protocol, study conduct and evaluation. The study should comply with Good Clinical Practices. Different sections of the report should be signed by responsible investigator(s).

It is essential that all the results should be presented in a clear way. Method of calculations of various parameters viz. AUC, $t_{1/2}$, K_{el}, etc. from raw data should be clearly stated. It is also necessary to include at least representative chromatographs.

Any dropout or withdrawal of subjects should be reported and deletion of data should be properly justified.

12.11 EXEMPTION

There are situations where bioequivalence study is not required. For example

1. If the product differs only in the strength, but in this case it is necessary that following conditions should be satisfied

   ♦ Drug pharmacokinetic pattern is linear.
   ♦ In lower and higher strength products ratio between active substance (drug) and excipients is the same.
   ♦ Manufacturing site for both higher and lower strength products is same.
   ♦ Both products have same dissolution rate.

2. If the minor changes have been done to formulation or method of manufacturing and if these changes can be convincingly proved to be irrelevant for the bioavailability of the drug.

3. The product is to be parenterally administered as a solution and such product(s) is/are already available in the market.

4. The product is an oral liquid in the form of solution e.g. elixir.

12.12 WHERE BIOEQUIVALENCE STUDY IS IRRELEVANT

In quite a few situations as listed below, bioequivalence studies are not required—

❖ The product is a gas for inhalation
❖ Products for local use and are intended to produce desired effect without systemic absorption

12.13 REGULATORY REQUIREMENTS FOR BIOEQUIVALENCE STUDIES

The guidelines by various regulatory authorities are now available over Internet. Students are advised to check the web site for respective regulatory authorities for the details. A summary of regulatory requirements of the American (US Food and Drug Administration, USFDA) and European (the European Agency for the Evaluation of Medicinal Products, EMEA) is given in Table 12.3

Table 12.3: Comparison of the regulatory requirements

	USFD	EMEA
Parameters on which to prove bioequivalnce	C_{max}, AUC_{0-t}, AUC_{∞}	C_{max}, AUC_{0-t}, AUC_{∞}.
Confidence Interval for C_{max}	Yes, 80-125	Yes, 80-125, (but if larger it can be justified)
Need for steady state	NO	Yes, if the formulation is of sustained release type
Need for a food effect study	Yes, only if the effect of food is specified in the labeling	For immediate release it is needed if there is a food effect reported with the Innovator product. It is needed for sustained release formulations.
Need for metabolite data	Supportive evidence	Yes if the drug is prodrug or if the metabolite contributes significantly to the efficacy for the product
Percentage of the AUC needs to be observed e.g. AUC_{0-t}/AUC_{∞} ratio)	>80%	>80%

12.14 GOOD CLINICAL PRACTICES IN BIOEQUIVALENCE

Good Clinical Practice (GCP) is an international ethical and scientific quality standard for designing, conducting, recording and reporting clinical trials that involve the participation of human subjects. Appropriate Guideline, preferably the ICH GCP Guidelines should be followed when generating bioequivalence data for the submission to regulatory authorities.

For each phase of the study GCP guidelines should be outlined, standard operating procedures (SOPs) should be formulated and data collection documents should be designed so as to maintain high standards of GCP.

Generally clinical SOPs should be formulated covering following steps of the bioequivalence study from the initiation up to the storage of samples:

> The study protocol
> Ethics committee approval
> Selection of staff and facilities
> Recruitment of subjects
> Obtaining trial materials
> Performing the actual study i.e. collection and recording of data
> Handling and storage of samples

These SOPs should establish the quality of clinical part of the study. They also help in performing the routine tasks and ensure that a standardized methodology is followed throughout the bioequivalence study. This helps in minimizing the variations.

A typical SOP should include following information:

> Title of the SOP, SOP number and effective date.
> Aim and objectives of the SOP.
> Detailed step by step instructions on how to carry out the procedure.
> List of all the materials and equipments needed for the procedure.
> Signatures of concerned people including Principal Investigator.

Data obtained during the procedure must be systematically collected so as to ensure accuracy, consistency, and integrity. Data collection documents e.g. logbooks, forms, clinical reports, case report forms etc. should properly maintained and archived. It is essential that a detailed blood analysis should be done during screening of the subjects for subject bank before the initiation and on completion of a bioequivalence study. Typically, blood analysis should contain following parameters.

> WBC count
> Haematocrit value
> Haemoglobin
> Sedimentation

> Blood sugar
> Serum creatinine
> Serum sodium concentration
> Serum potassium concentration
> Serum calcium concentration
> Serum bilirubin
> SGOT (Serum Glutmate Oxaloacetate Aminotransferase)
> SGPT (Serum Glutmate Pyruvate Aminotransferase)
> Alkaline phosphatase
> Total cholesterol
> Total protein

In addition subjects should be screened for Hepatitis, HIV and syphilis infections.

Many times following *non-compliances* are found in bioequiavlence studies and hence a special attention should be paid to these points:

> Subjects not receiving the drug products (test or reference) as per the randomization schedule.
> Biological samples compromised by improper identification, handling or storage.
> Improper reporting of adverse reactions e.g. vomiting and diarrhoea, which are known to affect absorption and elimination of drugs.
> Improper drug accountability records.
> Inadequate medical supervision and coverage.
> Protocol deviations *not reported* to the sponsor.
> Failure to adhere to the inclusion/exclusion criteria.
> Improper consent of subjects.
> Other situations in which the health and welfare of the subjects is not properly considered.

Bioequivalence studies are important scientific studies. They give the assurance to health care professionals that two formulations of the same drug (may be produced by different manufacturers) will have similar extent of efficacy and toxicity/adverse effects. At the same time designing an appropriate study can be a complicated task.

QUESTIONS

1. In brief explain bioequivalence study parameters.
2. Describe bioequivalence study protocol.
3. List the situations in which bioequivalence study can be exempted.
4. Explain following terms:
   (a) Bioequivalence
   (b) Bioequivalents
   (c) Bioavailability
   (d) Pharmaceutical equivalents
   (e) Therapeutic equivalents.
5. Write notes on:
   (a) Study design
   (b) Good clinical practices in bioequivalence.

13

Introduction to Bioanalysis

13.1 INTRODUCTION

Bioequivalence study of any drug involves mainly two parts, a clinical part and another is bioanalytical part. Previous chapter dealt with the clinical part of bioequivalence. In this chapter bioanalytical aspects of bioequivalence study will be introduced. Bioanalysis is increasingly gaining more and more importance. The scope of bioanalytical involvement in drug discovery and development is also becoming important. Linking Pharmacokinetic data with pharmacodynamic observations or investigating the fate of a drug in biological environment (metabolite profiling) are other examples besides bioequivalence where bioanalysis plays important role.

When blood samples are collected during a bioequivalence study, they are used either for collection of plasma or serum. Plasma can be obtained by simply centrifuging the blood containing anti-coagulant e.g. heparin, EDTA etc., at 2000 to 3000 rpm. Plasma can be collected by separating the supernatant after the centrifugation. For obtaining serum, blood is allowed to clot at room temperature and then centrifuged. The serum is separated and stored in storage vials. Blood plasma or serum is generally stored below -20°C. The plasma or serum is the one, which is used to extract drug for further determination. pH plays a very important role in extraction of drug from plasma. We shall therefore revise the basic concepts of pH and its importance.

13.2 BASIC CONCEPTS OF pH

An acid is any substance when added in water gives hydrogen ions:

$$HA + H_2O \rightarrow H_2O^+ + A^- \qquad \qquad ...13.1$$

Similarly a base ionizes in water to give hydroxyl ions:
$$B + H_2O \rightarrow BH^+ + OH^- \qquad \qquad ...13.2$$
Pure water ionizes slightly to produce H_3O^+ and OH^- ions:
$$2H_2O \rightarrow H_3O^+ + OH^- \qquad \qquad ...13.3$$
The dissociation constant K_W can then be defined as follows:
$$K_W = [H_3O^+] \cdot [OH^-] \qquad \qquad ...13.4$$
At 25°C $K_W = 1 \times 10^{-14}$. In pure water the concentration of H_3O^+ and OH^- is 1×10^{-7}, each.

Since it is not convenient to express the concentration in terms of actual figures such as 1×10^{-1} to 1×10^{-14}, a pH scale was proposed by Sprenson. *pH is defined as negative logarithm of hydrogen ion concentration*. Hence,
$$pH = -\log [H^+] \text{ or } -\log [H_3O^+] \qquad ...13.5$$
Using the definition of pH, the pH scale will be from 0 to 14. If the solution is acidic, its pH will range from 0 to 7, while a basic solution will have pH from 7 to 14.

The ionization of water is temperature dependent. It is therefore important to mention the pH at a given temperature.

pH of a solution changes if small quantities of acid or alkali are added to it. To avoid such changes in pH, buffers are used. A buffer is defined as a solution that resists change in pH when a small amount of acid or base is added. A buffer contains a mixture of a weak acid and its conjugate base or a weak base and its conjugate acid. In acetic acid- acetate buffer system, the equilibrium condition is given by,
$$HOAc \rightarrow H^+ + OAc^- \qquad \qquad ...13.6$$
The hydrogen ion concentration is given by,
$$[H^+] = K_a \cdot \frac{[HOAc]}{[OAc^-]} \qquad \qquad ...13.7$$
where,

    K_a = Dissociation constant.

Taking logarithm on both sides and simplifying the equation gives,
$$pH = pKa + \log \frac{[OAc^-]}{[HOAc]} \qquad \qquad ...13.8$$
This form of the equation is called as the Handerson-Hasselbach equation. This equation tells that when pH = pK_a, the concentration of ionized and unionized species in the solution is equal to each other.

This equation plays a very important role in the extraction of drug from plasma and HPLC method development for drugs.

13.3 EXTRACTION OF DRUG FROM PLASMA

Plasma is the most commonly used biological material in bioequivalence studies. Drug product, which is present in the plasma, is extracted using various methodologies. The most common methods used for the extraction of drug from plasma are—

1. Liquid-liquid extraction
2. Protein precipitation
3. Solid phase extraction
4. Direct plasma injection

13.3.1 Liquid-liquid Extraction

In liquid-liquid extraction, drug is extracted from plasma using a suitable organic solvent, and then concentrated followed by its analysis. The most commonly used solvents for liquid-liquid extraction are:

➢ Dichloromethane
➢ Hexane
➢ Tertiary butyl methyl ether
➢ Ethyl acetate
➢ Dioxane

Solvent is selected by taking into consideration the polarity of the drug molecule. If a drug is nonpolar, hexane is a preferred solvent. Whereas if drug molecule is moderately polar, dichloromethane is a preferred solvent. The general procedure is as follows.

Take 0.5 to 1 ml plasma and adjust the pH to desired value by adding small volume of buffer. Add appropriate quantity of internal standard and 5 to 10 ml of extraction solvent. The container usually is a stoppered glass tube, which is secured and loaded on a rotary extractor. The rotary extractor is set at 40 rpm. Extraction is carried out for 30 to 45 minutes. The tubes are then centrifuged and organic phase is transferred to conical tubes and evaporated under the stream of nitrogen. The residue is reconstituted in 100 to 200 μl of mobile phase and injected on HPLC.

Alternatively, instead of rotary extractor, the tubes are vortexed for 1 to 2 minutes followed by centrifugation.

Advantage of liquid-liquid extraction is that, the drug gets concentrated upon extraction and can be reconstituted in small volume

(100 to 200 μl). Hence even low concentration of drugs (even in ng/ml range) can be estimated with high accuracy.

Drugs are either acidic or basic. Each drug product has unique pK_a. Blood plasma pH ranges from 7.5 to 8.5. It is therefore important to know the pK_a of the drug and adjust the pH of plasma in such a way that the drug molecules are in unionized form. If the drug remains in ionized form, it will tend to partition into aqueous phase rather than getting extracted into organic phase. The Handerson-Hasselbach equation (Equation 13.8) becomes very important in adjusting the pH of plasma. If a drug is acidic, adjusting its pH equals to PK_a of -2 will ensure 100% unionized species into the organic phase. Reverse is true for basic molecule.

One has to remember that the organic solvents have density either higher or lower than plasma. If dichloromethane is used as extraction solvent, then plasma will form upper layer and dichloromethane the lower layer. If hexane is used, then plasma will form the lower layer and hexane the upper layer. While hexane can be transferred into another tube using pipette, it will be difficult to do the same for dichloromethane. A glass pipette attached to vacuum through a trap can be used to remove the plasma without creating mess. Figure 13.1 shows the schematic of such arrangement.

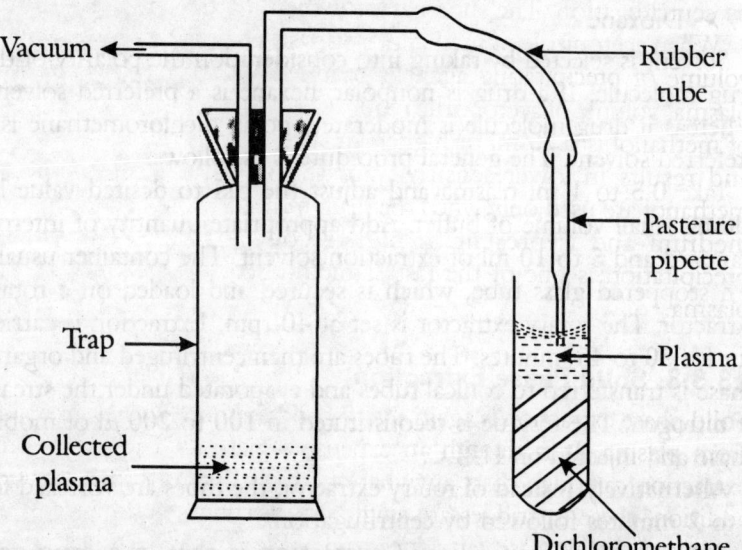

Fig. 13.1. Assembly for separation of lower layer of organic solvent

The above assembly can be readily made from available glass trap in the laboratory.

Liquid-liquid extraction is one of the most commonly used techniques for drug extraction from plasma. It gives concentrated drug solution, clean solution, does not load the HPLC column with impurities and is convenient. Care must be taken to avoid exposure of analyst to solvent vapors.

13.3.2 Protein Precipitation

Protein precipitation is the fastest method of drug extraction. This method is used when drug levels in plasma are relatively high (in $\mu g/ml$ range) and the drug molecule is stable in reagents used for protein precipitation. The most commonly used reagent for protein precipitation are—

> ➤ 10% trichloro acetic acid
> ➤ 10% perchloric acid
> ➤ Acetonitrile
> ➤ Methanol

0.5 ml plasma is pipetted into a polypropylene tube, internal standard may be added if required. 50 to 100 μl of 10% trichloro acetic acid or perchloric acid is added and the tube is vortexed followed by centrifugation. The supernatant is then injected on the HPLC.

When acetonitrile or methanol is used as precipitating agent, higher volume of precipitating agent is required. For example, for 0.5 ml plasma, volume of acetonitrile required is 0.5 ml or higher and volume of methanol is 0.75 ml or higher. In such cases the drug gets diluted and results in lower sensitivity of the method. Acetonitrile and methanol are used only when the drug molecule is not stable in acidic medium and is present in higher concentration. But protein precipitation is one of the fastest methods of drug extraction from plasma.

13.3.3 Solid Phase Extraction

Solid phase extraction is again a very good method for drug extraction from plasma. It is though an expensive method. Each solid phase extraction cartridge costs anywhere between Rs. 100 to Rs. 200. In addition, these cartridges are single use cartridges and hence cannot be reused. Solid phase cartridges come in various types e.g. C_{18}, C_{18}-cyano and mixed phase. The procedure followed is as below.

A solid phase cartridge is first conditioned with proper solvent, usually water and methanol. 0.5 ml of plasma is then loaded and a mild vacuum is applied. The drug present in the plasma gets adsorbed on the cartridge material and gets retained. The cartridge is then washed with 0.5 to 1.0 ml of water and is dried under vacuum. The drug is then eluted with mixture of water:methanol or water:acetonitrile into clean vials. The elute is then concentrated under nitrogen and is injected on HPLC column.

Although the procedure looks simple, it requires considerable efforts in method development and optimization of conditions. In addition it involves several operations and is time consuming. Now new fully automated solid phase extraction and injection on HPLC equipments are available. Though such equipments are expensive, they save time and are more accurate.

13.3.4 Direct Plasma Injection

In some cases, plasma can be directly injected onto HPLC columns. These are specially prepared HPLC columns and are commercially available. This is a recent development and hence not much information is available on their suitability and uses in bioanalytical field.

13.4 ANALYTICAL TECHNIQUES IN BIOANALYSIS

Many techniques are and have been used for bioanalysis. Now LC-MS and LC-MS/MS have taken over most of the other techniques in today's world. GC-MS and classical HPLC with UV or fluorescence detection still play important role in bioanalysis but are becoming less and less used techniques. These are important in cases where sensitivity of a technique is not an issue and also where the cost factor is involved.

HPLC analysis relies on following parameters:

➢ Retention time
➢ Peak area
➢ UV spectral character.

The biggest drawback of HPLC method is the lack of sensitivity and specificity. There are various examples where both the drug and its metabolite have the similar retention time and UV spectral character, and hence can mislead the analyst.

Gas Chromatography (GC), once a popular technique, now has lost its favorite position for bioanalysts. GC requires a tedious sample preparation, which makes it less economical. In addition, GC has limited use for polar drugs and thermo labile drugs. GC is still used for the detection of non-nitrogen containing drugs e.g. steroids and hormones. GC can be coupled with different detectors such as Electro Chemical Detector (ECD) or Mass Spectroscopy (MS). GC-MS is useful for the detection of compounds with high log P or compounds, which lack readily ionizable groups. But overall, use of GC techniques in bioanalysis is quite limited.

Now a days LC-MS/LS-MS/MS has taken over most of the bioanalytical work in pharmaceutical industries. Generally the preferred way of performing mass spectroscopy quantitation is by using MS/MS fragmentation. It is generally accomplished with a triple quadruple or ion trap mass spectrometer. One of the reason MS/MS is preferred is because many compounds have same intact mass. The first dimension of MS is often not satisfactory for the purpose of quantitation because of the lack of specificity, especially in the biological fluid. Hence it is always advisable to use second dimension of MS fragmentation, which provides unique fragment. Thus MS/MS, which provides combination of specific parent mass and unique fragment ion is preferable for the selective quantitation of a compound in biological fluid.

Following are commonly used mode of acquiring LC-MS data:

◆ **Total Ion Current (TIC):** The TIC is a plot of the total ion current in each MS scan plotted as an intensity point. It is a plot similar to HPLC-UV trace except that it can detect many more components such as UV transparent component. But identifying a particular compound can be very tricky as many compounds have the same mass and intact mass of a compound is not a unique identifier.

◆ **Selected Ion Monitoring (SIM):** In this, the MS is set to scan over a small range, usually one mass unit. The SIM plot is much more specific compared to TIC plot as it is a plot of ion current resulting from a very small range of mass. Still many times SIM plot shows more number of peaks with no unique identifier for a compound.

◆ **Selected Reaction Monitoring (SRM):** SRM produces a unique fragment ion and plot is usually simple consisting of single peak. Hence it is an ideal plot for the sensitive and specific quantitation. Thus it is the preferred method for mass spectrometric quantitation of plasma drug concentration.

13.5 BIOANALYTICAL METHOD VALIDATION

Bioanalytical method used for the quantitation of drug and its metabolites in biological fluids plays an important role in the evaluation and interpretation of pharmacokinetic data obtained in bioequivalence/bioavailability studies. Hence it is important that the bioanalytical methods used should be well characterized and validated so as to obtain reliable and reproducible results for satisfactory interpretations. Various parameters are taken into consideration for this purpose viz. stability of analyte in the biological fluid, accuracy, precision, specificity (i.e. selectivity), sensitivity and reproducibility.

Following guidelines should be taken into consideration for any bioanalytical method development and validation. *The term analyte expresses both drug or its metabolite*.

A. A detailed SOP (Standard Operating Procedure) of the analytical method should be written. SOP should include purpose of the method, list of reagents, test solutions including directions for preparation, storage and the expiration date. SOP should also cover instruments and parameters used in the method. SOP should be written in such a way that a qualified (skilled) person should be able to repeat the method.

B. In a method each item should be characterized in detail. The effect of variables such as materials, collection of samples, time lapse till final analysis, freeze-thaw of samples etc. should be characterized. It is also essential that same biological fluid as will be used for final study should be used for method validation. For example, if blood plasma is going to be used in the final study then method validation should also be done using blood plasma.

C. The method developed should state the concentration range over which the method can be satisfactorily used. Meaning, a standard curve should be prepared. Usually standard curve should consist of at least five different concentrations (excluding blank). Standard curve should cover the expected concentration range. It is essential that a standard curve should be generated for each analytical run and should be used to calculate unknown concentration of analyte in that particular run.

D. LOD (Limit of Detection) should be determined. LOD is the lowest concentration of analyte in biological fluid which can be determined by the method. Whereas, LOQ (Limit of Quantitation) is the lowest concentration on the standard curve which can be measured with accuracy and precision. Generally LOQ is measured by using five samples that are apart from standard curve and coefficient variation is determined.

E. Accuracy and precision of the method using known concentrations of analyte in biological fluid should be determined. For this purpose analysis of replicate sets of analyte samples of known concentrations are used. Generally five determinations per samples are done. It is important that three concentrations over the concentration range should be studied as follows:

❖ One concentration near the LOQ.
❖ One concentration near the center of concentration range.
❖ One concentration near the highest concentration of the concentration range.

The mean value should be within ± 15% of the actual value. But at LOQ it should not deviate by more than ± 20%. Also for precision, the mean value should not exceed 15% coefficient variation but for LOQ it should not exceed 20% coefficient of variation. These are called as Quality Control samples and they should be included in each run.

F. It is advisable that the specificity of the bioanalytical method should be determined using at least six different sources of the biological fluid. This means that if the drug concentration is to be determined in plasma then plasma from six different individuals should used for the determination of specificity of the method.

G. For bioanalytical methods where drug is extracted from biological fluid before the final analysis, it is essential that recovery of the drug should be established for the extraction procedure.

H. It is advisable that extrapolation below the lowest concentration and above the highest concentration on standard curve should not be done. Instead, if needed, the standard curve should be appropriately modified.

Following are some of the important parameters used in the validation of bioanalytical method.

1. *Accuracy*: It is the closeness between the analyte (drug or its metabolite) concentration determined by the method and the actual concentration.

2. *Precision*: It is the closeness between a series of measurements obtained from multiple samplings. Precision is usually expressed as the averages, Standard Deviation (SD) or Relative Standard Deviation (RSD). The RSD ranges define the intra-day precision and a normal acceptance criterion is that RSD should be less than 15%. Inter-day precision is assessed by calculating pooled RSD (or SD or averages) for the control samples assayed on different validation days. The normal acceptance criterion for inter-day precision is that pooled RSD should be less than 15%. It is important to note that a method can be precise but not accurate i.e. all the measurements may be close to each other but may not be close to actual concentration.

3. *Detection Limit*: It is the lowest amount of analyte, which can be detected (but not necessarily quantitated). In normal practice, it is calculated as the signal-to-noise ratio, which is equivalent to three (3) times the SD of the noise. Thus–

$$\text{Detection Limit} = \frac{3 \cdot \sigma}{S} \qquad \qquad ...13.9$$

where,

σ = SD of the noise.

S = Slope of the calibration curve.

4. *Quantitation Limit*: It is the lowest amount of analyte which can be detected by the method with acceptable accuracy and precision. In normal practice it is calculated as the signal-to-noise ratio, which is equivalent to ten (10) times the SD of the noise. Thus–

$$\text{Quantitation Limit} = \frac{10 \cdot \sigma}{S} \qquad \qquad ...13.10$$

where,

σ = SD of the noise.

S = Slope of the calibration curve.

5. *Linearity*: It is simply the range of concentrations of analyte for which the method gives the results which correlate to the actual amount of analyte in the biological sample.

6. *Robustness*: It is also called as *Ruggedness*. It is the measure of capability of a method to remain unaffected by small (but deliberate/purposeful) variations in the parameters of the method.

During method validation, special attention should be paid to following points to avoid *non-compliance* of the final report:

➤ The analytical laboratory should have scientifically sound data to support claims for the specificity of the assay employed in the study. Proper justification for non-interferences, both endogenous and exogenous e.g. metabolites, solvent contamination, etc. in measurement of the analytes.

➤ The analytical laboratory should have data to support the claims for the linearity of the assay employed in this study.

➤ The data demonstrating the sensitivity of the assay should be generated using the same instrumentation as that employed in the final bioanalysis of bioequivalence study samples.

➤ The data demonstrating the precision of the assay should be generated using the instrumentation employed in the final bioanalysis of bioequivalence study samples. The data should be generated for both standard and quality control samples and should include the consistency of precision of the standard and control samples carried through the assay procedure. Proper justification should be there for the precision based on the separation procedure, instrumentation, and analyte concentration levels in the biological fluids.

➤ The data should be available to demonstrate drug recovery for the measured analyte(s). It should include both analyte extraction efficiency from the biological fluid and recovery of the analyte(s) carried through the bioanalytical procedure.

➤ The stability of the drug should be determined both in the biological fluid and in the sample preparation medium under the same conditions as in actual analysis of the bioequivalence study samples.

➤ The data should be generated for the storage procedures (freezing and number of freeze/thaw cycles) demonstrating no adverse effect on drug stability for the period of time the samples were stored i.e. from sample collection till final analysis.

➤ The water quality specified for sample and reagent preparation should be consistent and readily available in the bioanalytical laboratory.

13.6 STABILITY OF THE ANALYTE IN BIOLOGICAL FLUID

Analyte needs to be stable in the biological fluid during collection, processing, storage or sample preparation. Stability will dictate as to how long a sample can be stored under specific conditions before bioanalysis can be performed reliably. Stability studies are essential so as to ensure following:

➤ Analyte does not degrade in the blood.
➤ Analyte does not degrade during processing to obtain plasma or serum.
➤ Analyte does not degrade under storage conditions (–80°C, –20°C, refrigerated or room temperature).
➤ Analyte does not degrade during extraction procedure.

Thus stability studies are essential to ensure that drug concentration determined in the biological sample is the true measure of the drug concentration at the time of sample collection. Usually stability studies are described as generally carried out.

Freeze–Thaw Cycle Stability

This is essential for the samples which are stored frozen (–80°C or –20°C) after the sample collection till its analysis. This stability study provides the data regarding stability of the analyte in biological fluid during freeze-thaw procedure. Usually two concentrations and three freeze-thaw cycles are studied and ideally the recovery of the analyte should be more than 90%. Generally for the freeze-thaw cycles stability control samples prepared for accuracy and precision are used. The control samples are stored frozen at desired temperature for 28 days and sampling is done at various time intervals viz. 1, 2, 4, 7, 11, 14, 21 and 28 days.

Ambient Temperature Stability

This is essential for the samples which are stored at room temperature after the sample collection till its analysis. In this case also control samples prepared for accuracy and precision are used. Usually, two concentrations are studied and samples are stored at room temperature for at least 4 hours with hourly sampling. The relative recovery should be more than 90% after 4 hours of storage at room temperature.

13.7 BIOANALYTICAL METHOD

After standardizing drug extraction procedure from biological fluid, method validation and stability studies, now the results obtained can be used to prepare a bioanalytical method. In general, a bioanalytical method comprises of following information in detail:

➤ Reagents and materials
➤ Instrumental details
➤ Preparation of standards
➤ Quality control samples
➤ Calculations
➤ Acceptance and rejection criteria

Following are commonly found non-compliances related to bioanalysis and hence special attention should be given:

◆ Inconsistencies between data reported to regulatory authorities and at the site of study.

◆ Inadequate validation of assay methodology with respect to specificity, linearity, sensitivity, precision, and reproducibility.

◆ Inadequate use of standard, scientifically sound quality control techniques, for example, appropriate standard curves and/or analyte controls covering the range of subjects' analyte levels.

◆ Non-inclusion of data points and no mention of sample rejection based on scientific reasoning in determination of assay method precision, sensitivity, accuracy, etc.

◆ Samples are allowed to remain for prolonged periods of time without proper storage.

◆ Improper maintainance of source data, e.g. source data written on scrap paper/filter paper/tissue paper etc and/or discarded in trash after transferring to analytical documents/laboratory book.

- ◆ Unskilled or inappropriately trained personnel for the conduction of analytical methodologies.
- ◆ Improper documentation of analytical findings.
- ◆ Improper written procedures for drug sample receipt and handling.
- ◆ Improperly written or no standard operating procedures.

Appendix I

REVIEW OF BASIC MATHEMATICS

Knowledge of basic mathematics is very essential for the proper understanding of various concepts in pharmacokinetics including absorption, distribution, metabolism and excretion. This appendix is meant as a review of basic mathematics involved in pharmacokinetics and not the in depth mathematical discussion.

First let us see how very small or large numbers can be expressed. In general, following form is used for the compact representation

$$Z \times 10^n \qquad \qquad ...I.1$$

where Z is a value between 1 and 10

  n can be a positive or negative integer

For example,

$$5120000 \equiv 5.12 \times 10^6$$
$$0.0000137 \equiv 1.37 \times 10^{-5}$$

Thus if the decimal point needs to be moved towards left so as to place it to the right of the first non-zero digit, then 'n' is positive. If decimal point needs to be moved towards right so as to place it to the right of the first non-zero digit then 'n' is negative. This can be seen clearly from above examples.

Many times equation I.1 is also expressed as follows:

  ZEn i.e. $Z \times 10^n$

For example,

$$5120000 \equiv 5.12 \times 10^6 \equiv 5.12E6$$
$$0.0000137 \equiv 1.37 \times 10^{-5} \equiv 1.37E\text{-}5$$

INDICES
Z^n

Here, Z is the number and it can be positive or negative and 'n' is the index i.e. the power to which a number is raised and it can be also positive or negative. Following are the rules that apply to indices:

Rule of Multiplication

$$Z^n \times Z^m = Z^{n+m} \qquad \qquad ...I.2$$

For example,

$$4^2 \times 4^3 = 4^5$$

But,

$$Z^n \times Y^m = \left(\frac{Z}{Y}\right)^n \times Y^{n+m} \qquad \qquad ...I.3$$

Rule of Division

$$\frac{Z^n}{Z^m} = Z^{n-m}$$

For example

$$\frac{4^3}{4^2} = 4^{(3-2)} = 4^1 = 4$$

But,

$$\frac{Z^n}{Y^m} = \left(\frac{Z}{Y}\right)^n \times Y^{n-m}$$

Rule of "Raising to a Power"

$$(Z^n)^m = Z^{n \cdot m}$$

It is important to remember following things about indices.

(i) Zero index

$$Z^0 = 1$$

Any number raised to zero is 1.

(ii) Negative Index

$$Z^{-n} = \frac{1}{Z^n}$$

Hence as n tends to infinity $A^{-n} \to 0$

(*iii*) Fractional Index

$$Z^{1/n} = \sqrt[n]{Z}$$

Logarithms

In a scientific notation 'log' indicates logarithm to the base 10. Logarithms to the base 10 are known as Common Logarithms. Basically, logarithms are a way of expressing a number in scientific notation. Thus,

$$Z = 10^n$$

hence   Log (Z) = n

Reverse transformation of a logarithm to original number can be done by using anti-logarithm tables.

Many times instead of using 10 as a base, a natural base (e) is used. The use of natural base is quite common in pharmacokinetics. The value of 'e' is:

$$e = 2.7182818$$

But e can be expressed as:

$$e = 1 + \sum_{x=1}^{\infty} \frac{1}{X!}$$

where,

$\quad$ X = integer ranging from 1 to ∞

$\quad$! = factorial.

For example, $5! = 5 \times 4 \times 3 \times 2 \times 1 = 120$

In general, if

$$Z = e^n$$

then,   ln (Z) = n

ln indicates the natural logarithm to the base 'e' and 'n' is the value of the natural logarithm of Z.

Natural logarithm is also known as Naperian Logarithm or Hyperbolic Logarithm. The reverse transformation of natural logarithm to original number can be done by using exponential tables. The relationship between common and natural logarithm can be expressed as:

$$\ln(Z) = 2.303 \times \log(Z)$$

or $$\log(Z) = 0.4343 \times \ln(Z)$$

Use of Logarithmic Tables

Although calculators and computers can readily give the logarithmic value of any number, it is essential to understand the overall process for proper understanding. (Please refer to Appendix II for logarithmic tables).

Find log of 543.2

♦ First express the number in scientifically compact notation thus
$$543.2 = 5.432 \times 10^2$$

♦ Look up 54 in left column of logarithm table

♦ In the middle columns (titled 0 to 9) look up column '3' and find the corresponding value in '54' row. The value is 7348

♦ In the right most columns (tilted "Mean Differences") look up the value in column '2' in the same row. The value is 2. Thus
$$7348 + 2 = 7350$$
hence
$$5.432 \times 10^2 = 100^{0.735} \times 10^2 = 10^{2.735}$$
And hence,
$$\log (543.2) = 2.735$$
Find log of 0.000432
$$0.000432 = 4.32 \times 10^{-4}$$

Follow the same process as described above to look up 43 and then 2 in logarithm table. The value is 6355. Thus
$$\text{Log} (0.000432) = \bar{4}.6355$$

Note that the number on left side of decimal point (called as 'characteristics') is nothing but the integer power to which 10 is raised. The number on right hand side of the decimal point is called as 'mantissa'.

Now look up antilog of 2.735.

Locate 0.73 and then 5 in antilog table. The value is 5433. Thus
$$\text{Antilog} (2.735) = 5.433 \times 10^2 = 543.3$$

Graphical Representation of Data

If
$$y = x^3$$

Then following data table can be obtained and a non-linear plot of the data is shown in Fig. AI.1.

x	y
0	0
2	8
4	64
6	216
8	512
10	1000

The slope of the line is defined as "the rate of change of y with respect to x varies with the value of x". For non-linear plot, the slope is not constant over the entire range.

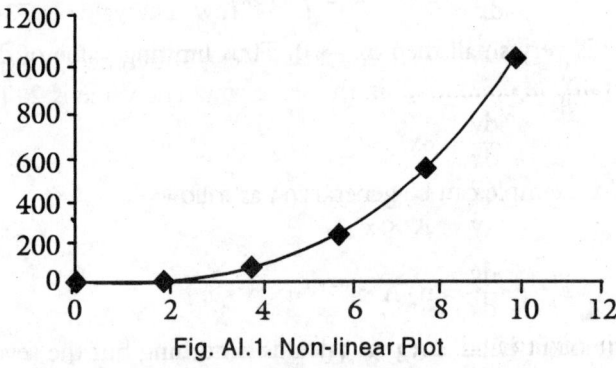

Fig. AI.1. Non-linear Plot

In a graph, dependent variable is usually on the Y-axis - vertical axis, also called a *ordinate*. Whereas, independent variable is usually on X-axis - horizontal axis, also called as *abscissa*. Hence usually Y-varies with respect to X and not other way. For example, in plasma concentration-time plot, plasma drug concentration is on Y-axis as it varies according to time, thus time is on X-axis.

A straight-line graph will be obtained only if the equation from which the plot is derived has following form:

$$y = mx + c$$

where,

        y = Dependent variable
        x = Independent variably
        m = slope of the straight line
        c = y-axis intercept i.e. y-value when x = 0.

Let us again use the expression $y = x^3$ to understand differentiation process. From differentiation the derivative of y with respect to x can be found.

$$y = x^3 \qquad \qquad ...I.4$$

Hence,

$$y + dy = (x + dx)^3 \qquad \qquad ...I.5$$

i.e. $\qquad y + dy = x^3 + 3x^2(dx) + 3x(dx)^2 + (dx)^3 \qquad ...I.6$

Subtract equation I.4 (original equation) from above equation (I.6). Thus,

$$dy = 3x^2(dx) + 3x(dx)^2 + (dx)^3 \qquad ...I.7$$

Divide both sides of the above equation (I.7) by dx, thus

$$\frac{dy}{dx} = 3x^2 + 3x(dx) + (dx)^2 \qquad \qquad ...I.8$$

But if dx is very small then $dx \to 0$. Thus limiting value of $dx = 0$. And hence,

$$\frac{dy}{dx} = 3x^2$$

The above example can be generalized as follows:

If $\qquad \qquad y = A \times x^n$

Then, $\qquad \frac{dy}{dx} = n \cdot A \cdot x^{n-1}$

On the other hand, integral calculus is nothing but the reversal of differential calculus. Integration is generally used to sum all smaller units (dy) so as to obtain whole value (y). Thus

$$\int dy = Y$$

$\int$ is the symbol of integration.

The derivative expression is

i.e. $\qquad \qquad \frac{dy}{dx} = A \cdot x^n$

$$dy = A \cdot x^n \cdot dx$$

Integration will give

$$y = \int dy = A \cdot x^n \cdot dx$$

$$= A \cdot x^n \cdot dx$$

$$= \frac{A \cdot x^{n+1}}{n+1} + A$$

A is called as constant of integration.

EXAMPLES OF BIOPHARMACEUTICAL CALCULATIONS
Problem 1
What is the V_d/kg of a drug whose total volume of distribution in a 60 kg person is 50 L?

Answer
Here, divide the total volume of distribution by body weight.

Thus, $\quad \dfrac{50}{60} = 0.833 \, \text{L} / \text{kg}$

V_d/kg of the drug. $= 0.833 \, \text{L/kg}$

Similarly, if V_d/kg of a drug and body weight of a person is known, then total volume of distribution can be easily calculated,

$$V_d/\text{kg} = 0.833 \, \text{L/kg}$$
$$\text{Body weight} = 60 \, \text{kg}$$

To obtain total volume of ditribution, multiply V_d/kg by body weight.

$$\text{Total } V_d = 0.833 \times 60$$
$$\text{Total } V_d = 49.98 \, \text{L}$$

Problem 2
Arterial blood concentration of a drug entering the kidney is 25 mg/L. Venous blood concentration is 15 mg/L. Blood flow to the kidney is 0.6 L per hour. Calculate kidney clearance rate of the drug.

Answer
Clearance rate = Extraction ratio*Blood flow,
First, calculate extraction ratio,

$$\text{Extraction ratio} = \frac{(C_{in} - C_{out})}{C_{in}}$$

$$= \frac{25 - 15}{25}$$

$$= \frac{10}{25}$$

$$= 0.4$$

Now clearance rate can be easily calculated as,

$$\text{Clearance rate} = \text{Extraction ratio} \times \text{Blood flow}$$
$$= 0.4 \times 0.6$$
$$= 0.24 \text{ L/hr}$$

Problem 3

Total volume of distribution of a drug in a 60 kg person is 80 L and the K_{el} is 0.3 hr^{-1}. What is the clearance of the drug?

Answer

$$\text{Clearance} = K_{el} \times V_d$$

First, calculate V_d (L/kg).

$$V_d = \frac{\text{Total volume of distribution}}{\text{Body weight}}$$

$$= \frac{80}{60}$$

$$= 1.333 \text{ L/kg}$$

Thus,

$$\text{Clearance} = 0.3 \times 1.333$$
$$= 0.399 \text{ L/hr/kg}$$

Problem 4

Elimination half-life of a drug is 5 hr. What is the K_{el}? Calculate the time required to reach 97% of steady state in terms of both, half-lives and hours.

Answer

Relationship between K_{el} and $t_{1/2}$ is:

$$K_{el} = \frac{0.693}{t_{1/2}}$$

$$= \frac{0.693}{5}$$

$$K_{el} = 0.139 \text{ /hour}$$

Time required to reach 97% of steady state is 5 half-lives:

Half-life	% of steady state
0	0
1	50
2	75
3	87.5
4	93.75
5	**96.875**

Time required in terms of hours = Number of half-lives × half-life

$$= 5 \times 5$$

$$= 25 \text{ hours}$$

Problem 5

Following information is known for a drug which follows one-compartment model,

Plasma drug concentration = 0.015 mg/ml
Drug concentration in urine = 0.008 mg/ml
Time period of urine collection = 300 min
Volume of urine collected = 150 ml

What is the renal clearance of the drug?

Answer

Refer page no. 183-184 for details

$$\text{Renal clearance } (Cl_{ren}) = \frac{C_4' \cdot V}{C_p \cdot t}$$

Where,

C_u' = Drug Concentration in urine
V = Volume of urine collected
t = Time for which urine was collected
C_p = Plasma drug concentration

Thus,

$$Cl_{ren} = \frac{0.008 \times 150}{0.015 \times 300}$$

$$= \frac{1.2}{4.5}$$

$$= 0.267 \text{ ml/min}$$

Problem 6

To achieve a steady state concetration of 20 mg/L of a drug having $V_d = 1.2$ L/kg and $t_{1/2} = 10$ hr, what should be the infusion rate? What will be the loading dose?

Answer

Refer page 188-189 for details of the calculation,

Steady state plasma concentration $C_{ss} = \dfrac{K_0}{K_{el.} V_d}$

Where,

         K_0 = Infusion rate
         K_{el} = Elimination rate constant
         V_d = Volume of distribution

First, calculate K_{el}

$$K_{el} = \frac{0.693}{t_{1/2}}$$

$$= \frac{0.693}{10}$$

$$= 0.0693 \text{ hour}$$

Now using the above equation for C_{ss}

$$20 = \frac{K_0}{0.0693 \times 1.2}$$

$$K_0 = 20 \times 0.0693 \times 1.2$$

$$K_0 = 1.66 \text{ mg/kg/hr}$$

Loading dose $= C_{ss} \times Vd$

$$= 20 \times 1.2$$

Loading dose $= 24$ mg/kg

Problem 7

Consider following information,

         Maintenance dose = 10 mg/kg
     Fraction of dose absorbed = 0.6
    Elimination rate constant = 0.2 /hr
     Volume of distribution = 1.5 L/kg,

What will be the dosing interval to achieve average steady state plasma drug concentration of 15 kg/L?

Answer

Refer page 238-239 for the details,

Average steady state plasma drug concentration $(C') = \dfrac{F \cdot X_0}{Cl \cdot \tau}$

Where,

$\quad$ F = Fraction of the dose absorbed

$\quad X_0$ = Maintenance dose

$\quad$ Cl = Clearance

$\quad \tau$ = Dosing interval

First calculate clearance

$$Cl = K_{el} \times V_d$$
$$= 0.2 \times 1.5$$
$$= 0.3 \text{ L/hr/kg}$$

Now using above equation for C',

$$15 = \frac{0.6 \times 10}{0.3 \times \tau}$$

$$\tau = \frac{0.6 \times 10}{0.3 \times 15}$$

$$= \frac{6}{4.5}$$

$$= 1.33 \text{ hr}$$

Thus, dosing interval is 1.33 hr.

LOGARITHMS

	0	1	2	3	4	5	6	7	8	9	1	2	3	4	5	6	7	8	9
10	0000	0043	0086	0128	0170						5	9	13	17	21	26	30	34	38
						0212	0253	0294	0334	0374	4	8	12	16	20	24	28	32	36
11	0414	0453	0492	0531	0569						4	8	12	16	20	23	27	31	35
						0607	0645	0682	0719	0755	4	7	11	15	18	22	26	29	33
12	0792	0828	0864	0899	0934						3	7	11	14	18	21	25	28	32
						0969	1004	1038	1072	1106	3	7	10	14	17	20	24	27	31
13	1139	1173	1206	1239	1271						3	6	10	13	16	19	23	26	29
						1303	1335	1367	1399	1430	3	7	10	13	16	19	22	25	29
14	1461	1492	1523	1553	1584						3	6	9	12	15	19	22	25	28
						1614	1644	1673	1703	1732	3	6	9	12	14	17	20	23	26
15	1761	1790	1818	1847	1875						3	6	9	11	14	17	20	23	26
						1903	1931	1959	1987	2014	3	6	8	11	14	17	19	22	25
16	2041	2068	2095	2122	2148						3	6	8	11	14	16	19	22	24
						2175	2201	2227	2253	2279	3	5	8	10	13	16	18	21	23
17	2304	2330	2355	2380	2405						3	5	8	10	13	15	18	20	23
						2430	2455	2480	2504	2529	3	5	8	10	12	15	17	20	22
18	2553	2577	2601	2625	2648						2	5	7	9	12	14	17	19	21
						2672	2695	2718	2742	2765	2	4	7	9	11	14	16	18	21
19	2788	2810	2833	2856	2878						2	5	7	9	11	13	16	18	20
						2900	2923	2945	2967	2989	2	4	6	8	11	13	15	17	19
20	3010	3032	3054	3075	3096	3118	3139	3160	3181	3201	2	4	6	8	11	13	15	17	19
21	3222	3243	3263	3284	3304	3324	3345	3365	3385	3404	2	4	6	8	10	12	14	16	18
22	3424	3444	3464	3483	3502	3522	3541	3560	3579	3598	2	4	6	8	10	12	14	15	17
23	3617	3636	3655	3674	3692	3711	3729	3747	3766	3784	2	4	6	7	9	11	13	15	17
24	3802	3820	3838	3856	3874	3892	3909	3927	3945	3962	2	4	5	7	9	11	12	14	16
25	3979	3997	4014	4031	4048	4065	4082	4099	4116	4133	2	3	5	7	9	10	12	14	15
26	4150	4166	4183	4200	4216	4232	4249	4265	4281	4298	2	3	5	7	8	10	11	13	15
27	4314	4330	4346	4362	4378	4393	4409	4425	4440	4456	2	3	5	6	8	9	11	13	14
28	4472	4487	4502	4518	4533	4548	4564	4579	4594	4609	2	3	5	6	8	9	11	12	14
29	4624	4639	4654	4669	4683	4698	4713	4728	4742	4757	1	3	4	6	8	9	10	12	13
30	4771	4786	4800	4814	4829	4843	4857	4871	4886	4900	1	3	4	6	7	9	10	11	13
31	4914	4928	4942	4955	4969	4983	4997	5011	5024	5038	1	3	4	6	7	8	10	11	12
32	5051	5065	5079	5092	5105	5119	5132	5145	5159	5172	1	3	4	5	7	8	9	11	12
33	5185	5198	5211	5224	5237	5250	5263	5276	5289	5302	1	3	4	5	6	8	9	10	12
34	5315	5328	5340	5353	5366	5378	5391	5403	5416	5428	1	3	4	5	6	8	9	10	11
35	5441	5453	5465	5478	5490	5502	5514	5527	5539	5551	1	2	4	5	6	7	9	10	11
36	5563	5575	5587	5599	5611	5623	5635	5647	5658	5670	1	2	4	5	6	7	8	10	11
37	5682	5694	5705	5717	5729	5740	5752	5763	5775	5786	1	2	3	5	6	7	8	9	10
38	5798	5809	5821	5832	5843	5855	5866	5877	5888	5899	1	2	3	5	6	7	8	9	10
39	5911	5922	5933	5944	5955	5966	5977	5988	5999	6010	1	2	3	4	5	7	8	9	10
40	6021	6031	6042	6053	6064	6075	6085	6096	6107	6117	1	2	3	4	5	6	8	9	10
41	6128	6138	6149	6160	6170	6180	6191	6201	6212	6222	1	2	3	4	5	6	7	8	9
42	6232	6243	6253	6263	6274	6284	6294	6304	6314	6325	1	2	3	4	5	6	7	8	9
43	6335	6345	6355	6365	6375	6385	6395	6405	6415	6425	1	2	3	4	5	6	7	8	9
44	6435	6444	6454	6464	6474	6484	6493	6503	6513	6522	1	2	3	4	5	6	7	8	9
45	6532	6542	6551	6561	6571	6580	6590	6599	6609	6618	1	2	3	4	5	6	7	8	9
46	6628	6637	6646	6656	6665	6675	6684	6693	6702	6712	1	2	3	4	5	6	7	7	8
47	6721	6730	6739	6749	6758	6767	6776	6785	6794	6803	1	2	3	4	5	5	6	7	8
48	6812	6821	6830	6839	6848	6857	6866	6875	6884	6893	1	2	3	4	4	5	6	7	8
49	6902	6911	6920	6928	6937	6946	6955	6964	6972	6981	1	2	3	4	4	5	6	7	8

LOGARITHMS

	0	1	2	3	4	5	6	7	8	9	1 2 3	4 5 6	7 8 9
50	6990	6998	7007	7016	7024	7033	7042	7050	7059	7067	1 2 3	3 4 5	6 7 8
51	7076	7084	7093	7101	7110	7118	7126	7135	7143	7152	1 2 3	3 4 5	6 7 8
52	7160	7168	7177	7185	7193	7202	7210	7218	7226	7235	1 2 2	3 4 5	6 7 7
53	7243	7251	7259	7267	7275	7284	7292	7300	7308	7316	1 2 2	3 4 5	6 6 7
54	7324	7332	7340	7348	7356	7364	7372	7380	7388	7396	1 2 2	3 4 5	6 6 7
55	7404	7412	7419	7427	7435	7443	7451	7459	7466	7474	1 2 2	3 4 5	5 6 7
56	7482	7490	7497	7505	7513	7520	7528	7536	7543	7551	1 2 2	3 4 5	5 6 7
57	7559	7566	7574	7582	7589	7597	7604	7612	7619	7627	1 2 2	3 4 5	5 6 7
58	7634	7642	7649	7657	7664	7672	7679	7686	7694	7701	1 1 2	3 4 4	5 6 7
59	7709	7716	7723	7731	7738	7745	7752	7760	7767	7774	1 1 2	3 4 4	5 6 7
60	7782	7789	7796	7803	7810	7818	7825	7832	7839	7846	1 1 2	3 4 4	5 6 6
61	7853	7860	7868	7875	7882	7889	7896	7903	7910	7917	1 1 2	3 4 4	5 6 6
62	7924	7931	7938	7945	7952	7959	7966	7973	7980	7987	1 1 2	3 3 4	5 6 6
63	7993	8000	8007	8014	8021	8028	8035	8041	8048	8055	1 1 2	3 3 4	5 5 6
64	8062	8069	8075	8082	8089	8096	8102	8109	8116	8122	1 1 2	3 3 4	5 5 6
65	8129	8136	8142	8149	8156	8162	8169	8176	8182	8189	1 1 2	3 3 4	5 5 6
66	8195	8202	8209	8215	8222	8228	8235	8241	8248	8254	1 1 2	3 3 4	5 5 6
67	8261	8267	8274	8280	8287	8293	8299	8306	8312	8319	1 1 2	3 3 4	5 5 6
68	8325	8331	8338	8344	8351	8357	8363	8370	8376	8382	1 1 2	3 3 4	4 5 6
69	8388	8395	8401	8407	8414	8420	8426	8432	8439	8445	1 1 2	2 3 4	4 5 6
70	8451	8457	8463	8470	8476	8482	8488	8494	8500	8506	1 1 2	2 3 4	4 5 6
71	8513	8519	8525	8531	8537	8543	8549	8555	8561	8567	1 1 2	2 3 4	4 5 5
72	8573	8579	8585	8591	8597	8603	8609	8615	8621	8627	1 1 2	2 3 4	4 5 5
73	8633	8639	8645	8651	8657	8663	8669	8675	8681	8686	1 1 2	2 3 4	4 5 5
74	8692	8698	8704	8710	8716	8722	8727	8733	8739	8745	1 1 2	2 3 4	4 5 5
75	8751	8756	8762	8768	8774	8779	8785	8791	8797	8802	1 1 2	2 3 3	4 5 5
76	8808	8814	8820	8825	8831	8837	8842	8848	8854	8859	1 1 2	2 3 3	4 5 5
77	8865	8871	8876	8882	8887	8893	8899	8904	8910	8915	1 1 2	2 3 3	4 4 5
78	8921	8972	8932	8938	8943	8949	8954	8960	8965	8971	1 1 2	2 3 3	4 4 5
79	8976	8982	8987	8993	8998	9004	9009	9015	9020	9025	1 1 2	2 3 3	4 4 5
80	9031	9036	9042	9047	9053	9058	9063	9069	9074	9079	1 1 2	2 3 3	4 4 5
81	9085	9090	9096	9101	9106	9112	9117	9122	9128	9133	1 1 2	2 3 3	4 4 5
82	9138	9143	9149	9154	9159	9165	9170	9175	9180	9186	1 1 2	2 3 3	4 4 5
83	9191	9196	9201	9206	9212	9217	9222	9227	9232	9238	1 1 2	2 3 3	4 4 5
84	9243	9248	9253	9258	9263	9269	9274	9279	9284	9289	1 1 2	2 3 3	4 4 5
85	9294	9299	9204	9309	9315	9320	9325	9330	9335	9340	1 1 2	2 3 3	4 4 5
86	9345	9350	9355	9360	9365	9370	9375	9380	9385	9390	1 1 2	2 3 3	4 4 5
87	9395	9400	9405	9410	9415	9420	9425	9430	9435	9440	0 1 1	2 2 3	3 4 4
88	9445	9450	9455	9460	9465	9469	9474	9479	9484	9489	0 1 1	2 2 3	3 4 4
89	9494	9499	9504	9509	9513	9518	9523	9528	9533	9538	0 1 1	2 2 3	3 4 4
90	9542	9547	9452	9557	9562	9566	9571	9576	9581	9586	0 1 1	2 2 3	3 4 4
91	9590	9595	9600	9605	9609	9614	9619	9624	9628	9633	0 1 1	2 2 3	3 4 4
92	9638	9643	9647	9652	9657	9661	9666	9671	9675	9680	0 1 1	2 2 3	3 4 4
93	9685	9689	9694	9699	9703	9708	9713	9717	9722	9727	0 1 1	2 2 3	3 4 4
94	9731	9736	9741	9745	9750	9754	9759	9763	9768	9773	0 1 1	2 2 3	3 4 4
95	9777	9782	9786	9791	9795	9800	9805	9809	9814	9818	0 1 1	2 2 3	3 4 4
96	9823	9827	9832	9836	9841	9845	9845	9854	9859	9863	0 1 1	2 2 3	3 4 4
97	9868	9872	9877	9881	9886	9890	9894	9899	9903	9908	0 1 1	2 2 3	3 4 4
98	9912	9917	9921	9926	9930	9934	9939	9943	9948	9952	0 1 1	2 2 3	3 4 4
99	9956	9961	9965	9969	9974	9978	9983	9987	9991	9996	0 1 1	2 2 3	3 3 4

ANTILOGARITHMS

	0	1	2	3	4	5	6	7	8	9	1	2	3	4	5	6	7	8	9
.00	1000	1002	1005	1007	1009	1012	1014	1016	1019	1021	0	0	1	1	1	1	2	2	2
.01	1023	1026	1028	1030	1033	1035	1038	1040	1042	1045	0	0	1	1	1	1	2	2	2
.02	1047	1050	1052	1054	1057	1059	1062	1064	1067	1069	0	0	1	1	1	1	2	2	2
.03	1072	1074	1076	1079	1081	1084	1086	1089	1091	1094	0	0	1	1	1	1	2	2	2
.04	1096	1099	1102	1104	1107	1109	1112	1114	1117	1119	0	1	1	1	1	2	2	2	2
.05	1122	1125	1127	1130	1132	1135	1138	1140	1143	1146	0	1	1	1	1	2	2	2	2
.06	1148	1151	1153	1156	1159	1161	1164	1167	1169	1172	0	1	1	1	1	2	2	2	2
.07	1175	1178	1180	1183	1186	1189	1191	1194	1197	1199	0	1	1	1	1	2	2	2	2
.08	1202	1205	1208	1211	1213	1216	1219	1222	1225	1227	0	1	1	1	1	2	2	2	3
.09	1230	1233	1236	1239	1242	1245	1247	1250	1253	1256	0	1	1	1	1	2	2	2	3
.10	1259	1262	1265	1268	1271	1274	1276	1279	1282	1285	0	1	1	1	1	2	2	2	3
.11	1288	1291	1294	1297	1300	1303	1306	1309	1312	1315	0	1	1	1	2	2	2	2	3
.12	1318	1321	1324	1327	1330	1334	1337	1340	1343	1346	0	1	1	1	2	2	2	2	3
.13	1349	1352	1355	1358	1361	1365	1368	1371	1374	1377	0	1	1	1	2	2	2	3	3
.14	1380	1384	1387	1390	1393	1396	1400	1403	1406	1409	0	1	1	1	2	2	2	3	3
.15	1413	1416	1419	1422	1426	1429	1432	1435	1439	1442	0	1	1	1	2	2	2	3	3
.16	1445	1449	1452	1455	1459	1462	1466	1469	1472	1476	0	1	1	1	2	2	2	3	3
.17	1479	1483	1486	1489	1493	1496	1500	1503	1507	1510	0	1	1	1	2	2	2	3	3
.18	1514	1517	1521	1524	1528	1531	1535	1538	1542	1545	0	1	1	1	2	2	2	3	3
.19	1549	1552	1556	1560	1563	1567	1570	1574	1578	1581	0	1	1	1	2	2	3	3	3
.20	1585	1589	1592	1596	1600	1603	1607	1611	1614	1618	0	1	1	1	2	2	3	3	3
.21	1622	1626	1629	1633	1637	1641	1644	1648	1652	1656	0	1	1	2	2	2	3	3	3
.22	1660	1663	1667	1671	1675	1679	1683	1687	1690	1694	0	1	1	2	2	2	3	3	3
.23	1698	1702	1706	1710	1714	1718	1722	1726	1730	1734	0	1	1	2	2	2	3	3	4
.24	1738	1742	1746	1750	1754	1758	1762	1766	1770	1774	0	1	1	2	2	2	3	3	4
.25	1778	1782	1786	1791	1795	1799	1803	1807	1811	1816	0	1	1	2	2	2	3	3	4
.26	1820	1824	1828	1832	1837	1841	1845	1849	1854	1858	0	1	1	2	2	3	3	3	4
.27	1862	1866	1871	1875	1879	1884	1888	1892	1897	1901	0	1	1	2	2	3	3	3	4
.28	1905	1910	1914	1919	1923	1928	1932	1936	1941	1945	0	1	1	2	2	3	3	4	4
.29	1950	1954	1959	1963	1968	1972	1977	1982	1986	1991	0	1	1	2	2	3	3	4	4
.30	1995	2000	2004	2009	2014	2018	2023	2028	2032	2037	0	1	1	2	2	3	3	4	4
.31	2042	2046	2051	2056	2061	2065	2070	2075	2080	2084	0	1	1	2	2	3	3	4	4
.32	2089	2094	2099	2104	2109	2113	2118	2123	2128	2133	0	1	1	2	2	3	3	4	4
.33	2138	2143	2148	2153	2158	2163	2168	2173	2178	2183	0	1	1	2	2	3	3	4	4
.34	2188	2193	2198	2203	2208	2213	2218	2223	2228	2234	1	1	2	2	3	3	4	4	5
.35	2239	2244	2249	2254	2259	2265	2270	2275	2280	2286	1	1	2	2	3	3	4	4	5
.36	2291	2296	2301	2307	2312	2317	2323	2328	2333	2339	1	1	2	2	3	3	4	4	5
.37	2344	2350	2355	2360	2366	2371	2377	2382	2388	2393	1	1	2	2	3	3	4	4	5
.38	2399	2404	24010	2415	2421	2427	2432	2438	2473	2449	1	1	2	2	3	3	4	4	5
.39	2455	2460	2466	2472	2477	2483	2489	2495	2500	2506	1	1	2	2	3	3	4	5	5
.40	2512	2518	2523	2529	2535	2541	2547	2553	2559	2564	1	1	2	2	3	4	4	5	5
.41	2570	2576	2582	2583	2594	2600	2606	2612	2618	2624	1	1	2	2	3	4	4	5	5
.42	2630	2636	2642	2649	2655	2661	2667	2673	2679	2685	1	1	2	2	3	4	4	5	6
.43	2692	2698	2704	2710	2716	2723	2729	2735	2742	2748	1	1	2	2	3	4	4	5	6
.44	2754	2761	2767	2773	2780	2786	2793	2799	2805	2812	1	1	2	3	3	4	4	5	6
.45	2818	2825	2831	2838	2844	2815	2858	2864	2871	2877	1	1	2	3	3	4	5	5	6
.46	2884	2891	2897	2904	2911	2917	2924	2931	2938	2944	1	1	2	3	3	4	5	5	6
.47	2951	2958	2965	2972	2979	2985	2992	2999	3006	3013	1	1	2	3	3	4	5	5	6
.48	3020	3027	3034	3041	3048	3055	3062	3069	3076	3083	1	1	2	3	4	4	5	6	6
.49	3090	3097	3105	3112	3119	3126	3133	3141	3148	3155	1	1	2	3	4	4	5	6	6

ANTILOGARITHMS

	0	1	2	3	4	5	6	7	8	9	1	2	3	4	5	6	7	8	9
.50	3162	3170	3177	3184	3192	3199	3206	3214	3221	3228	1	1	2	3	4	4	5	6	7
.51	3236	3243	3251	3258	3266	3273	3281	3289	3296	3304	1	2	2	3	4	5	5	6	7
.52	3311	3319	3327	3334	3342	3350	3357	3365	3373	3381	1	2	2	3	4	5	5	6	7
.53	3388	3396	3404	3412	3420	3428	3436	3443	3451	3459	1	2	2	3	4	5	6	6	7
.54	3467	3475	3483	3491	3499	3508	3516	3524	3532	3540	1	2	2	3	4	5	6	6	7
.55	3548	3556	3565	3573	3581	3589	3597	3606	3614	3622	1	2	2	3	4	5	6	7	7
.56	3631	3639	3648	3656	3664	3673	3681	3690	3698	3707	1	2	3	3	4	5	6	7	8
.57	3715	3724	3733	3741	3750	3758	3767	3776	3784	3793	1	2	3	3	4	5	6	7	8
.58	3802	3811	3819	3828	3837	3846	3855	3864	3873	3882	1	2	3	4	4	5	6	7	8
.59	3890	3899	3908	3917	3926	3936	3945	3954	3963	3972	1	2	3	4	5	5	6	7	8
.60	3981	3990	3999	4009	4018	4027	4036	4046	4055	4064	1	2	3	4	5	6	6	7	8
.61	4074	4083	4093	4102	4111	4121	4130	4140	4150	4159	1	2	3	4	5	6	7	8	9
.62	4169	4178	4188	4198	4207	4217	4227	4236	4246	4256	1	2	3	4	5	6	7	8	9
.63	4266	4276	4285	4295	4305	4315	4325	4335	4345	4355	1	2	3	4	5	6	7	8	9
.64	4365	4375	4385	4395	4406	4416	4426	4436	4446	4457	1	2	3	4	5	6	7	8	9
.65	4467	4477	4487	4498	4508	4519	4529	4539	4550	4560	1	2	3	4	5	6	7	8	9
.66	4571	4581	4592	4603	4613	4624	4634	4645	4656	4667	1	2	3	4	5	6	7	9	10
.67	4677	4688	4699	4710	4721	4732	4742	4753	4764	4775	1	2	3	4	5	7	8	9	10
.68	4786	4797	4808	4819	4831	4842	4853	4864	4875	4887	1	2	3	4	6	7	8	9	10
.69	4898	4909	4920	4932	4943	4955	4966	4977	4989	5000	1	2	3	5	6	7	8	9	10
.70	5012	5023	5035	5047	5058	5070	5082	5093	5105	5117	1	2	4	5	6	7	8	9	11
.71	5129	5140	5152	5164	5176	5188	5200	5212	5224	5236	1	2	4	5	6	7	8	10	11
.72	5248	5260	5272	5284	5297	5309	5321	5333	5346	5358	1	2	4	5	6	7	9	10	11
.73	5370	5383	5395	5408	5420	5433	5445	5458	5470	5483	1	3	4	5	6	8	9	10	11
.74	5495	5508	5521	5534	5546	5559	5572	5585	5598	5610	1	3	4	5	6	8	9	10	12
.75	5623	5636	5649	5662	5675	5689	5702	5715	5728	5741	1	3	4	5	7	8	9	10	12
.76	5754	5768	5781	5794	5808	5821	5834	5848	5861	5875	1	3	4	5	7	8	9	11	12
.77	5888	5902	5916	5929	5943	5957	5970	5984	5998	6012	1	3	4	5	7	8	10	11	12
.78	6026	6039	6053	6067	6081	6095	6109	6124	6138	6152	1	3	4	6	7	8	10	11	13
.79	6166	6180	6194	6209	6223	9237	6252	6266	6281	6295	1	3	4	6	7	9	10	11	13
.80	6310	6324	6339	6353	6368	6383	6397	6412	6427	6442	1	3	4	6	7	9	11	12	13
.81	6457	6471	6486	6501	6516	6531	6546	6561	6577	6592	2	3	5	6	8	9	11	12	14
.82	6607	6622	6637	6653	6668	6683	6699	6714	6730	6745	2	3	5	6	8	9	11	12	14
.83	6761	6776	6792	6808	6823	6839	6855	6871	6887	6902	2	3	5	6	8	9	10	13	14
.84	6918	6934	6950	6966	6982	6998	7015	7031	7047	7063	2	3	5	6	8	10	11	13	15
.85	7079	7096	7112	7129	7145	7161	7178	7194	7211	7228	2	3	5	7	8	10	12	13	15
.86	7244	7261	7278	7295	7311	7328	7345	7362	7379	7396	2	3	5	7	8	10	12	13	15
.87	7413	7430	7447	7464	7482	7499	7516	7534	7551	7568	2	3	5	7	9	10	12	14	16
.88	7586	7603	7621	7638	7656	7674	7691	7709	7727	7745	2	4	5	7	9	11	12	14	16
.89	7762	7780	7798	7816	7834	7852	7870	7889	7907	7925	2	4	5	7	9	11	13	14	16
.90	7943	7962	7980	7998	8017	8035	8054	8072	8091	8110	2	4	6	7	9	11	13	15	17
.91	8128	8147	8166	8185	8204	8222	8241	8260	8279	8299	2	4	6	8	9	11	13	15	17
.92	8318	8337	8356	8375	8395	8414	8433	8453	8472	8492	2	4	6	8	10	12	14	15	17
.93	8511	8531	8551	8570	8590	8610	8630	8650	8670	8690	2	4	6	8	10	12	14	16	18
.94	8710	8730	8750	8770	8790	8810	8831	8851	8872	8892	2	4	6	8	10	12	14	16	18
.95	8913	8933	8954	8974	7995	9016	9036	9057	9078	9099	2	4	6	8	10	12	15	17	19
.96	9120	9141	9162	9183	9204	9226	9247	9268	9290	9311	2	4	6	8	11	13	15	17	19
.97	9333	9354	9376	9397	9419	9441	9462	9484	9506	9528	2	4	7	9	11	13	15	17	20
.98	9550	9572	9594	9616	9638	9661	9683	9705	9727	9750	2	4	7	9	11	13	16	18	20
.99	9772	9795	9817	9840	9863	9886	9908	9931	9954	9977	2	5	7	9	11	14	16	17	20

POWERS, ROOTS AND RECIPROCALS

n	n^2	n^3	$\sqrt{n}$	$\sqrt[3]{n}$	$\sqrt{10n}$	$\sqrt[3]{10n}$	$\sqrt[3]{100n}$	$\dfrac{1}{n}$
1	1	1	1	1	3.162	2.154	4.642	1
2	4	8	1.414	1.260	4.472	2.714	5.848	.5000
3	9	27	1.732	1.442	5.477	3.107	6.694	.3333
4	16	64	2	1.587	6.325	3.420	7.368	.2500
5	25	125	2.236	1.710	7.071	3.684	7.937	.2000
6	36	216	2.449	1.817	7.746	3.915	8.434	.1667
7	49	343	2.646	1.913	8.367	4.121	8.879	.1429
8	64	512	2.828	2.000	8.944	4.309	9.283	.1250
9	81	729	3.000	2.080	9.487	4.481	9.655	.1111
10	100	1000	3.162	2.154	10.0	4.642	10.000	.1000
11	121	1331	3.317	2.224	10.488	4.791	10.323	.09091
12	144	1728	3.464	2.289	10.954	4.932	10.627	.0833
13	169	2197	3.606	2.351	11.402	5.066	10.914	.07692
14	196	2744	3.742	2.410	11.832	5.192	11.187	.07143
15	225	3375	3.873	2.466	12.247	5.313	11.447	.06667
16	256	4096	4.000	2.520	12.649	5.429	11.696	.06250
17	289	4913	4.123	2.571	13.038	5.540	11.935	.05882
18	324	5832	4.243	2.621	13.416	5.640	12.164	.05556
19	361	6859	4.359	2.668	13.784	5.749	12.386	.05263
20	400	8000	4.472	2.714	14.142	5.848	12.599	.0500
21	441	9261	4.583	2.759	14.491	5.944	12.806	.04762
22	484	10648	4.690	2.802	14.832	6.037	13.006	.04545
23	529	12169	4.769	2.844	15.166	6.127	13.200	.04348
24	576	13824	4.899	2.884	15.492	6.214	13.389	.04167
25	625	15625	5.000	2.924	15.811	6.300	13.572	.0400
26	676	17576	5.099	2.962	16.125	6.383	13.751	.03846
27	729	19683	5.196	3.000	16.432	6.463	13.925	.03704
28	784	21952	5.292	3.037	16.433	6.542	14.095	.03571
29	841	24389	5.385	3.072	17.029	6.619	14.260	.03448
30	900	27000	5.477	3.107	17.321	6.694	14.422	.03333
31	961	29791	5.568	3.141	17.607	6.768	14.581	.03226
32	1024	32768	5.657	3.175	17.889	6.840	14.736	.03125
33	1089	35937	5.745	3.208	18.166	6.910	14.888	.03030
34	1156	39304	5.831	3.240	18.439	6.980	15.037	.02941
35	1225	42875	5.916	3.271	18.708	7.047	15.183	.02857
36	1296	46656	6.000	3.302	18.974	7.114	15.326	.02778
37	1369	50653	6.083	3.332	19.235	7.179	15.467	.02703
38	1444	54872	6.164	3.362	19.494	7.243	15.605	.02632
39	1521	59319	6.245	3.391	19.748	7.306	15.741	.02564
40	1600	64000	6.325	3.420	20.00	7.368	15.874	.0250
41	1681	68921	6.403	3.448	20.248	7.429	16.005	.02439
42	1764	74088	6.481	3.476	20.494	7.489	16.134	.02381
43	1849	79507	6.557	3.503	20.736	7.548	16.261	.02326
44	1936	85184	6.633	3.530	20.976	7.606	16.386	.02273
45	2025	91125	6.708	3.557	21.213	7.663	16.510	.02222
46	2116	97336	6.782	3.583	21.448	7.719	16.631	.02174
47	2209	103823	6.856	3.609	21.679	7.775	16.751	.02128
48	2304	110592	6.928	3.634	21.909	7.830	16.869	.02083
49	2401	117649	7.000	3.659	22.136	7.884	16.985	.02041
50	2500	125000	7.071	3.684	22.361	7.937	17.100	.020

POWERS, ROOTS AND RECIPROCALS

n	n^2	n^3	$\sqrt{n}$	$\sqrt[3]{n}$	$\sqrt{10n}$	$\sqrt[3]{10n}$	$\sqrt[3]{100n}$	$\frac{1}{n}$
51	2601	132651	7.141	3.708	22.583	7.990	17.213	.01961
52	2704	140608	7.211	3.733	22.804	8.041	17.325	.01923
53	2809	148877	7.280	3.750	23.022	8.093	17.435	.01887
54	2916	157464	7.348	3.780	23.238	8.143	17.544	.01852
55	3025	166375	7.416	3.803	23.452	8.193	17.652	.01818
56	3136	175616	7.483	3.826	23.664	8.243	17.758	.01786
57	3249	185193	7.550	3.849	23.875	8.291	17.863	.01754
58	3364	195112	7.616	3.871	24.083	8.340	17.967	.01724
59	3481	205379	7.681	3.893	24.290	8.387	18.070	.01695
60	3600	216000	7.746	3.915	24.495	8.434	18.171	.01667
61	3721	226981	7.810	3.936	24.698	8.481	18.272	.01639
62	3844	238328	7.874	3.958	24.900	8.527	18.371	.01613
63	3969	250047	7.937	3.979	25.100	8.573	18.469	.01587
64	4096	262144	8.000	4.000	25.298	8.618	18.566	.01562
65	4225	274625	8.062	4.021	25.495	8.662	18.663	.01538
66	4356	287496	8.124	4.041	25.690	8.707	18.758	.01515
67	4489	300763	8.185	4.062	25.884	8.750	18.852	.01493
68	4624	314432	8.246	4.082	26.077	8.794	18.945	.01471
69	4761	328509	8.307	4.102	26.268	8.837	19.038	.01449
70	4900	343000	8.367	4.121	26.458	8.879	19.129	.01429
71	5041	357911	8.426	4.141	26.646	8.921	19.220	.01408
72	5184	373248	8.485	4.160	26.833	8.963	19.310	.01389
73	5329	389017	8.544	4.179	27.019	9.004	19.399	.01370
74	5476	405224	8.602	4.198	27.203	9.045	18.487	.01351
75	5625	421875	8.660	4.217	27.386	9.086	19.574	.01333
76	5776	438976	8.718	4.236	27.568	9.126	19.661	.01316
77	5929	456533	8.775	4.254	27.749	9.166	19.747	.01299
78	6084	474552	8.832	4.273	27.928	9.205	19.832	.01282
79	6241	493039	8.888	4.291	28.107	9.244	19.916	.01266
80	6400	512000	8.944	4.309	28.284	9.283	20.000	.01250
81	6561	531441	9.000	4.327	28.460	9.322	20.083	.01235
82	6724	551368	9.055	4.344	28.636	9.360	20.165	.01220
83	6889	571787	9.110	4.362	28.810	9.398	20.247	.01205
84	7056	592704	9.165	4.380	28.983	9.435	20.328	.01190
85	7225	614125	9.220	4.397	29.155	9.473	20.408	.01176
86	7396	636056	9.274	4.414	29.326	9.510	20.488	.01163
87	7569	658503	9.327	4.431	29.496	9.546	20.567	.01149
88	7744	681472	9.381	4.448	29.665	9.583	20.646	.01136
89	7921	704969	9.434	4.465	29.833	9.619	20.724	.01124
90	8100	729000	9.487	4.481	30.000	9.655	20.801	.01111
91	8281	753571	9.539	4.498	30.166	9.691	20.878	.01099
92	8464	778688	9.592	4.514	30.332	9.726	20.954	.01087
93	8649	804357	9.644	4.531	30.496	9.761	21.029	.01075
94	8836	830584	9.695	4.547	30.659	9.796	21.105	.01064
95	9025	857375	9.747	4.563	30.822	9.830	21.179	.01053
96	9216	884736	9.798	4.579	30.984	9.865	21.253	.01042
97	9409	912673	9.849	4.595	31.145	9.899	21.327	.01031
98	9604	941192	9.899	4.610	31.305	9.933	21.400	.01020
99	9801	970299	9.950	4.626	31.464	9.967	21.472	.01010
100	10000	1000000	10.000	4.642	31.623	10.000	21.544	.0100

Index